SENSING HEALTH

DIGITAL CULTURE BOOKS

The Digital Culture Books series is committed to liberatory and transformational scholarship that critiques and works toward repairing historical and ongoing harm and imagines more just and equitable futures. With this series, the University of Michigan Press is seeking books that apply the insights and tools of intersectional feminist studies, queer studies, critical race studies, critical ethnic studies, critical disability studies, and related fields to the study of digital culture. As part of the series' focus on the digital and the Press's commitment to accessibility, books will be published simultaneously in print and open access e-book versions with multimedia capabilities.

TITLES IN THE SERIES

Sensing Health: Bodies, Data, and Digital Health Technologies
Mikki Kressbach

Collecting Lives: Critical Data Narrative as Modernist Aesthetic in Early Twentieth-Century U.S. Literatures
Elizabeth Rodrigues

SENSING HEALTH

Bodies, Data, and Digital Health Technologies

MIKKI KRESSBACH

UNIVERSITY OF MICHIGAN PRESS
ANN ARBOR

Published in the United States of America by the
University of Michigan Press
Printed and bound by CPI Group (UK) Ltd, Croydon, CR0 4YY

First published February 2024

A CIP catalog record for this book is available from the British Library.

Library of Congress Cataloging-in-Publication Data

Names: Kressbach, Mikki., author. | Michigan Publishing (University of Michigan), publisher.
Title: Sensing health : bodies, data, and digital health technologies / Mikki Kressbach.
Other titles: Bodies, data, and digital health technologies | Digital culture books.
Description: Ann Arbor, Michigan : University of Michigan Press, 2024. | Series: Digital culture books | Includes bibliographical references (pages 247–267) and index.
Identifiers: LCCN 2023035008 (print) | LCCN 2023035009 (ebook) | ISBN 9780472076598 (hardcover) | ISBN 9780472056590 (paperback) | ISBN 9780472904013 (ebook)
Subjects: LCSH: Activity trackers (Wearable technology)—Psychological aspects. | Self-care, Health. | Women—Health and hygiene. | Women—Mental health.
Classification: LCC RA776.95 .K74 2024 (print) | LCC RA776.95 (ebook) | DDC 613/.04244—dc23/eng/20231101

LC record available at https://lccn.loc.gov/2023035008
LC ebook record available at https://lccn.loc.gov/2023035009

DOI: https://doi.org/10.3998/mpub.12744203

The University of Michigan Press's open-access publishing program is made possible thanks to additional funding from the University of Michigan Office of the Provost and the generous support of contributing libraries.

Digitalculturebooks, an imprint of the University of Michigan Press, is dedicated to publishing work in new media studies and the emerging field of digital humanities.

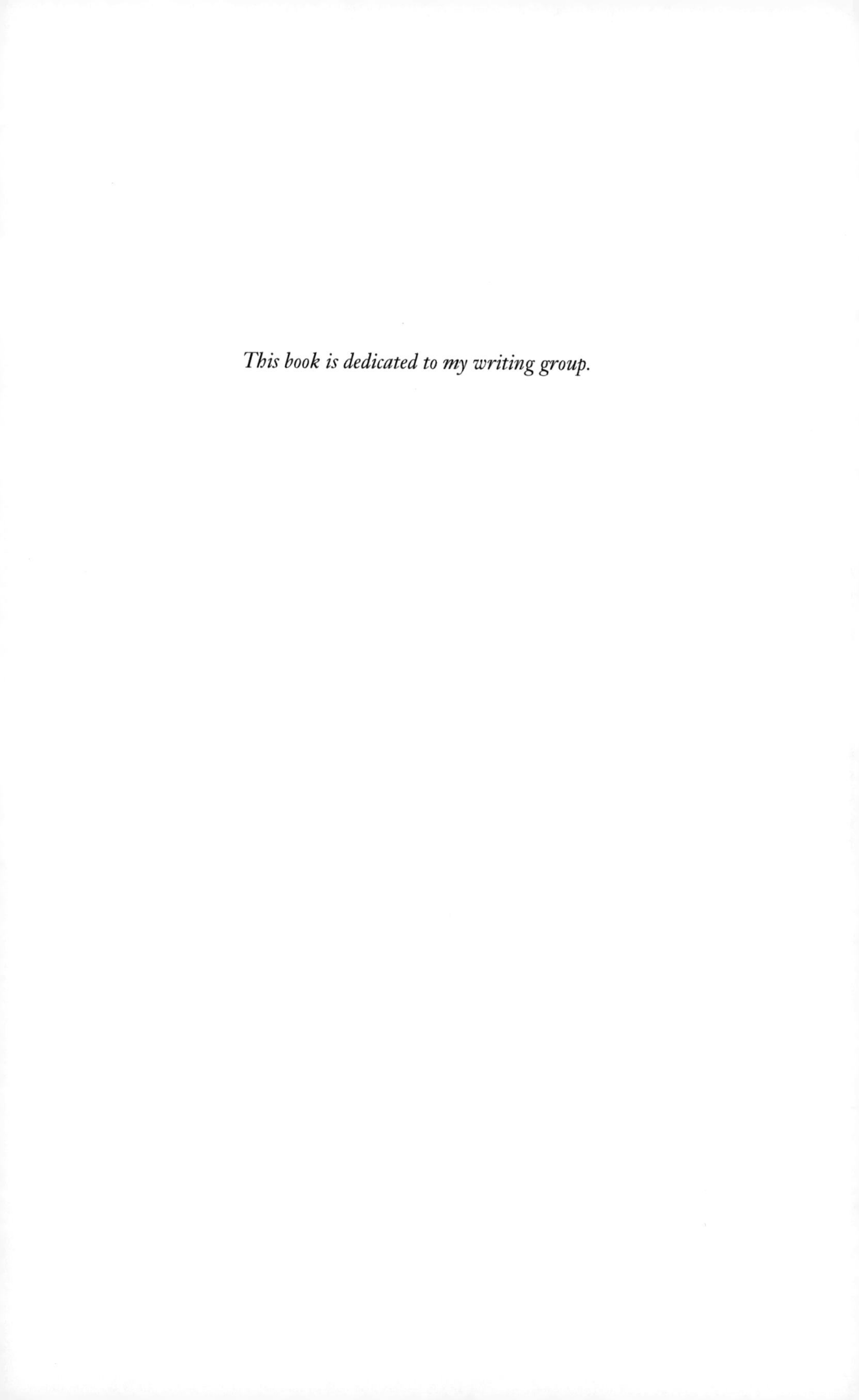

This book is dedicated to my writing group.

Contents

Digital materials related to this title can be found on the Fulcrum platform via the following citable URL: https://doi.org/10.3998/mpub.12744203

Figures

Acknowledgments

This book is a collaboration misattributed to a single author. It is a project that would not have been completed without the support and feedback of my colleagues, friends, and mentors. First and foremost, this book is dedicated to my writing group. What started as a group of graduate students in Cinema and Media Studies at the University of Chicago has grown into a group of colleagues and friends who have supported one another through writing dissertations, navigating the challenges of the academic job market, and publishing their first books. It has been a privilege to learn from this group over the years. Membership has changed over the years, but I'm grateful for the group's members who supported me during graduate school, including Hannah Frank, Matt Hubbell, Ian Jones, Tyler Schroeder, and Ling Zhang. However, I owe my greatest thanks to the group's most dedicated members, Will Carroll, Nicole Morse, and Jordan Schonig, who have read every single page of this manuscript (multiple times). I cannot express how much their weekly feedback and overall emotional support helped shape this book. They have been there every week helping me map out arguments, troubleshoot sentences, debate theoretical minutiae, and calm my anxieties. Perhaps most usefully, they provide a source of relief by funneling all of our energy into absurd theorizations of pop culture and cinephilia. They are my coauthors. There would be no book without them. I would not be the scholar or writer I am without them.

I want to thank my colleagues and mentors at Michigan State University (MSU) and Loyola Marymount University (LMU), who continually offered their professional support for this project. Josh Yumibe served as a mentor in the early stages of this project, when I was still testing out methodologies, arguments, and audiences. He encouraged me to develop my class, Ordinary Media, which was the first time I incorporated wearable devices in the classroom. Josh also allowed me to test out early arguments for chapter 3 in an invited talk on fitness technology and data. I'm thankful for the feedback of Justus Nieland, Kaveh Askari, and Ellen McCallum, who not only attended the talk but provided essential support during my time at MSU, and pushed this project to consider a range of historical and theoretical perspectives. The community at MSU gave me the confidence to break from my dissertation project and pursue new research that I found exciting and invigorating. At LMU, I was welcomed and supported by my incredible department, including Miranda Banks, Rick Hadley, Carla Marcantonio, Anupama Prabhala, and Sue Scheibler. Even amid the challenges and isolation of COVID-19, they were my greatest champions, providing a solid and supportive foundation to complete this project. I feel so fortunate to have a department that wholeheartedly believes in me and this book and has given me the space to pursue a project that steps far beyond the boundaries of film and media studies. I want to thank Miranda and Anu, in particular, for repeatedly showing up to provide emotional and professional support during the end stages of this project, when I faced some of the toughest personal challenges of my life. At a time when I needed it most, they provided the calming voice of reason and took on extra academic labor when they were already overburdened with work.

Writing an interdisciplinary book requires juggling a number of audiences, each with a different set of stakes and methodological frameworks. I want to thank my editor, Sara Cohen, for her incredible help in navigating this daunting task. She was able to provide a fresh perspective on the introduction and helped me shape a project that (I hope) speaks to audiences across the sciences, social sciences, and humanities, while still holding on to the values and methodologies of my home discipline. Her thorough feedback helped me craft the framework for this project and allowed me to see the book from an outside perspective. I'm also thankful for her excellent communication and organizational skills, which helped keep the project on track.

While this book project emerged at the end of my time as a graduate student at the University of Chicago, the courses I taught and conversations with fellow graduate students were hugely influential in shaping the trajectory of the project. I want to thank Jean-Thomas Trembley for providing the opportunity and incentive to branch out into digital health through his special issue on breath and media for the *New Review of Film and Television*. Jean-Thomas's excellent editorial feedback helped me work through very early arguments for this book. His creative thinking and presence in my graduate courses were always a source of inspiration, and the fourth chapter of this book is indebted to his work as an editor and peer. I was also fortunate enough to receive the Tave Teaching Fellowship, which gave me the opportunity to teach Popular Science and New Media, where with University of Chicago undergraduates I was able to explore digital health and some of its central methodologies. Over the course of ten weeks, I tested out phenomenological description, close analysis, and various philosophical and theoretical frameworks. Consequently, I learned alongside my students, locating points of interest, frictions, and challenges. The nineteen undergraduates in the course showed unwavering enthusiasm and often helped educate me on emerging media technologies. Their final projects showed unmatched creativity and gave me invaluable insight and inspiration for the core arguments for this project. Their voices appear in chapter 3 and served as a launching point for student-based research.

I'd also like to extend thanks to all of the students who have taken my classes on health and technology in the last five years. While they may not realize it, their contributions to class discussions and thoughtful writings were an endless source of inspiration. I specifically want to thank Ivan Medina-Mendez and Thomas Streed from my Ordinary Media class at MSU, who were not only excellent students but fantastic collaborators. Ivan's and Thomas's contributions to our pedagogy article on phenomenological description were essential to developing my lessons on description in the classroom, and to my own research. I also want to thank those students enrolled in my fall 2020 Science, Medicine and Digital Media class, who showed immense dedication to our virtual sessions week after week. Their experiences with digital health during the COVID-19 outbreak offered a new and enlightening perspective on my work at a critical stage of development. Phenomenological descriptions from students at MSU and LMU shaped the third chapter of this book, and I cannot thank them enough for their scholarly work.

The first, third, fourth, and fifth chapters have benefitted from feedback and discussion at conferences over the years, including the annual Society for Cinema and Media Studies conference, the Chicago Film Society, the Health Humanities Consortium, World Picture, and the Society for Literature, Science, and the Arts. I want to thank all of my former panelists and audiences for their generous time and feedback. In particular, I would like to thank Katherine Contess, Diane Negra, Scott Richmond,

Andrea Charise, and Kirsten Ostherr for their invigorating conversation and questions. Diane specifically gave me the encouragement to submit an early version of the first chapter to *Television and New Media*, where it now appears in article form. At LMU, I have also had the opportunity to present versions of the third chapter and introduction in partnership with the health and society minor. I want to thank Rachel Washburn for giving me the opportunity to share my work with faculty across the school and students engaged in critical health studies.

This project has also been generously supported by grants from LMU. I received the School of Film and Television Fellowship, which allowed me the time to complete the final draft of the book, and the Academic Technology Grant, which provided funding to purchase wearable devices for my class. Without this financial support, I would not have had the opportunity to explore my research with my students and develop the critical examples of phenomenological description that appear in chapter 3.

I have to thank my friends who provided essential respite from this project over the years. This book was written during a period of immense grief and loss. I often lost myself in this project, using it as a way to get away from the difficulties of my personal life. My friends continually helped pull me out of this space, providing relief in the form of meals, laughter, film and television viewing, and continuous support. Thank you to Jordan Schonig for constantly distracting me with deep analysis of made-for-streaming romantic comedies and with reality-TV-viewing parties. Jordan, I would not have made it without your daily commentary on the absurdity of academia. A big thanks must go out to Will Carroll for introducing me to the dangerous world of K-dramas. Our watch parties were such an excessive and addictive indulgence. Ian Jones provided endless distractions in the form of brain-breaking tweets, repulsive gifs, and videos of things moving real good. I would not have survived the last few years without my dedicated *Bachelor* watch group. Kristin Mahoney, Liz Mahoney, Lyn Goeringer, Yalena Kelinsky, and Brian, thank you for helping me on my journey. I want to thank David Clawson for bringing me along on some indulgent vacations. These escapes were essential to my mental health, and I look forward to future "writing retreats" around the world. Finally, my friends outside of academia provided some of the very few opportunities I had to truly step outside of work. A massive thanks to Tiffany Chow, my friend, sister, and forever-all-you-can-eat companion. Thank you for listening to me complain about things that are completely inconsequential and foreign to you, and for eating all the things with me. And thanks to Zach Hartline for putting up with us.

Finally, I want to thank my late friend, Hannah Frank. Hannah passed away before I began this project, but the lessons I learned from her undoubtedly shaped the final version of this work. Her friendship and support helped me become the scholar I am today. Throughout the writing process, I found myself asking, "What Hannah would think?" Her memory helped guide me, and it's hard to imagine that this book is here and she is not. Hannah, I miss you every day.

Introduction

Sensing Health

A gentle vibration on my wrist, like the press of a thumb, triggers an almost automatic reaction. My arm raises from a resting position, tucked at my side, swiveling so my elbow settles into the crease between my leg and pelvis, about two feet below my tilted head, perfectly aligned with the direction of my gaze. With the rotation of my wrist, a message emerges from the bottom of the screen of my Apple Watch: a small icon showing three concentric circles in red, green, and blue sits next to a header labeled "Activity." Below, text in a bold white font tells me, "You can still do it. 16 calories and you'll close your Move ring, Mikki. A brisk, 5-minute walk should do it" (Fig. 1). I raise my right hand and with a slight push on the dial to the right of the screen, the message scrolls down to reveal a statistic in boldface, comparing the number of calories I've burned to the set daily goal. A tiny bar graph visualizes spikes in my activity, showing tall lines early in the morning and tapering off as the day continues. As I glance at the screen, I can feel my upper body tense, pulling my shoulders toward my ears, muscles contracting inward. The sudden disruption of my relaxed, prone body with the tensing of muscles across my chest and back leads me to shift my hips back and forth, and stretch my legs forward as if my lower half is trying to resist the pull of my upper body at the screen's instructions. I have to actively will my shoulders to sink back down into the pillow behind my head, stretching my head to the left and right to release the tension across my collarbone. As I feel my body sink further into the couch, I think to myself, "sixteen calories is nothing, you don't have to move."

8:23
ACTIVITY
Close your rings
Kevin, you're so close to closing your Move ring. A brisk, 12-minute walk should do it.
Coaching
Wearing an Apple Watch feels like having a personal trainer on your wrist. It keeps track of how you're progressing toward your daily goals, and gives you a nudge to close your rings at the end of each day.

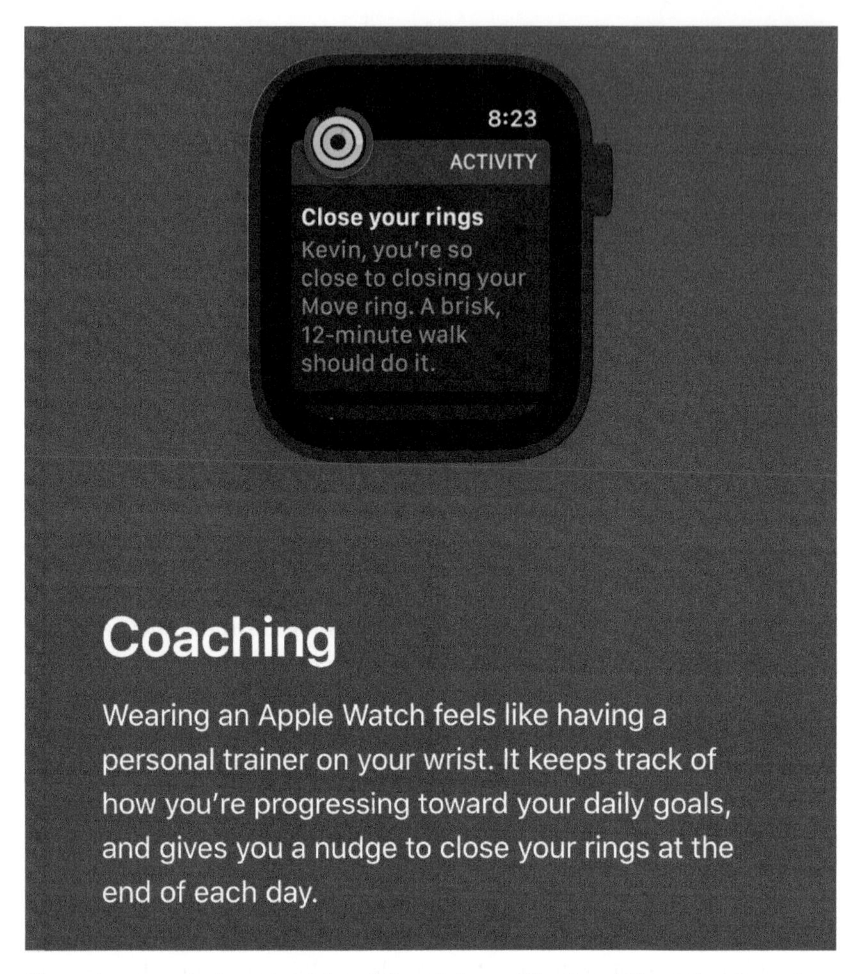

Fig. 1. An example from Apple's website of the notification delivered at the end of a user's day. Apple describes the daily reminders as "coaching," which includes a quantified suggestion for activity and data visualizations. ("Close Your Rings," Apple, accessed February 2023, https://www.apple.com/watch/close-your-rings/.)

My habitual responses to the Apple Watch are partly related to how my body has learned the vibration patterns of the device; with a single, sharp pulse to my wrist, I may lift the screen to my gaze and watch the text message pop up on the screen, or the repeated vibration against my skin may cause me to stop all my actions and see who is calling on my phone. However, the imperative to move—to burn more calories in pursuit of a daily goal—cannot be reduced to a Pavlovian training of my body. The power of the message described above lies in the way it prompts not only a reaction but also a reflection on my body, my actions, and by extension, my health.

The statistics outlined on the Apple Watch interface are meant to implicitly reflect my health—or at the very least, my efforts to perform, pursue, or maintain health. The Apple Watch is a common example of a smartwatch, which combines a range of features typically supported by a smartphone, including messaging to calendar and geolocation services, with health- and fitness-tracking features. The smartwatch is perhaps one of the most recognizable examples of digital health technology, or the growing market of health-related material technologies and the algorithms and analytical methods they use and support. Digital health technologies include a wide range of commercial and medical products, from digital patient records to popular wearable technologies, but all roughly aim "to support health systems in all countries in health promotion and disease prevention . . . by improving the accessibility, quality, and affordability of health services" to promote "patients' wellbeing."[1] Popular digital health technologies like smartwatches locate these improvements in personal data tracking. Through sensors and algorithms, devices and platforms claim to grant access to a range of metrics, including heart rate, steps or distance traveled, and blood oxygen levels, and offer a tracking system to monitor the data over time. The data-tracking system is designed as a way to maintain or improve physical and mental well-being. Mobile technologies and networked platforms have become essential tools for the development of digital health: from digitized patient records to crowd-sourced diagnostics, to the health-monitoring apps that now come standard on Apple and Android smartphones. Across all of these technologies, health is defined both explicitly and implicitly, whether through quantified measurements or supporting medical information. These standards are reinforced through features such as biofeedback, or goal-based systems that frame behaviors and vitals in relation to the platform's biostatistical health standards. Collectively, the data, supplementary information and visualizations, and tracking features claim to provide individuals with a representation of their health. Apple Watch, for example, reinforces a standard of health maintenance based on achieving a daily calorie count. This measure is communicated through a combination of vibration mechanisms and interface design that organizes statistical information and suggests strategies for maintaining and improving health. But where do these definitions of health come from, and how can they affect an individual's perception of their body, health, and behaviors?

This book addresses this question by approaching digital health technologies as aesthetic experiences. By "aesthetics," I am not referring to the Kantian association with beauty or judgment, but instead invoke its Greek origin, *aisthetikos*, which describes that which is perceptible to the senses.[2] Aesthetics includes visual, auditory, and haptic forms of perception, all of which are central to the design and experience of digital health technologies. As the opening description illustrates, digital health technologies involve material technologies, data tracking, and feedback systems as well as a range of sense perceptions and embodied reactions. The definition of "health" emerges through an embodied *experience* of the Apple Watch, not simply through the biomedical data it provides. Indeed, the power and complexity of digital health technologies lie in the way the platforms and devices become embedded in day-to-day life, circling wrists or populating the screens of phones, supposedly monitoring and supporting an individual's well-being. Consequently, the technology's definition of health is found in the familiar and small interactions, the push notifications, reminders, visualizations, and statistics that pop up throughout the day. Like the experience of health itself, these encounters often fade into the background or go unnoticed. But their power often lies in their ordinariness, the ways these articulations of health are communicated through the most basic ephemeral encounters with technology: the glimpses, glances, and vibrations that occur throughout the day. Pinpointing the definition or experience of health is thus a challenge as it becomes dispersed across a range of ephemeral encounters with screens or devices.

To capture and analyze the aesthetic experiences of digital health technologies, I turn to the descriptive methods of film and media studies, a discipline challenged with understanding the relationship between the aesthetic forms of time-based audiovisual texts and mediated experiences. My approach combines two separate but interwoven modes of description. I first focus on descriptions of the technology's design and interactive features as a way to analyze the visual and haptic rhetoric of health. I then turn to phenomenological description as a way to capture the corresponding bodily reactions and sense perceptions created through the structures of the device or platform. By combining these two modes of description, I consider the rhetoric and design of digital health platforms and interfaces as well as the range of sensuous experiences that collectively inform how individuals understand their bodies and health. These two modes of description offer a way to grasp and analyze how health is communicated to individuals, and the specific configurations of the body and lived experiences they generate.

Digital health technologies combine the features of mobile and digital technologies with biomedical preventative approaches to health that have developed over the last half-century. For example, Apple Watch has a default daily exercise goal of thirty minutes per day, in line with public health campaigns and official recommendations from the CDC.[3] However, the emphasis on quantifiable measures of health ultimately reinforces a highly reductive, individualistic understanding of what it means to be fit, healthy, and well. Like Apple Watch, digital health technologies often foreground numbers tied to weight and physical ability, like the number of calories I burn or minutes I exercise, and efface any social and environmental determinants of health. Rather than considering how, for example, socioeconomic conditions or genetics may shape my health, I'm urged to continually examine my day through the lens of data, accumulating, improving, and conforming to the structures of the device imposed on me by the technology. Moreover, many of these devices and platforms are only financially accessible to those with expendable income, or they are made available through private insurance companies that ask for data sharing in exchange for reduced healthcare costs.[4] For example, Apple Watch pricing starts at $279 and requires a corresponding smartphone to access the full range of features.[5] As a result, scholars have critiqued digital health for reinforcing preventative models for health that emphasize the ideology of bodily control, optimization, and improvement.[6] Through a focus on numbers, and structures that encourage the improvement of metrics, digital health technologies promote a model of health that prioritizes individual self-surveillance and controlling the body and behaviors as a form of health maintenance.

At the same time, a user's perception and understanding of health cannot be reduced to the goals or structures of the technology. As I describe above, I do feel the pressure to conform my body and habits to the structures of the device. Failure to accumulate those numbers can feel like a failure to be healthy or even a failure of the self. But my opening description cannot be reduced to a narrative of mindless conformity at the hands of technology. I ultimately resist the call of the device, choosing not to align my actions with the watch's recommendations. Descriptions of the experience of digital health show that these technologies often create complicated relationships between the body and health. While the technologies reinforce preventative definitions of health that emphasize improvement, this does not necessarily mean that individuals conform their habits to the data on screen or ignore their bodies in favor of numbers.[7] More often than not, the digital health experience incorporates moments of conformity and resistance, bodily alienation, and reflexivity.[8]

As a practice concerned with the specificity of subjective experience, phenomenological description can highlight the way individual bodies navigate the biomedical structures of technology. At the same time, phenomenological description cannot offer a generalizable account of the experience of digital health. The descriptions instead reveal how approaching digital health as aesthetic experiences can be used to explore the tensions between technologies and bodies, and the multiplicity of experiences generated through the platforms and devices. Put another way, my use of description acknowledges and critiques the biomedical structures of digital health technology while remaining attentive to the lived experiences of users.

The use of description in this book presents both practical and philosophical possibilities for the study, design, and use of digital health technologies. First, description can help researchers, designers, and users cultivate digital media literacies to understand the role of emerging technologies in a changing health and media landscape.[9] By describing specific encounters with technology, it showcases how particular design choices and interactive features shape the perception and meaning of health. Accounts tracing the relationship between design and experience can be used by scholars in the social sciences and humanities studying the impact of digital health technologies, as well as designers invested in developing technologies that move away from biomedical frameworks for health. However, this literacy is not limited to the study of digital health. As I show, the act of description itself prompts critical reflection on the part of the describer. As digital health becomes integrated into institutions and official medical treatment regimens, it will be harder for individuals to opt out or resist the biomedical definitions of health promoted via the platforms and devices. It will become imperative for individuals to develop digital literacy skills to question, resist, and reflect on the structures of health and bodies that many commercial technologies promote. The practice of description prompts an individual to translate their experiences into language and may be capable of encouraging a more attentive and critical relationship to the experiences generated through digital health technologies. As a contribution to what Kristin Ostherr calls, "the digital health humanities," my use of description can thus help expand the study of media and technology in the health humanities, which has largely been informed by traditions in literary analysis.[10]

Second, the practice of describing digital health technologies can be used to expand the philosophy and theory of health. While health may remain "absent" or in the background, for the most part, I suggest that description reveals how technologies may be capable of bringing to the fore a sense of the body's affordances and relationship to the world. The practice of describing often shows moments of friction and bodily attunement that escape the biomedical binary between health and illness—moments of what I call "feeling health." Drawing on philosophical work in medical phenomenology, I question whether descriptive accounts can be used to move away from a strictly biomedical approach to health, in favor of a spectrum model that describes how the sense of possibility and "ability" fades or diminishes in illness. This phenomenology of health does not suggest that "ability" or capacity is measured by external (biomedical) standards, but is instead dependent on an individual's subjective being-in-the-world.[11] Likewise, a spectrum model of health is not meant to suggest that bodily reflexivity and attunement is a moral good that can replace the exclusionary structures of biomedical definitions of health. Description instead provides a method for nuancing and clarifying how health is made meaningful and felt for individual bodies as they engage with digital health technologies.

The practice of describing the aesthetic experience of digital health technologies can thus be applied across a variety of practical and academic contexts. Scholars and practitioners analyzing the use and function of digital health may find the sections of close aesthetic description particularly useful, while those interested in developing critical reading practices may benefit from description as a method of self-reflection, and scholars interested in theories and philosophies of health may find the discussions of description and embodiment a useful resource for developing definitions of health alongside biomedical frameworks. As I show throughout this book, digital health technologies generate complex and contradictory experiences and understandings of the body. It's only by attending to the "mundane frictions," moments of resistance, reflexivity, and ambivalence, alongside moments of conformity that one can grasp how digital health technologies shape the perception of health.[12] By approaching digital health as aesthetic experiences, this book offers strategies for capturing, reading, critiquing, and theorizing the veritable configurations of the body and the embodied experiences they generate.

Describing (Digital) Health

Studies of digital health technologies have largely overlooked the role of aesthetics and design in favor of analyzing corporate rhetoric. Both sociological and humanist studies tend to focus on how language and the structures of commodification construct and exploit an imagined ideal user.[13] The marketing campaigns, quantified structures, gamified components, and price points of digital health all collectively imagine a single, unified fantasy of the ideal user. The advertisements for many devices showcase active, able bodies of young professionals who have incorporated the technology into the flows and rhythms of their busy, everyday lives. The companies rarely acknowledge disability (save for an occasional wheelchair user) or the range of environments and social conditions, such as parenting or types of work, that may prohibit conforming to the structures of the device.[14] Instead, the simplicity of meeting a daily numerical goal is held up as the pathway to health. From the prices of the technologies to the reduction of health to calorie counts and exercise, and even the way the reminders and notifications implicitly assume how a workday is structured, digital health technologies (and fitness and wellness culture, more generally) imagine an ideal user who inhabits a middle- or upper-class white lifestyle.[15] The fantasy of the digital health subject is supported through datafication of the body and behaviors that are compared to biostatistical norms. Scholars have thus argued that digital health technologies function as tools for normalization, "compelling" individuals to meet criteria that do not take into account nonnormative bodies or lived experiences.[16]

While such accounts provide essential critiques of how the language of healthism, neoliberal values, and biomedical authority are perpetuated via digital health, they ultimately overlook the power of the visuals and feedback features and risk homogenizing the digital health experience. Digital health technologies implicitly communicate a definition of health through a combination of visual and linguistic rhetoric and feedback features, and how individuals use, understand, and experience those interactions varies from person to person. Approaching digital health as an aesthetic experience helps provide an account of digital health that acknowledges how biomedical approaches to health are reinforced through design and feedback features while remaining open to the veritable sense experiences of the individuals who use the technologies.[17]

However, the ephemerality of the digital health technology experience poses an analytical challenge. How does one translate into written form the experience of a push notification or audio feedback during a workout? Close visual analysis of an interface may reveal the rhetorical power of visualization, or analyzing the rhetoric of an advertisement may reveal the goals of a product, but these processes alone cannot capture the lived experience of interacting with the device. Thus, I approach digital health as scholars approach film and other moving-image media: as aesthetic experiences generated through a combination of formal properties, viewing conditions, and embodied sensations. By "aesthetic experience," I don't mean to suggest that digital health objects are experienced as artworks or even that they provoke experiences of beauty (the two major concepts that drive philosophical aesthetics). Rather, my use of "aesthetic" more broadly names a mode of experience that is attuned to the particularities of sensation, both bodily and perceptual. While the description of these particularities is most commonly associated with academic disciplines concerned with the analysis of artworks, such as film and media studies, all kinds of objects provoke aesthetic experiences and thus demand close description of them. In film and media studies, description functions as the method for quoting the ephemeral properties of a text as well as a means for analyzing the experience of cinema.[18] That is, description functions as a way to trace the relationship between the formal structures of a text—e.g., editing, cinematography, lighting—and the mediated experience of such techniques. Because the discipline uses description as the grounds for analysis, scholars have argued that film and media studies has been highly influenced by phenomenological methods and modes of thinking.[19] Though the use of description by scholars in the discipline is not always explicitly operating through traditions of phenomenology, description functions as a tool for capturing and elucidating the aesthetic experience of moving images.[20] Thus, while I distinguish between descriptions of the device and platform design and phenomenological descriptions of the experiences of digital health technologies, these two strategies are ultimately intertwined and continuous with one another. In this respect, my use of description resembles the methods of medical phenomenology, which combines the close, firsthand description of one's experience with analysis to make broader claims about the body, health, and medicine. This book brings film and media studies' analytical methods into conversation with medical phenomenology to show how design choices and technological features inform the experience and perception of health.

The practice of embodied description has been an essential resource for interrogating the relationship between generalized models of "the subject" and the experiences of individual bodies. Medical phenomenology and disability studies, for example, are both invested in how medically determined norms for health are often at odds with bodies and experiences.[21] Indeed, the distinction between medically defined disease and the subjective experience of illness has been advanced through the intersection of phenomenology and disability, particularly through the work of S. Kay Toombs. Through her phenomenological descriptions of multiple sclerosis, she highlights the disconnect between her lived experience and medical interpretations of her illness.[22] While traditions of phenomenology in philosophy originally aimed to theorize a universal subject, the method of phenomenological description has been adopted by feminist, and later disability, queer, and critical-race scholars, who see phenomenology as a way to identify the points of friction, tension, and impossibility that some individuals face as they move about the world. Across these disciplines, phenomenology interrogates the norms of society, showing the way certain bodies, identities, or actions may be at odds with the socially constructed "natural" order. Most famously, Simone de Beauvoir adopted phenomenology to explore how the feminine subject was constructed through the interaction between a world structured by patriarchy and the female body.[23] Frantz Fanon took the phenomenological investment in the "I can" of the subject, to theorize the "I cannot" of the Black subject, whose race continually "interrupts" the possibility of "being-at-home" in the world.[24] Rather than providing universal theories of the subject, the application of phenomenology in these fields has demonstrated the tension between normalizing structures and particular bodies, illustrating that there is no single, universal body or subject.

My use of description follows these traditions by highlighting the complicated relationship between the experiences of the individual body and the structures of digital health technology. As an able-bodied, middle-class, cis, half-Asian woman, I have the economic and physical privileges to purchase the digital health technologies discussed throughout this book and to pursue the fitness and wellness goals they promote. I am also an active person who (for the most part) derives some pleasure or stress relief from exercising, and these physical and mental affordances undoubtedly shape my embodied experiences of digital health technologies. I also live in a major urban city, where I can readily access outdoor spaces year-round, pursue a range of physical activities, and acquire or participate in the latest fitness and wellness trends and technologies. Thus, in many ways, I am the target market for the digital health market.

At the same time, there are ways I do not "fit" the model of the imagined ideal user seen across digital health advertisements and websites. I am a half-Asian woman who does not have the ideal "healthy," toned, and thin body promoted by health and fitness companies, and I know that no amount of exercise will ever change that fact. Exercise and physical activity have never come easy to me due to unchangeable aspects of my anatomy: my short legs and knock-knees make me slow, often awkward, and prone to injury. I am not necessarily what someone imagines when they think of the ideal "healthy subject." Thus, despite my able-bodiedness and socioeconomic and environmental privileges, my body continues to be at odds with the rational, biomedical fantasy of the devices. My descriptions reveal the tensions and complexity of these experiences as I oscillate between moments of fluidity and friction, between falling into the biomedical imperatives of the device and critical questioning.[25]

My descriptions cannot be read as simply disciplining the body in pursuit of a quantified measure of health. In other words, description shows there is nothing disembodied about digital health technologies;[26] these devices and platforms continually prompt individuals to reflect on the body and their movements through the world. I examine whether that reflection or reflexive encounter encourages objectification, self-alienation, or neoliberal subjugation. The answer is almost always, yes and no. These technologies do not become seamlessly integrated into everyday life; they trigger frictions, questions, and skepticism. Description often shows that digital health presents multiple configurations of the body—technological, biomedical, sensorial—that overlap and contradict one another.[27] However, I do not claim that one perspective defines digital health, but instead emphasize how description reveals that such frameworks for health and the body coexist in the experience of these devices and platforms.[28]

The oscillation between absorption and friction in the experience of digital health can be explained through phenomenological approaches to the body, particularly the work of Maurice Merleau-Ponty, who has shown that the body is experienced as both a subject and an object. Through the practice of description, Merleau-Ponty argues that individuals experience the body from a first- and third-person perspective: as the conduit for sensations and actions, but also as fleshy material that can be measured, observed, and examined. For example, in one of his most famous examples, he uses the experience of touching one's left and right hands. This action creates the simultaneous sensations of being touched and touching. In other words, the hand appears as both the object of sensation as well as the active agent of sensation itself.[29] Thus, for phenomenologists, the experience of the body is never static, but continually shifts between subject and object as individuals move through the world. Indeed, an awareness of the materiality of the body can emerge at any time, from the presence of an itch to the experience of pain.

A phenomenological approach to the body allows space for the presence of multiple experiences of the body through digital health. The body can appear continuous with the device, as when the weight of the watch circling the wrist helps maintain the swing of the arm as an individual takes a walk. Or the body can appear strangely objectified as the numbers and visualizations transform it into the focus of biomedical observation. The subject-object body from phenomenology helps account for how these technologies often create moments and encounters that remind one that they both *have* and *are* a body. These are moments when the technology merges with human experience, but also reminds one that one is a fleshy body with affordances and limitations. I suggest that the act of describing such oscillations between subject and object can help theorize an embodied understanding of health to move beyond the preventative, biomedical framework.[30]

However, an embodied understanding of health—an understanding of what it means *to feel* healthy—poses experiential and philosophical challenges. Health is most often only noticed in its absence, when one becomes sick or encounters physical and emotional barriers that interrupt the flow of everyday life. Biomedicine emphasizes homeostatic models of health, where the "normal functioning" of the body (often measured through quantifiable tests) is contrasted with the disruption of illness.[31] Medical phenomenology has reinforced this understanding by aligning health with the unconscious experience of the body. Drew Leder's account of the "absent body" describes how health, like the body, recedes from our awareness in our movements through the world, only to appear in injury or illness.[32] Indeed, as I move throughout my day, I am rarely conscious of my body's functioning. I do not sense my steps, my breath, or my body's internal functions; instead, my perception is directed toward my actions, completing the basic tasks of my day. My "healthy" body is a vehicle for action but remains in the background of my consciousness.

"Feeling healthy" thus appears to be an oxymoron, inaccessible in one's day-to-day movements through the world. However, for phenomenologists trained to describe the backgrounds of experience as much as the intentional objects of perception, the body is always present. Even when individuals are not conscious of their bodies—when the body functions unconsciously as the agent of touch—their body remains the conditions for the possibility of that experience.[33] For Merleau-Ponty, careful descriptions of sensations and actions function as a way to show the presence of the body at all times as it moves between the background and foreground of consciousness.

Thus, while health may remain "absent" or in the background, description can show how digital health technologies may bring a sense of the body's affordances and relationship to the world to the fore. Through her phenomenology of pregnancy, Iris Marion Young has already contested the uniformity of health as "equilibrium" (a state only experienced by the ideal young adult male body) by pointing to the natural cycles of women's bodies as an example of how health is often punctuated by moments of disturbance and irregularity.[34] Likewise, scholars in disability studies have complicated the assumption of a binary between health and illness by examining experiences of health within illness, or arguing that adjusting to living with chronic illness can be understood as a form of health. These scholars argue that the illness experience—and by extension, the health experience—are constituted through the interaction of subject and world, and thus are continually shifting and being shaped by subjective experiences and engagements with the world.[35] Following these accounts, I turn to the work of medical phenomenologist Frederick Svenaeus to suggest that health cannot be reduced to absence. Drawing on Heideggerian phenomenology, he posits a definition of health that is related to the moments when one feels one's bodily capacities to navigate the environment and perform tasks, or one's subjective faculty for action.[36] He argues that health can be understood through a spectrum model that acknowledges how individuals' bodies shift through experiences of health and illness.

The complicated, reflexive experiences of the body are rarely discussed as components of the ordinary experience of fitness, health, or wellness.[37] I bring Svenaeus's spectrum model into conversation with descriptions of digital health to theorize the moments of bodily attunement and reflexivity that cannot be explained as the rationalization of the body through quantification or as instances of self-alienation.[38] As these technologies become embedded into the fabric of day-to-day life, they create interruptions and reminders to reflect on the body. Sometimes quantification, biofeedback, and other forms of bodily analysis may encourage one to objectify the body, but at other moments, these encounters may draw attention to bodily sensations, remind one of one's bodily capacities, or prompt one to sense one's body as one moves through the world. The descriptions of digital health technologies offer examples of such experiences and suggest that descriptions may reveal moments when health can be felt.

Defining Health

Digital health technologies promote a framework for health that has emerged over the last century through a constellation of changes in medical research, healthcare policy, and economics, and through technological advances. All of these factors have collectively shaped an ideology of health associated with individual health management and prevention. While medicine has traditionally defined health through the homeostatic model, where health is understood as the absence of disruptions to the body's biological functions, the vernacular understanding of the term is more closely aligned with the concept of preventative care. The rising rates of chronic illness in the United States in the twentieth century prompted a major shift in medical approaches to healthcare. Heart disease and other chronic "lifestyle diseases" are conditions that emerge from everyday habits and behaviors, such as diet and physical activity. While genetics and environmental conditions factor into the development of these diseases, they are considered to be largely preventable. In response, medicine has placed greater emphasis on strategies for prevention, focusing on habits and behaviors—"lifestyle choices"—that supposedly reduce the risk of illness.[39] Thus, today, health isn't simply the disease-free body; instead, every body becomes a site of risk for chronic disease that must be monitored and maintained to prevent future illness.[40] Health becomes located in the everyday habits and behaviors that seemingly shape one's future well-being.

Fitness and wellness have emerged as key approaches to support a preventative model of health. Chronic illness prevention is often focused on factors that contribute to the development of disease, such as weight and diet. Fitness, in particular, is framed as an essential resource for disease prevention as a way to manage weight and strengthen the cardiovascular system.[41] The twentieth century saw the rise of institutional initiatives, including the establishment of physical education programs, public health campaigns, and the rise of the commercial fitness industry and gym culture, all of which promote fitness as a critical tool to support and maintain health.[42] Just as fitness integrates physical activities and behaviors into a definition of health, the concept of wellness incorporates an ever-expanding array of environmental, social, psychological, and economic factors. As a relatively novel approach to health, wellness has grown in popular discourse since WWII through popular self-help literature, the rise of alternative medicine, and New Age health. Wellness is typically associated with a more expansive and holistic definition of health, and brings broader social, economic, and environmental conditions, as well as considerations of mental health, into a definition of an individual's well-being. Wellness practices, from yoga to meditation to special diets, and other therapeutic forms of care, are largely understood as tools to ensure the future holistic health of the individual. In other words, wellness is an aspirational concept that imagines an anticipated state of the body. Wellness is thus something pursued and performed through *choices* that supposedly decrease the "risk" (and cost) of preventable diseases.[43] Wellness is not a state one attains or achieves, however, but a receding goal that influences one's present.

Quantification has been a central tool for the incorporation of fitness and wellness into contemporary preventative understandings of health. One of the challenges for preventative medicine has been convincing individuals to change their daily habits, behaviors, and choices that ideally reduce risk, but cannot necessarily guarantee good health. Quantification helps translate prevention into seemingly tangible numbers, visualizations, and goals. As elements of the body and daily life become quantified, they can be monitored, maintained, and improved on, and the data can be used to set standards, norms, and targets. It gives individuals clearly defined parameters for understanding how their daily habits and choices inform the future goal of "health." The same framework has been used to expand health to consider environmental, social, and psychological factors that shape individual health and well-being. By quantifying components of fitness and wellness, from stress and anxiety to physical exertion, the range of behavioral, emotional, and physical factors are rendered legible and traceable by biomedical means.[44] Over the last century, quantified measures of health, wellness, and fitness, including BMI (body mass index), blood pressure, calorie intake, exercise minutes, stress ratings, and steps walked have all become standards for monitoring and assessing health and well-being.

The application of quantification to an expanded definition of health is related to the expansion of biomedicine, or what has been called the medicalization of "life itself."[45] Biomedicalization explains the contemporary expansion of medical authority through technoscientific developments, economic and political policies that have given rise to privatized medical-industrial systems, and the expansion of "risk" and surveillance through emerging technologies and medical advancements.[46] Within the biomedical paradigm, medicine and medical approaches to the body and daily life are increasingly viewed not as a resource for treatment, but as a tool for "transformation."[47] The methods and frameworks for biomedicine are "speculative, anticipatory,"[48] and do not necessarily aim to "restore" health, but instead serve as a way to improve on and optimize the self. Biomedical frameworks, such as quantification, surveillance, and risk, have supported and promoted the incorporation of fitness and wellness into preventative models of health, effectively expanding medical jurisdiction across a growing range of bodies, habits, and behaviors.[49]

The expansion of biomedical power through forms of health surveillance, maintenance, and anticipation of risk, has paradoxically been upheld by the shift toward the rhetoric and ideology of individual responsibility.[50] In other words, health, fitness, and wellness are increasingly understood as personal and private concerns to be managed and maintained by individuals, rather than healthcare practitioners or medical institutions. Quantification and other forms of surveillance support the ideology of individual responsibility by suggesting that by counting, tracking, and completing daily numerical fitness and wellness efforts, individuals have greater control over their health. Numerical frameworks for fitness, wellness, and health create the perception that illness and indeed the health of the body can be controlled through individual actions and choices.

Individualized approaches to preventative health are largely framed through economic incentives, such as reduced healthcare costs associated with chronic illness. For example, the Department of Health and Human Service's 2018 *Guide to Physical Activity*, 2nd ed., begins with an explicit message about the relationship between fitness, preventative health, and spending:

> Today, about half of all American adults—117 million people—have one or more preventable chronic diseases. Seven of the ten most common chronic diseases are favorably influenced by regular physical activity. Yet nearly 80 percent of adults are not meeting the key guidelines for both aerobic and muscle-strengthening activity, while only about half meet the key guidelines for aerobic physical activity. This lack of physical activity is linked to approximately $117 billion in annual health care costs and about 10 percent of premature mortality.[51]

Quantified forms of health maintenance, from exercising thirty minutes a day to a 2,000-calorie diet, appear to place the tools of preventative medicine in the hands of individuals, reducing the risk of future illness and the cost of healthcare. However, it simultaneously suggests that responsibility falls on the individual, who can and should work to maintain and manage their own health.

Thus, biomedicalization supports an ideology of health closely aligned with the logic of late capitalism.[52] As "patient-consumers," individuals are encouraged to engage in preventative health through daily fitness and wellness practices, consumer choices, and quantified forms of surveillance to prevent an anticipated illness.[53] The preventative model of health is thus deeply classed because it assumes all individuals are equally capable of accessing the tools for health monitoring and are capable of maintaining their health through fitness and wellness efforts. There is no consideration of how physical, environmental, and socioeconomic privileges may shape who can and cannot engage in preventative health practices. Indeed, the individuals most often at "risk" are those who face broader environmental and social challenges that impede health maintenance. As numerous scholars have shown, the burden of healthcare cost and maintenance is unevenly distributed, falling on populations that exist at the margins.[54] However, the ideology of individual responsibility effaces these realities, suggesting that disease or illness is a personal failing.[55]

Digital health technologies inherit and expand the biomedical, preventative framework for health, wellness, and fitness. By offering new ways to quantify, track, and monitor health fitness and wellness, digital health technologies reinforce the ideology of individual responsibility and self-care associated with biomedicine and neoliberal capitalism.[56] Through datafication, digital health technologies also increasingly conflate prevention and improvement. Most platforms incorporate elements, such as daily quantified goals, community competitions, and reminders that continually push individuals to meet new statistical standards, accumulate more steps, burn more calories, move a bit more, and stand a bit more, all in pursuit of health. Structured like a game or competition, accretion masks the fact that health, within these parameters, is not something that anyone can achieve or attain.[57] Instead, individuals who ascribe to these systems end up caught up in a never-ending cycle of accumulation and improvement; and by extension, health becomes framed through the logic of capital.

Moreover, as Olivia Banner has argued, digital health technologies are part of a contemporary biomedical marketplace, where through datafication bodies are fragmented into pieces, converted into value, and bought and sold according to the logic of capital. She terms this system "communicative biocapitalism," and argues that digital health creates new avenues for the production of health data, which can in turn be used to create new markets for capitalist exploitation.[58] Digital health websites and platforms use the data-mining practices of Web 2.0 to expand this marketplace by converting health communication—conversations around health, bodies, and wellness—into new sources for profit.[59] This expansion is facilitated and promoted through digital health platforms that draw on the rhetoric of self-care and empowerment, encouraging users to take their medical care into their own hands.

This is all the more true of popular digital health technologies, which are first and foremost consumer products, designed, developed, and sold by major corporations. While companies like Apple and Fitbit may employ medical experts and borrow from the rhetoric and authority of biomedicine, most products are produced outside of medical or academic research labs.[60] Moreover, companies generate profits not simply by selling technologies, but through data-mining practices. The data collected through digital health technologies thus do not simply serve as a personal and private mechanism for the collection and analysis of health data, but instead function as a source of profit for companies that capitalize on user data and communication.[61] All of these economic processes are masked through the language of "you." Digital health marketing campaigns and slogans often foreground the personal—the individual—health benefits to promote the idea that their technologies can endow users with power and control over their bodies while effacing the literal costs and markets they may create through self-tracking practices.

The expansion of preventative health through datafied surveillance has led many scholars to argue that digital health technologies are tools for neoliberal subjugation. Scholars have argued that digital health technologies expand biomedical surveillance, effectively extending the "medical gaze," once confined to the clinic, to the habits, spaces, and routines of everyday life.[62] The platforms and devices use quantification and tracking to offer individuals an ever-widening range of elements to monitor, reinforcing the sense that the body and health can be controlled through personal actions and choices. Situated within a contemporary biomedical marketplace that emphasizes individual "choice" and "freedom," digital health technologies reinforce the diffusion of medical power across an assemblage of authorities, including healthcare providers, technologies, and the individuals themselves. Within this context, biomedical power is not felt as an exterior pressure imposed on an individual; instead, the practices of self-monitoring appear to be self-motivated choices executed by responsible individuals in pursuit of health.[63]

Within the quantified, anticipatory logic of preventative health and digital health technologies, the body becomes increasingly fragmented and obfuscated. Digital health technologies offer more and more specific methods of health monitoring, and as a result, the holistic body is replaced by discrete data sets. For example, as I look at the "Health" app on my phone, my body, health, and behaviors are transformed into discrete data sets, ranging from heart-rate averages to progressively granular information such as "walking asymmetry" or respiratory rate. The data provided by my phone claim to offer something "more" than is phenomenologically available to me. My attention moves away from my body as a whole toward the "revelations" about my body that are only accessible via the app. As a result of such claims, scholars have argued that digital health technologies encourage individuals to understand themselves as data.[64] This argument has largely been made through the study of the "quantified self movement," an international community that provides forums and events to share self-quantification practices, technologies, and findings, all united around the epistemology of "self-knowledge through numbers."[65] Social-scientific studies of the community have argued that members understand themselves through numbers and the technoscientific frameworks provided by technology and algorithms.[66] As such, they have largely criticized digital health for objectifying the body, claiming that digital health and other quantification technologies extend the dehumanizing practices of datafication through the logic of preventative health.[67]

Digital health technologies are undoubtedly designed to reinforce preventative health and neoliberal values and systems of subjugation. At the same time, it shouldn't be assumed that companies automatically get what they want: that individuals automatically conform to the rules of the device and come to understand their bodies and health according to their biomedical standards.[68] While companies may imagine an ideal user, this does not determine individual experience or application. This is perhaps most clearly evident in the high attrition rates for digital health technologies as individuals lose interest or become frustrated by the structures of the device.[69] But phenomenological descriptions also reveal how ordinary and everyday use of digital health is littered with skepticism, doubt, and resistance.

Health cannot be fully explained by pointing to the goals of digital health companies or the ideology of biomedicalization. Bodies are not seamlessly integrated into and understood through technology: they struggle with, exceed, and often escape the technical structures imposed on them. The meaning of health only emerges through the experiences and encounters with the biomedical frameworks supported by the technologies and platforms. Examining digital health as a collection of aesthetic experiences offers a way to understand how biomedical iterations of health have become ingrained into day-to-day lives and how such definitions are navigated and interpreted by those who use them.

Organization

Each chapter is focused on a "genre" or type of popular digital health technology. These classifications range from clearly defined categories, such as wearable fitness trackers, to technologies that collect similar types of data and operate through similar feedback structures, such as posture and running wearables that track the position of the body and provide real-time feedback. These groupings help pinpoint the specific aesthetic features and analytical frameworks for health, fitness, and wellness. The grouping of technologies also roughly corresponds to contrasting approaches to the body that are supported through datafication and design features: the technology aims to either improve the body or observe the body. Technologies aimed at improvement use strategies such as goals, rewards, and challenges to encourage individuals to increase the quantity or frequency of their actions in pursuit of "health." Observational technologies place greater emphasis on tracking the body over time as a way to reveal physiological processes inaccessible to human perception. Despite these conceptual differences, many of these technologies share common features, such as goal-based design, reminders and push notifications, and data-visualization analysis. But there are significant differences in how concepts like wellness or fitness are employed to promote their definition of health that by extension create unique experiences and understandings of the body.

The chapters in this book move progressively from discussions of design and digital literacy toward more philosophical discussions of how to define health. Every chapter combines descriptions of the interfaces and feedback features with phenomenological descriptions of my experiences, but the early chapters place more emphasis on the design to first establish how aesthetics construct definitions of "health." With this foundation, the subsequent chapters place greater emphasis on phenomenological description to illustrate how researchers and users can use descriptive practices to examine the lived experiences of digital health and develop a philosophical alternative to preventative, biomedical understandings of the healthy body.

Digital health is a rapidly developing market. It is possible that many of the technologies discussed in this book will no longer be available or will have become entirely eclipsed by a novel device or platform by the time of publication. However, this book highlights aesthetic and biomedical structures and a method of analysis that is not confined to the case studies I describe. As a result, the chapters offer blueprints for how digital health technologies operate and understand health that can be applied to emerging and future platforms and devices.

The first chapter explores the aesthetics of popular menstrual- and fertility-tracking apps, Clue and Flo. Through descriptions of the interface design and analytics features of these apps, I argue that these technologies encourage individuals to understand their lives through their menstrual cycles. Menstrual-tracking apps often market themselves as tools for female empowerment by encouraging women to understand their bodies and health through self-tracking. Locating the interface design features in the history of the biomedicalization of menstruation, I show how the use of data visualization and euphemistic and humorous iconography encourages menstrual concealment and bodily management. Rather than dismissing these technologies, I advocate for collaborations between data scientists, designers, and humanists to revise the way these technologies express medical authority and rethink how they can be used to explore populations and conditions that have historically been overlooked in medical research.

The second chapter examines the aesthetics of "sextech" and the sexual wellness industry. In recent years, there has been an explosion of sex toy companies aimed at empowering women through the language of sexual health and wellness. Often created by and for women, sex tech are marketed as tools to help women understand their bodies and improve sexual wellness. Through the analysis of the Lioness smart vibrator, I examine how quantification and biofeedback are being used to incorporate sexual pleasure into the language of health and wellness. By situating these devices in the twentieth-century history of sexology, I explore how sextech inherits and promotes a logic of sexual equality that relies on quantification. The emphasis on numbers and data visualizations frame pleasure and sexual liberation through the neoliberal logic of accumulation: "more is better." At the same time, the datafication of pleasure may also present opportunities for the destigmatization of women's bodies and sexuality and can create reflexive relationships to the body that resist the rhetoric of "equilibrium" surrounding health that has led to the medicalization of pregnancy, menstruation, and menopause. I end by questioning how design can be used to create sustained and careful attention to bodily sensations, which can perhaps generate accounts of the body that acknowledge the natural excess, cycles, and pleasures that punctuate the experience of health.

The third chapter focuses on the aesthetic experience of fitness-tracking technologies. I begin by charting the history of the integration of fitness into health, noting the major methodologies, values, and biomedical paradigms that have influenced the design of fitness-tracking technologies. I analyze how these technologies promote a preventative model of fitness and health through descriptions of the Fitbit and Apple Watch interfaces and feedback features. Drawing on discourses of data visualization, I provide an account of how authority and objectivity are communicated through common visualization strategies from biomedicine and the ephemeral feedback features of mobile technologies. Then, using IRB-approved research I've collected from former students, I examine phenomenological descriptions of their experiences with Fitbit to complicate the assumption that these technologies lead to objectification and self-alienation. While experiences varied, their accounts illustrate how the act of description itself encouraged critical reflection on the biomedical definitions of health and fitness promoted by the device.

The fourth chapter analyzes the aesthetics of meditation and breathing technologies to demonstrate how quantification can be used to conflate health and wellness. I begin by offering a brief history of the emergence of wellness to trace how health has increasingly shifted toward a preventative performance of lifestyle management. With a focus on Herbert Benson's pivotal studies on meditation and "the relaxation response," I examine how contemporary breathing and meditation technologies use the logic of quantification and biofeedback to reinforce the biomedicalization of wellness. Through descriptions of design features of the Muse meditation headband and the Breathesync app, I demonstrate how design emphasizes the preventative logic of health in wellness and privilege bodily management over experience and sensation. While these technologies may reinforce neoliberal configurations of health in wellness, I turn to phenomenological descriptions of Apple Watch's Mindfulness app to explore how the use of vibration and feedback features holds the possibility of returning us to an embodied understanding of health. I end by introducing the work of Svenaeus, who advocates for a phenomenological approach to health focused on the body in a state of equilibrium, rather than emphasizing the anticipation of illness.

The fifth chapter continues to develop the concept of "feeling health" through descriptions of wearables that offer real-time feedback on movements and activities. These devices range from belts to clips to smart socks, and collect biometric data on heart rate, cadence, and body position to provide visual and aural feedback on the body as it moves. I begin with descriptions of the popular boutique fitness class, Orangetheory Fitness, which uses connected heart rate monitors to encourage participants to work within specific heart rate zones, to analyze how technology is used to navigate the challenge of quantifying "intensity." Orangetheory uses wearables to render the subjective perception of intensity objective to give individuals more "control" over their bodies as they work through the class. Placing this alongside the Rate of Perceived Exertion (RPE) scale, I argue that the visual feedback undermines the reflexive possibilities of quantification created through RPE. I then turn to the aesthetics of technologies that use haptic and audio feedback, including the UprightGO posture wearable and the Moov fitness tracker, which is designed to help individuals improve their running form. Through phenomenological descriptions of these devices, I explore how continuous feedback creates sustained attention to the body located in a surrounding environment. Building off the previous chapter, I focus on Moov to develop the concept of "feeling health," or the lived experience of health. I argue that the device's use of quantification and feedback reveals how technology can create moments when individuals feel the affordances of the body as it moves through the world, or health as a "homelike being-in-the-world."

A Note on Language

Throughout this book, I use "user" and "individual" to distinguish between the subject imagined by digital health companies and the actual people who use and experience them. "User" appears when I discuss the goals of the company, and "individual" appears in descriptions of the actual encounters and experiences with the platforms and devices. This distinction borrows from Ramesh Srinivasan's ethnographic studies of technology, where he argues that scholars need to move away from the dehumanizing, universalizing term "user" in favor of embracing "the diverse knowledge systems, values, and protocols" that shape an individual's experience and interpretations of technology.[70] The language of "user" perpetuates the abstraction of human interactions with technologies, and "the longer we speak about digital technologies as disembodied, the longer we perpetuate myths that disrespect the power and potential of communities and cultures world-wide."[71] I primarily invoke the language of "individuals" to foreground the subjectivity of experience and ideally bring back the body and the human in discussions of digital health design. I believe this is a small, but important step toward seeing the multiple ways in which individuals sense, experience, and interpret digital health technologies in their day-to-day lives.

CHAPTER 1

Life as Cycle

The Datafication of Menstrual Health

On August 10, 2018, the US Food and Drug Administration (FDA) announced the approval of the first mobile app for contraception.[1] Developed in Switzerland by Elina and Raoul Berglund, Natural Cycles combines daily self-reported data and a basal smart thermometer to predict a user's ovulation window. Marketed primarily toward cisgender heterosexual women, the app tracks qualitative and quantitative information about the user's menstrual cycle. The basal thermometer provides an "indirect" measure of hormones, which is combined with self-reported data, processed through the app's algorithm, and interpreted as a "green" or "red" day, indicating whether a user should use contraception. Like other predictive algorithms, Natural Cycles is designed to learn a user's behavioral and bodily patterns over time: through dedicated daily self-tracking, the user is rewarded with the knowledge that they can engage in sexual activity without contraception.[2] The FDA's announcement followed the European Commission's (CE) approval in 2017, with both organizations citing the support of the largest scientific study ever conducted on natural contraception, which surveyed 15,000 women over eight months, and revealed the app and smart thermometer to be 93 percent effective under typical use,[3] a full 6 percent higher than the average contraceptive pill.[4]

Natural Cycles is part of the growing "femtech" industry, which primarily targets cis women through the language of "empowerment," health, and wellness. For example, the Berglunds claim their product helps women avoid hormone-based contraception and become more "aware and in control of their bodies than ever before . . . to empower women to take control of their fertility."[5] And like other femtech products, technology and biomedical frameworks for health are at the center of these goals. The Natural Cycles' website foregrounds the FDA and European Commission certification standards, scientific studies to support the statistics on contraception, and Elina Berglund's background in science and engineering. Other fertility and pregnancy apps similarly appeal to science, technology, and data to suggest that their products align with official medical recommendations and standards for reproductive health. But as scholars have recently shown, many of the seemingly neutral, technoscientific structures embedded in pregnancy and fertility apps reinforce heteronormative, gendered understandings of pregnancy and fertility. Gareth M. Thomas and Deborah Lupton, Rachael Louise Healy and Maria Novotny, and Les Hutchinson all provide accounts of how pregnancy and fertility apps' tracking features often assume heterosexual, partnered users, emphasize statistical norms and medicalized risk, and promote self-surveillance of the pregnant/fertile body.[6] These arguments demonstrate that despite the language of "freedom" offered by pregnancy and fertility apps, these technologies often use data and tracking features to promote a vision of the pregnant body as a site of risk that needs careful monitoring and must conform to a medical timeline and a set of biomedical health norms.

Feminist health studies has repeatedly shown how the pregnant (and potentially pregnant) body has been a site of control and regulation by medicine for the last two centuries.[7] The expansion of medical power over the feminine body has been facilitated by the growth of the fertility industry, which is projected to be valued at nearly $50 billion by 2030.[8] With decreasing fertility rates, healthcare plans increasingly cover fertility-related procedures and testing, particularly for those with top-tier plans. However, even with these additional forms of support, fertility testing and procedures like in vitro fertilization (IVF) and egg freezing remain financially inaccessible to many Americans.[9] Digital health technologies like Natural Cycles aim to address this growing market of consumers with fertility concerns who lack the healthcare coverage to support more traditional forms of medical observation and intervention. While Natural Cycles profits from the growth of the fertility industry and medicalization, the expansion of medical power is masked by the rhetoric of "freedom" and the invocation of the "natural." For example, Natural Cycles' website foregrounds the promise of "hormone-free" birth control, and in a personal letter on the page, Berglund contrasts her product with fertility support that is commonly "invasive . . . I . . . wanted to take a break from hormonal birth control to give my body a chance to get back to its natural state well before a pregnancy."[10] At the same time, the website stresses the science behind their technology and FDA approval. This medical authority is framed as a tool for users who no longer have to rely on the health-care system to receive fertility support: "skip the pharmacy, no prescription needed."[11] Through self-surveillance features, the device claims to free the user from the structures of the medical system, but ostensibly extends biomedical methods for monitoring and regulating the body to the consumer.

While many "femtech" products expand and adapt biomedical monitoring systems associated with fertility and pregnancy, scholars and critics have overlooked how these apps influence individuals' perception of menstruation and the menstrual cycle more generally. There is a great deal of overlap between menstrual trackers, pregnancy apps, and fertility technologies; indeed, many of the apps include pregnancy sections or can be switched to "pregnancy mode" if the user becomes pregnant. However, this chapter will primarily explore menstrual-tracking apps to build on these fertility-related discussions by examining how biomedicalized and datafied models of the menstrual cycle can influence individuals' understanding of their cycles, bodies, and overall health.[12]

Like many of the technologies discussed throughout this book, menstrual-tracking apps promote the idea that self-tracking produces "empowerment" through self-knowledge and control over the body. The most popular apps, including Flo and Clue, are advertised as tools to understand the menstrual cycle and enable "you to take control of your health and learn more about your unique self."[13] Users "learn about themselves" by logging daily emotional and physical symptoms in addition to information about their periods, which ideally allows them to understand the impact of their cycle on their day-to-day lives and overall health. Thus, knowledge is constructed by transforming users' emotional, physical, and social experiences into data, rendering their symptoms trackable and comparable over time. In other words, these apps encourage women and people who menstruate to understand menstruation—and by extension, their health—through the framework of biomedicine and big-data analysis, which stress the value of regulation, statistical norms, and correlation.

Popular and scholarly criticism of menstrual technologies has largely remained focused on the inaccuracy of prediction algorithms as well as the affinity for pink interfaces and gendered address.[14] While most remain focused on how feminized iconography and word choice target straight women, this chapter considers how the self-tracking and data-analytic features reinforce discourses of menstrual concealment and biomedical bodily alienation. I begin with descriptions of the interface aesthetics of Flo and Clue to show how their design encourages menstrual suppression through the use of euphemistic humor and iconography. While menstrual-tracking apps aim to make menstruation more transparent by educating women and people who menstruate about cycle phases and symptoms, I argue that their aesthetics rely on humorous and euphemistic icons to stand in for bodily processes that are socially considered as abject or disgusting. Jokes and euphemisms have historically served as a way to "talk around" menstruation, framing it as an unclean or impolite topic that should remain concealed or hidden. Menstrual-tracking app design extends this logic, reinforcing the perception that menstruation remains a "sensitive" or taboo subject.

I then describe the aesthetics of the cycle visualizations and analytics sections to consider how these apps use and promote the biomedical model of menstruation. Most menstrual-tracking apps use hormone-based models of the menstrual cycle, which break down the process into four primary phases. A visualization of this model almost always serves as the homepage for the app and is central to the data archive and analysis features. The four phases of the cycle are visually placed alongside self-tracking features to reinforce the perceived connection between sex hormones, menstrual cycle phases, and bodily experience. By situating menstrual-tracking apps in the history of premenstrual syndrome (PMS), I show how this visual model promotes an understanding of the hormonal body as the cause of distress or disturbances to the cyclical norm, leading to a separation between the "true self" and the menstrual body. The analytic sections are meant to show clear connections between emotional and physical experiences and phases of the menstrual cycle, which can lead individuals to understand their lives through their fluctuating hormones. Much like discourses of PMS, the hormonal body emerges as the locus of distress, which can lead individuals to invalidate their emotions or blame hormonal fluctuations for any physical or emotional discomfort. By giving such explanatory power to biological processes that remain out of the individual's control, these apps frame the body as an unruly and uncontrollable cause of a range of complex emotional and physical experiences.

While this chapter illustrates how the existing aesthetics and tracking features risk reinforcing biomedical bodily alienation and stigmas surrounding menstruation, I end by considering how the technologies might be adjusted to promote a more reflexive understanding of menstrual health. Reproductive health research increasingly relies on big-data methods and analytics to determine what constitutes "healthy" in the scientific and public spheres alike. In response, many scholars warn that hyper-reliance on data threatens to efface social and cultural context, a tendency particularly dangerous for the fields of health and medicine.[15] At the same time, the recent phenomenological, ethnographic work of Laetitia Della Bianca illustrates the multiple forms of embodiment and selfhood that emerge through datafied and self-tracking practices that resist simply reading menstrual-tracking technologies as tools for the medicalization of the reproductive body. She argues that fertility tracking "processes shape multiple distributions of the self, through which users align multiple elements, including their embodied self, datafied cycle, relations with others, biomedical knowledge, experiential knowledge, bodily sensations, and others."[16] Sociological studies likewise question the complex set of embodied experiences that emerge in PMS, showing how medical recognition of psychological and physiological experiences can serve as a critical source of validation, particularly for those who have historically been overlooked or dismissed due to gendered stereotypes. So, while data can often obscure or suppress individual experiences and cultural and social context, it nonetheless holds immense epistemological value for intuitions, the public, and individuals alike. In their study of PMS and women's experiences, Jane Ussher and Janette Perz ask how to remain critical of the social and scientific constructions of menstrual distress without dismissing the lived experiences of those who suffer from premenstrual symptoms.[17] Likewise, through phenomenological descriptions of my experiences with menstrual-tracking apps I ask how to remain critical of the biomedical, determinist structures of these apps while still recognizing that they can serve as critical tools for people who menstruate to make sense of their embodied experiences and sense their body's natural fluctuations and changes throughout a menstrual cycle. With these concerns in mind, I end with a call for collaborations between humanists, scientists, and designers to redesign these apps to support reflexive relationships to the body and promote research on historically underexplored issues of sexual and reproductive health.

Managing Excess and Excretion

With more than 153 million users worldwide, Flo is the "#1 app for women's health."[18] Flo's central interface is focused on the period count-

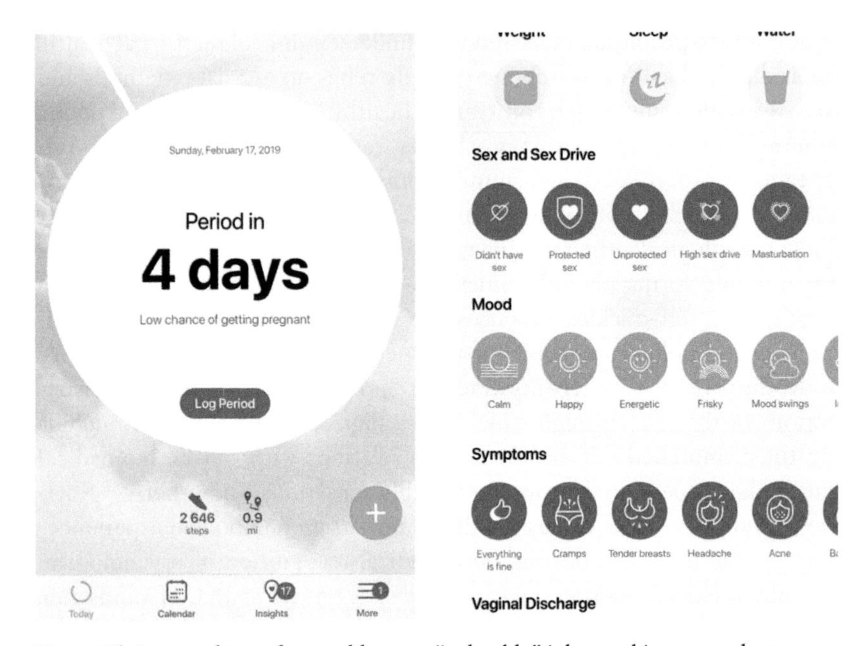

Fig. 2. Flo's central interface and log use "palatable" jokes and iconography to visualize symptoms and the cycle timeline. (Flo Health, Inc., "Flo," Apple App Store, vers. 4.31, 2019, accessed March 2019.)

down (Fig. 2), where a large circle floats over the background of fluffy pink clouds counting down the days to ovulation. The text below informs the individual of their risk of getting pregnant, and a red button allows them to log the dates of their latest period. Most of the interactions occur through the daily log, accessible through the small turquoise "plus-sign" icon on the bottom right of the screen. Selecting the icon reveals a pop-up window where individuals are meant to log daily activities and emotional and physical symptoms. In addition to spaces to input weight, sleep hours, and water consumption, the log interface is broken down into categories ranging from "sex and sex drive" to "mood" and "physical activity." Each offers a variety of cute, emoji-like icons with corresponding labels that can be selected and logged on a given day. For example, "sad" is coupled with a tiny rain cloud, and a balloon represents "bloating." Like most menstrual-tracking apps, Flo uses polite symbols to track bodily abjection, including various droplet icons to stand in for the heaviness of flow, an animated toilet with a lock representing constipation, and a roll of toilet paper for diarrhea. The visualization of symptoms becomes increasingly abstract as it represents the range of options for vaginal discharge, presenting qualities such as "sticky" and "creamy" through white and purple circles.

Menstrual-tracking apps are often deemed progressive for acknowledging the variety of symptoms that surround menstruation.[19] For example, Flo gives as much emphasis to diarrhea—a less openly discussed condition—as it does to bloating or cravings. By placing diarrhea, nausea, and constipation alongside more commonly recognized menstrual symptoms, these apps employ the logic of "period talk," which seeks to demystify the range of emotional and physical processes associated with menstruation and empower individuals by "[allowing] the speaker to draw on a well-established and pervasive axiom of perceived silence. In the disruption of this silence, the speaker can explore, disrupt and test the gender norms that surround menstruation, and more generally."[20] Flo and other menstrual-tracking apps would seem to disrupt this silence by acknowledging the presence and persistence of fluids and excretion, undermining the highly sanitized rhetoric of hygiene that surrounds menstruation. Ideally, by "talking about" these symptoms, menstrual-tracking apps work to undo some of the shame associated with menstrual abjection.

Indeed, Clue, an app celebrated for its progressive gender-neutral color scheme and address, claims that its use of language and iconography is explicitly designed to break the silence and linguistic suppression that have historically been upheld by menstrual euphemisms: "Clue bypasses cultural discomfort by speaking plainly and refusing the use of euphemisms. Sex is called 'sex,' not 'the baby dance.' Menstrual bleeding is called 'bleeding,' not 'Aunt Flo.'"[21] Clue is one of the few apps that continually revises its log iconography to offer the most transparent and neutral representations of behaviors and bodily processes to avoid gender stereotypes and menstrual shame. For example, its website details the decision to change its sex icons to address a more inclusive audience. Originally, sexual activity was visualized through two contrasting images of lounging stick figures with the "protected sex" figure wearing a tie. Following complaints that the figure coded masculine and reinforced heteronormativity, Clue revised the icons to an image of a flip-flop sandal for "unprotected sex" and rain boots for "protected," which were designed to be humorous, "but with emotional intelligence."[22]

Despite Clue's efforts, the app's design and emphasis on humor tie it to menstrual jokes and euphemisms, which are often used to reinforce the idea that menstruation is a taboo subject. Sociological studies have illustrated how euphemisms, jokes, metaphors, and other linguistic codes support the perception that menstruation (and by extension the menstruating body) should remain "hidden" because it is "disgusting," "unclean," and "dirty."[23] Euphemistic references to blood, an unwelcome guest ("Aunt Flo"), and distress ("the curse") all subtly support the perception that menstruation is both unwelcome and unpleasant for both the person who menstruates and the public alike. While vulgar and graphic references ("shark week") directly support the perception of menstrual abjection, polite euphemisms likewise uphold the sense that menstruation is a topic that should not be discussed directly or publicly. Even terms like "period" help create distance between the speaker and referent, reinforcing the idea that menstruation is a "sensitive topic" that requires both linguistic and physical concealment.[24]

Both Flo and Clue's use of cute or humorous icons might be compared to menstrual jokes: they transform the symptoms and experiences that were once perhaps considered gross or uncomfortable into funny, palatable animations that often dance and wiggle on selection. Numerous scholars have argued that menstrual jokes and euphemisms serve as ways to discuss the taboo topic, and consequently reveal both stereotypical and subversive[25] understandings of menstruation and femininity.[26] In her analysis of Tampax's "Mother Nature" campaign, Camilla Røstvik describes how Tampax's marketing company drew on feminist cultural analysis of menstruation to create humorous advertisements for their products. The series of print and video ads depicted menstruation as "Mother Nature," a middle-aged "she-devil, decked out in green Chanel and high heels," being fought off by strong "Alpha girls" using Tampax products. The visual gags and funny taglines promoted a more diverse image of young, female menstruators, but simultaneously reinforced negative stereotypes of menstruation and femininity through the characterization of the Mother Nature character.[27] Whether they aim to intervene in or reinforce existing understandings of menstruation, both euphemisms and jokes operate as ways to indirectly address the unfamiliar or uncomfortable topic. For example, in her discussion of menstrual jokes, Victoria Newton describes how humor is used to navigate the unknown: "Joking about a subject which is not fully understood dissipates anxieties, but also offers a method of talking about something that [the speaker] and others are experiencing, without divulging how much they do or do not actually know."[28]

Menstrual jokes and euphemisms can function as a socially acceptable way to address menstruation without the speaker revealing their relationship to the taboo subject, offering a "safe" space for discussion. The funny icons of Flo or Clue may similarly offer a source of relief:

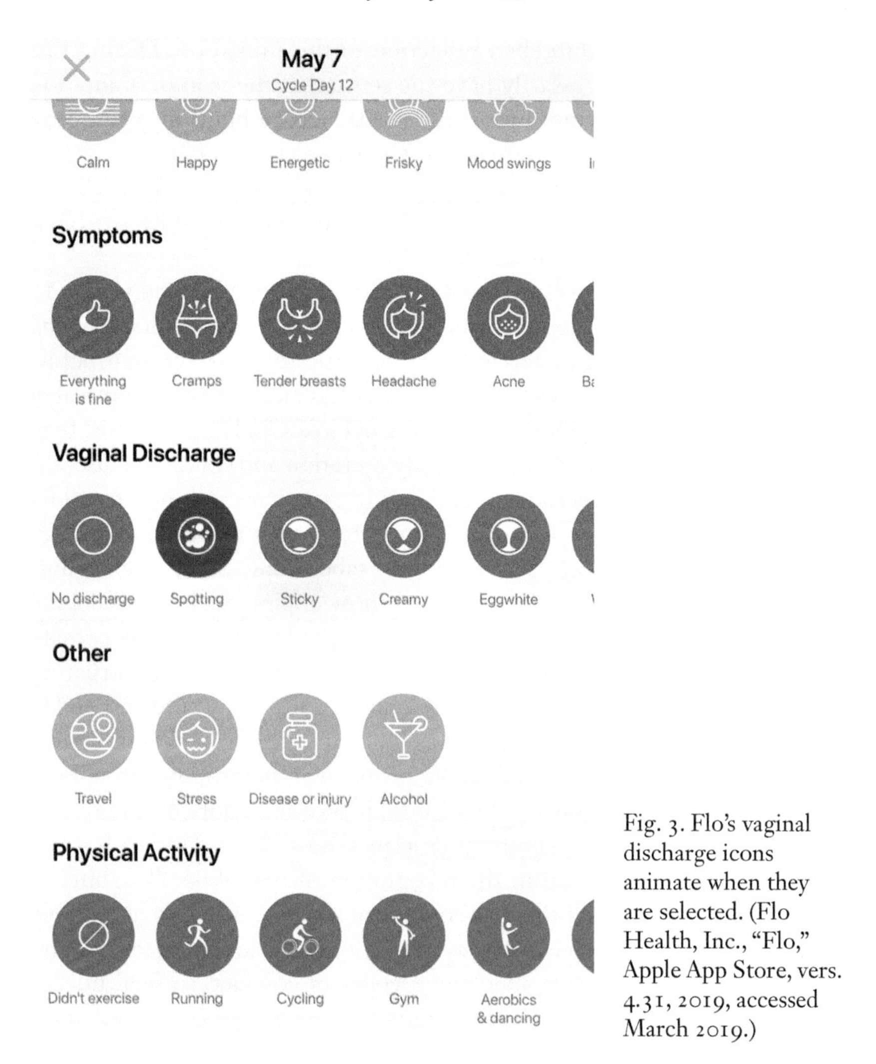

Fig. 3. Flo's vaginal discharge icons animate when they are selected. (Flo Health, Inc., "Flo," Apple App Store, vers. 4.31, 2019, accessed March 2019.)

individuals can track the presence of these symptoms while remaining at a mediated distance through the visual abstraction of their experiences. For example, opening Flo's log prompts me to reflect on my emotional and physical experiences. I swipe through the "vaginal discharge" options and select "no discharge," an icon showing a white circle over a purple background (Fig. 3). This prompts a tiny white circle to burst from the center of the icon, momentarily filling it in and contracting inward. I find this encounter both strange and satisfying as my attention very quickly moves from my own embodied reflection to the animation. During this interaction, I don't necessarily have the sense that the icon or animation reflects the physical symptom or my experience; rather, I'm focused on the sense of gratification that comes when a selection effectively transforms bodily abjection into an animated abstraction. Vaginal discharge no longer seems to refer to my own bodily excess, but the oddly satisfying array of moving, circular animations.

In the case of Flo and Clue, the discreet animations allow individuals to indirectly acknowledge forms of menstrual abjection. But confined to the private space of the app interface, they do little to break through public or even personal pressures to keep bodily excess and excretions concealed and controlled. Consequently, like menstrual jokes and euphemisms, they reinforce the social suppression of bodily excretion and continued discomfort with the ordinary emotional and bodily experiences of menstruation. Though jokes and other forms of "period talk" may break down certain social barriers that prevent acknowledging taboo topics, they often simultaneously reinforce the concealment of those topics. Sociologist Sophie Laws describes linguistic codes that are both produced by and perpetuate "menstrual etiquette," the set of practices and rules around menstruating bodies and public menstrual discourse. She argues that polite and coded language for menstruation perpetuates the etiquette of cleanliness, discretion, and concealment that encourage people who menstruate "to uphold the taboos against themselves through their own behaviors of silence and concealment."[29] Newton similarly describes how the humor of a menstrual joke is often located in the recognition of the taboo: "laughing at it, we are acknowledging that the content of the joke is not an acceptable thing to mention, or do, in everyday life. Thus the joke reinforces existing gendered power structures, ideologies, codes of conduct, societal norms, and values."[30] Indeed, sociological studies on perceptions of menstruation among women and girls have reported the use of humor as a key strategy "to manage their unease, to talk around menstruation."[31] The log interfaces of these apps operate through a similar structure; the tiny toilets and balloons politely poke fun at the presence of the symptom, while still reinforcing the fact that these are topics not to be discussed directly; combining acknowledgment with abstraction and humor, they suggest that these natural bodily processes should remain suppressed.[32]

The emphasis on symbols and polite iconography is related to an investment in discretion: iconography helps distance individuals from their bodily excess and helps encode this process into a private symbolic system.

This practice is not new; rather, menstrual-tracking apps are an extension of analog systems of menstrual tracking that typically take the form of personal calendars and notation systems. Many individuals who menstruate keep track of their menstrual cycles through visual or linguistic codes. For example, a dot or an "x" can serve as a way to mark the days of a menstrual cycle on one's personal calendar. Menstrual-tracking apps essentially digitize this notation system to ideally offer a more private and consolidated space for monitoring.

However, in the largest study to date on menstrual- and fertility-tracking apps, Epstein and colleagues found that participants often still expressed fear of menstrual disclosure through their tracking apps.[33] Like calendars, phones operate in a semipublic space, vulnerable to wandering eyes, and participants noted this through their discussion of the relationship between the app's design and sense of privacy: "I used to be embarrassed when other people looked at my phone and saw a bright pink tracking app."[34] The fear of the prying eye "decoding" the pink app on her interface led this participant to switch to Clue, an app that explicitly avoids feminine iconography. Clue's app icon shows a series of red overlapping circles that form a flower or atom-shaped graphic on a white background. The name, "Clue," similarly obscures the program's relationship to menstruation, which allowed her to "feel more secure in letting other people handle my phone." Others echoed her sentiment, detailing attempts to rename their trackers or to suggest that apps use a more neutral design approach: "no one will guess what it is because it looks like an average app."[35]

Across accounts from participants, there is a persistent fear of others discovering that they are menstruating or that they track their menstrual cycles. Numerous scholars have discussed how people who menstruate, particularly cis women, have been conditioned to conceal menstruation. Studies of advertising and menstrual hygiene products, ethnographies of adolescent girls and women, and phenomenologies of menstruation have all demonstrated how society has encouraged the suppression of menstrual acknowledgment.[36] Across these accounts, scholars emphasize how women, from their "earliest awareness of menstruation," are essentially told "do not discuss your menstruation. . . . Keep the signs of your menstruation hidden."[37] For feminist scholars, this imperative is essential to upholding the regulation of feminine bodies, encouraging women to police their behaviors and appearance under the guise of "personal hygiene."[38] Femininity thus comes to be defined as the absence of the abject fluids that emerge in ordinary life, leading women to reject and resent their body's natural processes.[39]

The analysis of the log interfaces and participant accounts places menstrual-tracking apps in the history of consumer menstrual technologies, in which retailers and companies have continuously struggled to "promote and sell products that people are embarrassed to be seen buying."[40] The menstrual hygiene industry has been central to upholding the perception that menstruation and the menstruating body are abject and require careful management and concealment. But by stigmatizing all signifiers of menstruation, including their own products, companies undermine conspicuous consumption practices.[41] In the 1920s, companies aimed to solve the menstrual-market paradox by selling wrapped boxes of their products, allowing individuals to discreetly purchase their products at their local stores without any anxiety or embarrassment. Reflecting on these practices in 1958, one Kotex executive remarked, "to some extent, I think we led women to feel that packaging is related to this whole subject by deliberately hiding it, making it something that has a social stigma attached to it."[42] As the testimony from Epstein and colleagues' study suggests, menstrual-tracking apps face similar challenges, despite the language of transparency and empowerment. Both Clue and Flo, for example, disguise their primary function through abstract icons: the Flo icon that appears on the dashboard of a smartphone features a white feather over a pink background, and Clue's generic icon likewise resists any connection to menstruation. Thus, while menstrual-tracking apps sell themselves as essential tools for individuals to learn and demystify the menstrual cycle, in practice they often function as tools for concealment—new forms of wrapping that mask menstrual disclosure.

Though concealment most immediately refers to managing markers of abject menstrual fluid, from avoiding leaks and stains to the use of products designed to be discreet and uphold standards of Western cleanliness, it extends to the suppression of *any* symbolic, physical, or social markers of menstruation. Menstrual jokes and euphemisms are examples of menstruation being concealed linguistically, providing a verbal means to reassert the menstrual taboo and reinforce its suppression. menstrual-tracking apps allow individuals to continue to suppress symbolic and linguistic markers of menstruation, not only through the use of euphemistic humor but through the emphasis on discretion and privacy. So, while apps like Clue and Spot On (Planned Parenthood's menstrual-tracking app) employ a gender-neutral color scheme in an attempt to address a more inclusive audience, they are consequently also useful tools for menstrual concealment.[43] Indeed, Clue's name and app icon avoid any direct reference to menstruation, offering the ideal means to conceal menstrual monitoring.

Descriptions of these apps' log and design features reveal how they reinforce the perception that menstruation is an entirely private experience of self-management.[44] The tracking features of the log interface are meant to provide discreet means of tracking symptoms and, ideally, of anticipating bodily excretion and excess. Tracking over time supposedly allows individuals to predict, manage, and perhaps suppress bodily excess and excretion, privately and personally. The logs function as a way to monitor physical and emotional changes, and by detecting patterns, they may allow individuals to better conceal traces of their menstrual status.

Biomedical Cycles

Logging personal data over time through these apps results in a substantial archive of daily behaviors, physical symptoms, moods, and activities. For both Clue and Flo, this archive informs the predictive algorithm and is meant to give individuals a resource to track patterns and disruptions in their cycle, monitor average cycle or period length, and anticipate upcoming periods. For example, individuals can scroll through the calendar section of the app to locate the beginning of their last cycle, or even go forward several months ahead to see when they may expect future periods. Some have anecdotally reported using these features to plan their vacations or activities around predicted windows. And like other analog forms of menstrual tracking, the app is most often used to monitor late periods as an indicator of pregnancy.[45]

Menstrual-tracking apps use biomedical hormone-based models of the menstrual cycle to predict future windows for menstruation, ovulation, and PMS. The biomedical model breaks the typical menstrual cycle down into four primary phases—menstruation, follicular, ovulation, and luteal—each designated by shifts in hormone levels that are understood to trigger corresponding physiological reactions in the ovaries, fallopian tubes, and uterus. The information collected through menstrual-tracking apps is processed through an algorithm based on this biomedical model to predict specific windows for ovulation and menstruation. While researchers have ascribed particular hormone levels and ratios to each corresponding phase, it's incredibly difficult for menstrual-tracking apps and research studies alike to know for certain whether individuals are currently in the follicular, ovulation, or luteal phase. Indeed, research on the menstrual cycle has faced the challenge of studying the effects of these three phases precisely because they often lack identifiable physiological changes:[46] the exact phase can only be identified through daily hormone-level testing.[47] Instead, the biomedical model and menstrual-tracking apps use approximate windows to gauge these phases, based on the model twenty-four- to thirty-eight-day cycle, with ovulation typically occurring fourteen days following the first day of menstruation. Clue's "information" section explains that the "fertile window" includes the six days before ovulation and twenty-four hours after, but warns that pregnancy can happen outside of this predictive window.[48] In addition to the four-phase model, Clue offers examples of more accurate ways to help determine ovulation—including monitoring discharge, basal temperature, and at-home luteinizing-hormone testing—but it warns users that the app does not currently incorporate this kind of data "into its predictive algorithm for your fertile window."[49] This warning is meant to clarify that the cycle phase breakdown is not personalized (outside of menstruation) to the individual user, but instead is based on statistical models for typical hormone fluctuation patterns.

Despite warning individuals that the biomedical model may not align with their unique menstrual phases, the interface design of menstrual-tracking apps often reinforces the four-stage model. For example, Clue's home screen features a circular arrow graphic, which is segmented and color-coded to designate specific phases. The start of the arrow graphic is shaded red to designate menstruation, and the middle section is shaded blue to designate the "fertile window." Clue does not label the follicular and luteal phases, but the inclusion of the fertile-window section visually breaks the cycle graphic into four distinct sections. These phases are then accompanied by supporting information sections that provide short summaries of each of the four phases, including descriptions of the hormonal processes and any possible physiological changes.[50] Flo's calendar view of the menstrual cycle similarly breaks down the cycle into color-coded phases: red designating the menstruation phase, blue the fertile phase (Fig. 4). Both of these interfaces use bold color-contrasting models to communicate the biomedical model, encouraging individuals to consider menstruation as part of an ongoing four-phase process.

Though these models are most immediately used to predict menstruation and ovulation, they simultaneously support a cycle-based approach to overall health. Menstrual-tracking apps often promote the idea that the menstrual cycle functions "as a vital sign . . . [it] can tell you about your health and wellness just like your blood pressure, heart rate, or pulse."[51]

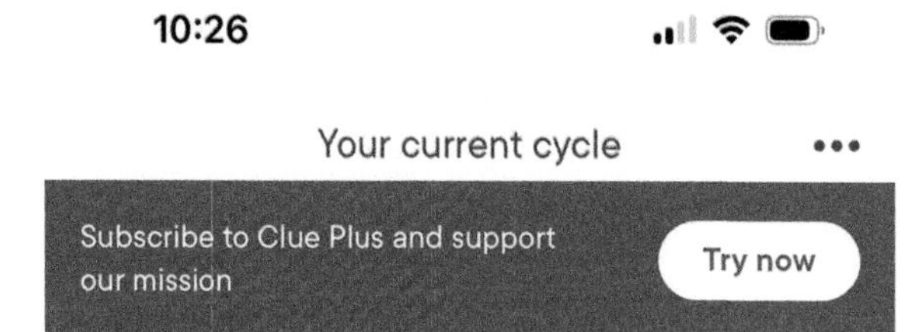

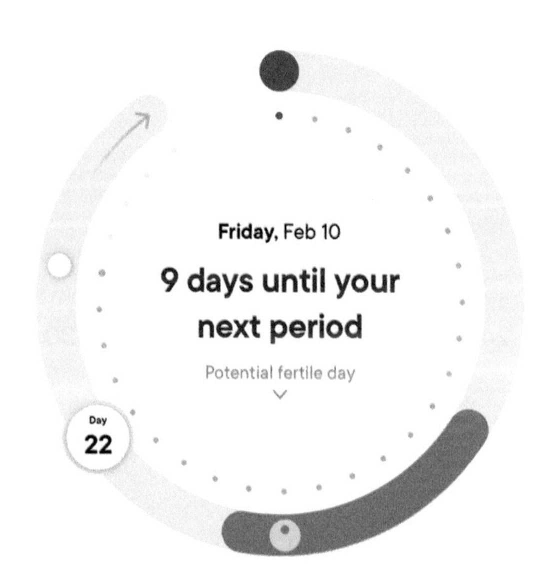

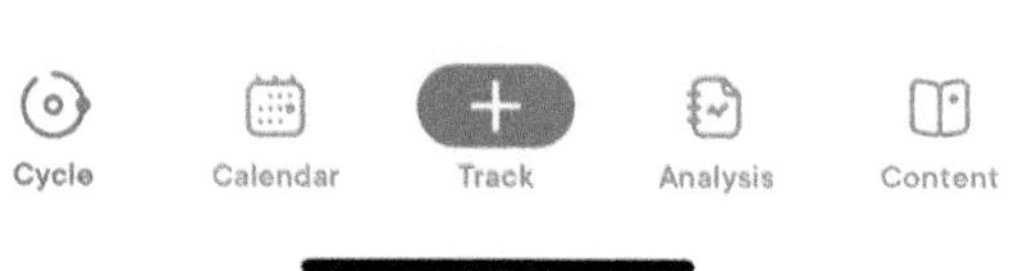

Fig. 4. Clue's central interface color-codes the menstrual and ovulation phases of the cycle to visually segment the cycle into the four phases. (BioWink, "Clue," vers. 103.0, accessed February 2023.)

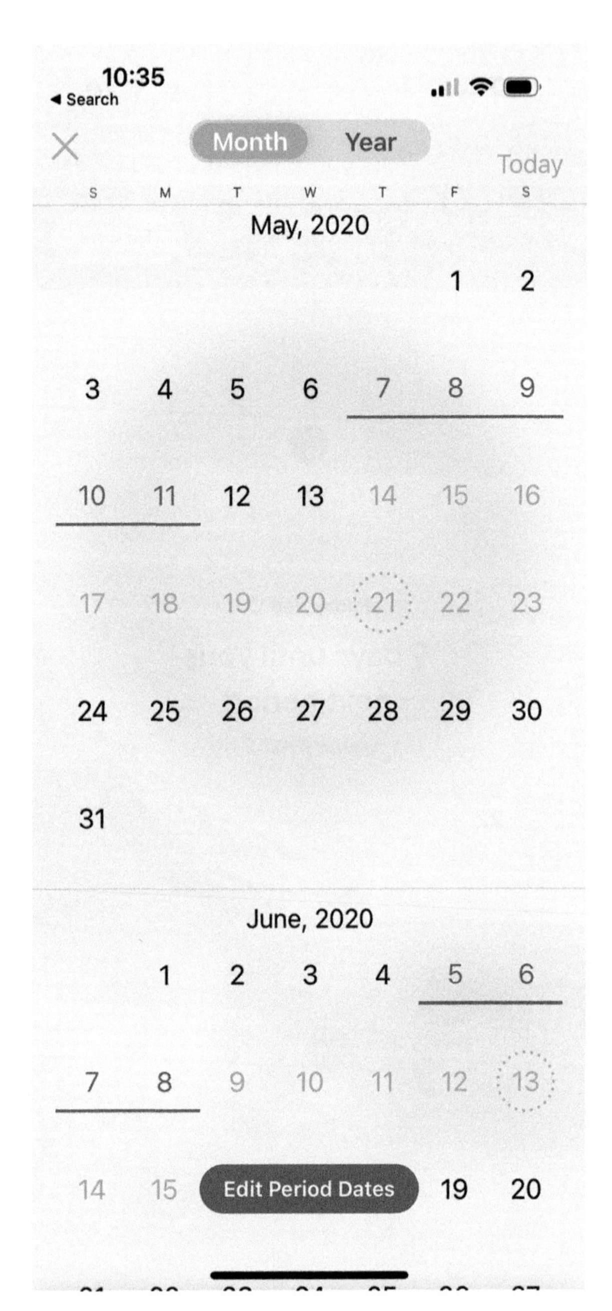

Fig. 5. Flo's calendar view marks ovulation and menstruation days to visually separate the cycle into four phases. (Flo Living, "Flo," vers. 4.31, accessed July 2021.)

Company websites and supporters of this understanding often stress how changes to the menstrual cycle can indicate a range of issues, including immunological problems, hormonal imbalances, nutritional deficiencies, and allergies.[52] Individuals are encouraged to track as much information as possible to not only learn how their body reacts throughout a cycle, but also to use the four phases as a baseline to monitor any changes or disruptions. The cycle, according to Clue, is an essential barometer of overall health: "[it] can let you know when everything is working as usual, when your body is going through a change, or when something is not as it should be."[53] Numerous health institutions claim that regular periods are an indication that "your body is working normally," while deviations from this norm "may be a sign of a serious health problem."[54] Atypical emotional and physical reactions are meant to serve as potential indicators of other health issues: "ovulatory disturbances . . . are an important but clinically silent risk factor for ill health."[55] App developers and medical researchers have framed menstrual-tracking apps as critical tools to support this mode of health monitoring, and ultimately support ongoing research into the effects of all four phases of the menstrual cycle.[56] Indeed, by datafying the symptoms, they seem to offer an accurate and accessible way to monitor correlations between an individual's cycle and their physical and emotional well-being.[57]

However, some sociological studies have criticized this biomedical framework, arguing that these apps set norms and baselines that fail to consider the diversity of cycle timelines and experiences.[58] While most cycles do last twenty-four to thirty-six days, scientists and physicians note the range of factors that can cause disruption to this model, including stress, diet, or social circumstances that do not necessarily indicate a major health problem. The highly regulated, cyclical structures of the algorithm cannot account for these types of deviations; instead, they focus on whether a menstrual cycle is early or late, and frame variations in a cycle as an indicator of pregnancy (or of a potential health problem). Lupton and Healy have argued that the use of the biomedical model of menstruation reinforces the idea that menstruation is a function of fertility. As a result, these apps appear to extend historical models of menstruation, where the menstrual cycle is described as a process that aims to result in pregnancy.[59] In this context, the appearance of menstruation risks being understood as a "failed pregnancy," a breakdown in the function of the system.[60] Locating fertility tracking apps in a broader cultural concern around women's infertility, Celia Roberts and Catherine Waldby claim the use of quantification and biomedical models of fertility renders it an asset, or "a material resources controlled and managed by the woman herself with the expectation of future value."[61] This leaves the reproductive body vulnerable to commodification, supporting the expansion of markets devoted to monitoring, preserving, and supporting the promise of a future healthy and successful pregnancy.[62]

While the medical model supports understanding menstruation through pregnancy, it also promotes regularity *throughout* the menstrual cycle, framing *any* violation of the norm as a potential problem. Thus, this model risks expanding the medicalization of the reproductive body, as the follicular and luteal phases increasingly come to be understood through the logic of illness. The emphasis on regularity across the cycle phase risks promoting an extension of the homeostatic model of health, where health is understood as consistency, uniformity, and regularity. While a cycle-based model of health acknowledges the shifts and changes that occur during a menstrual cycle, those shifts are part of a larger pattern that functions as the norm or standard—a vital sign—by which an individual should gauge their overall health.

More recently, menstrual-tracking apps' cycle models have faced criticism for their ties to natural family planning practices associated with the Catholic Church. Fox and colleagues locate the apps in a history of analog cycle-tracking technologies that have been used by religious institutions as a form of natural birth control. Only in the 1980s did these models begin to strip off their religious associations, promoting monitoring as a method to resist pharmaceutical and medicalized models of contraception.[63] Drawing on feminist health principles, more recent, secular supporters of cycle- or fertility-awareness models often claim that this approach is essential to counteracting bodily alienation. Cycle awareness functions as a kind of "body literacy," as individuals learn to read and interpret the "signs and signals of [their] menstrual cycle."[64] Closely monitoring the body's slight changes, from discharge to energy levels and muscle tension, encourages individuals to become increasingly attuned to daily shifts in their bodies. Menstrual advocates frame this practice as a form of "cultural resistance," a way for people who menstruate to "rely less on institutionalized health care and more on their own resourcefulness."[65] Cycle awareness thus directly counteracts the mind-body split "that is ultimately damaging to women's health locus of control . . . and makes them vulnerable to cultural bias . . . and medical misogyny."[66] At the same time, the secular form of cycle awareness is often supported by medical practitioners who see this practice not as resistance to institutional care, but as a supplement. Remaining attuned to and tracking shifts across the duration of the menstrual cycle helps individuals advocate for themselves as they learn about the biomedical model of menstruation and its effect on their bodies.[67]

The awareness-based model of health monitoring contrasts with many of the goal-based self-tracking technologies discussed throughout this book. In goal-based tracking, data archives are used to provide benchmarks for improvement, while incentive and deadline structures encourage individuals to modify their behaviors accordingly. Control through these self-tracking technologies entails using data to change present behaviors to meet future outcomes. Menstrual-tracking apps, by contrast, are not designed to allow people who menstruate to change or influence their actual menstrual cycles. Rather, self-tracking is largely "observational": "In menstrual cycle tracking . . . women primarily *observe* what they are tracking with little or no control. . . . Rather than trying to change the outcome of being tracked, women track to learn how to adjust their thoughts and behaviors around it . . . observing can help explain symptoms and even identify causes."[68] Indeed, Epstein and colleagues found that the primary function of the app for most individuals was not contraception or getting pregnant, but a desire to gain an understanding of overall health that emerges from the patterns and correlations discerned through the archival and analytic features of the apps. For example, studying the personal archive may reveal a pattern of bloating on the second day of a period, or mood swings during ovulation. Observing these types of patterns will ideally allow individuals to anticipate emotional and bodily changes, and even to make small adjustments to habits or behaviors accordingly.

In other words, "control" is not located in the physiological process of the menstrual cycle, but in the ways that individuals adjust or manage their social and behavioral patterns around their cycle. In her ethnographic study of fertility-tracking apps, Della Bianca found that individuals used self-tracking and data as mediators for their experiences, to interpret, navigate, and understand shifts in their bodies according to their cycles.[69] This approach to menstrual management has also been found in studies that explore women's perception of PMS symptoms. In their 2012 study, Jane Ussher and Janette Perz found that women who monitored and anticipated their PMS symptoms often developed coping and management strategies for any emotional or physical changes. Women described how they would modify their behaviors, including decreasing stressors or removing themselves from social situations to reduce situations that result in premenstrual anger or irritation. Locating these testimonies in a broader cultural analysis of menstrual discourse, Ussher and Perz describe this strategy as a form of self-silencing supported by "monitoring and regulating their environment, in order to regulate their premenstrual emotional reactions."[70] In other words, the testimony suggests that individual responses—self-silencing—functioned as a "solution" for social and cultural norms that deem PMS distress as a problem.

The biomedical model of the menstrual cycle offers a structure to support these monitoring and self-management systems, which are only further reinforced and expanded through menstrual-tracking apps. By breaking the cycle into four visually distinct phases, and providing supplementary information about the physiological and chemical changes in the body, these apps promote a biomedical way of seeing menstruation. Combined with self-tracking, menstrual-tracking apps provide a system through which individuals can monitor their behaviors and reactions to hormonal shifts, and make adjustments accordingly. In other words, menstrual-tracking apps promote the biomedical model as a tool for self-management, where menstrual awareness can be mobilized to control and suppress the threat of social disruption.

Life as Cycle

While the cycle visualizations help support a biomedical way of seeing menstrual health, the analytic sections of menstrual-tracking apps encourage a biomedical way of understanding the body more generally, and indeed of understanding life itself. Almost all menstrual-tracking apps include analytic sections that offer statistical information on cycles and timeline features designed to reveal patterns and correlations. Flo's "graphs and reports" section, for example, organizes the data according to a range of categories, including cycle length, period length, and intensity. Each of these options offers a visualized breakdown of a single month's data, mapping the cycle through a horizontal bar, color-coded to indicate the various phases. Individuals have the option to view these graphs alongside the logged emotional and physical symptoms (Fig. 6). For each month, a cycle timeline spans the width of the screen, sectioned off in red for days menstruating and blue for ovulation, with a list of symptoms below and corresponding yellow dots to mark the days they were logged. Looking at these visualizations, individuals can easily see connections between the phases of their cycle and logged symptoms. A cluster of yellow "headache" dots

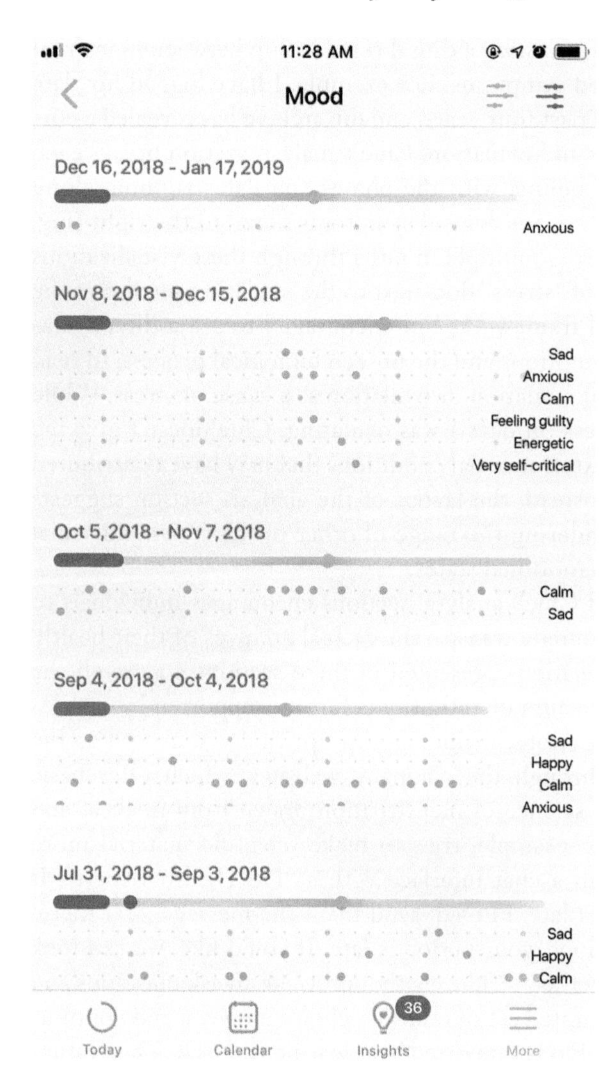

Fig. 6. Flo's analytics section maps emotions alongside cycle phases to reveal correlations. (Flo Health, Inc., "Flo," vers. 4.31, 2019, accessed November 2019.)

below the period section suggests a connection, or the repeated appearance of "craving" dots two days before ovulation may reveal a correspondence between the cycle phase and this symptom.

While the design of Flo's interface may suggest clear connections between a user's cycle and symptoms, it's very difficult to know for sure whether these behavioral and emotional patterns can be linked to specific phases of the menstrual cycle. Though scholars and journalists continually warn that "correlation is not causation," the design of these apps encourages individuals to *assume* a causal relationship between menstrual cycle phases and logged symptoms. For example, I have logged my data in my Clue app for the past four years, and my archive has revealed a correlation between stress and ovulation. Clue's analysis section breaks each cycle into a vertical timeline, with the phases and dates running along the left side of the screen, and logged symptoms noted to the right (Fig. 7). Comparing data across multiple months through these visualizations has revealed a pattern of "stress" dots next to the ovulation section of the timeline. In this visual framework, I'm encouraged to see a direct relationship between my emotions and the unseen biological process: to read stress as an indicator of ovulation or ovulation as a cause of stress. While I may have logged stress on days I was ovulating, Clue doesn't give me the choice to include exterior social conditions that may have contributed to this experience.[71] Instead, the layout of the analysis section suggests causality without considering the range of other professional and social factors that shape my emotional states.

Looking at Flo and Clue's analytic sections encourages individuals to see the patterns as seemingly transparent, factual archives of their health. By extension, the correlations presented in these sections appear all the more authoritative. The aura of authority is further supported by supplementary information sections, including pop-up windows, as well as the wealth of resources through the company websites, which offer basic information about the science of menstruation drawn from medical and scientific texts. Flo, for example, tries to make scientific material more "approachable" through a chat interface with a "Flo Health Expert." If an individual's period is late, Flo will send them the message: "Hi there! Based on Flo's predictions, your period is late. If you'd like, we can look for a possible cause together."[72] The chatbot proceeds to ask questions and offer the individual a limited set of multiple-choice answers, and continually reminds them that Flo is supported by scientific research. This feature aims to simulate the experience of chatting with a medical representative, reinforcing the sense that the information and interfaces the apps provide are informed by reproductive health experts. Clue, which describes itself as "scientific and straightforward,"[73] foregrounds its partnerships with academic institutions and medical researchers, proudly displaying university crests and links to published studies using data collected through the app. While the lengthy terms and conditions, and the fine print of some supplementary information sections, state that companies are not sources of medical authority and encourage individuals to consult their physicians,

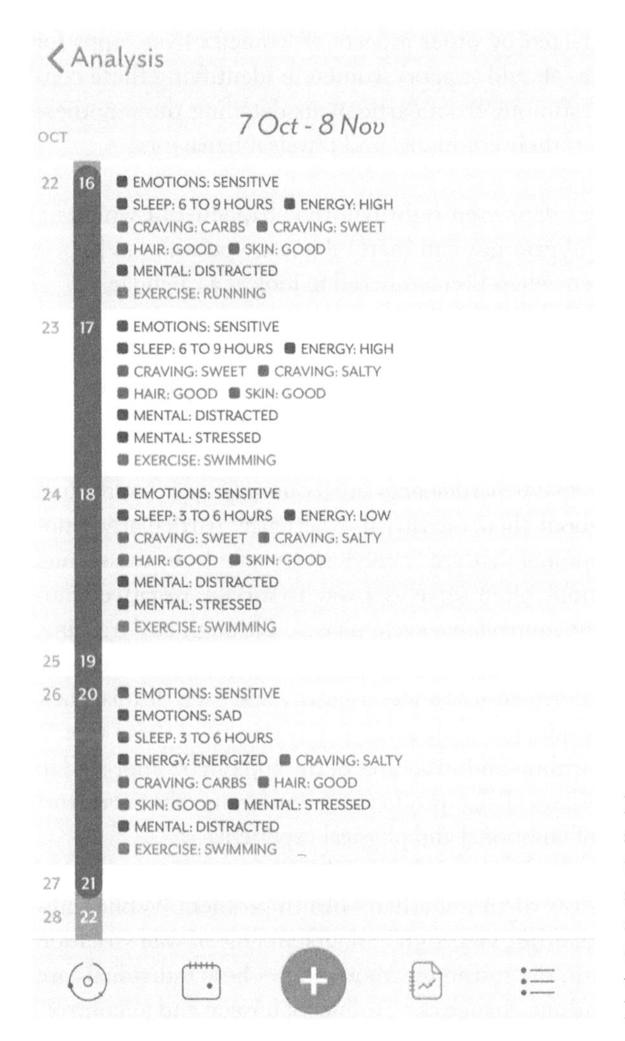

Fig. 7. Individuals scroll vertically through Clue's analytics timeline to see cycle correlations. (Biowink, "Clue," vers. 5.13, accessed November 2019.)

they all simultaneously rely on the aesthetics and rhetoric of biomedicine to assert their value.

The aura of science and medicine, in combination with the analytics sections of menstrual-tracking apps, supports a biomedical way of understanding bodies, behaviors, and emotions. The organization of the archival sections not only breeds awareness of the four phases, but encourages individuals to understand the relationship between their cycles and personal experiences. Epstein and colleagues frame the correlations and patterns that emerge through these apps as transparent self-knowledge: "Menstrual cycles affect and are affected by other aspects of women's lives. Apps for tracking menstrual cycles should support women in identifying these connections."[74] They cite testimony from participants detailing the way these apps helped them explain their emotional and physical behaviors:

> I was consistently . . . depressed right before it happened. I would be really unhappy and grumpy, and then I'd get my period. . . . [K] eeping track of it, then, when I remembered to look at a calendar, I'd be, "oh, this is why I feel like this."[75]
>
> Sometimes I'm really emotional and irrational and I can look at my tracker, see that my period is due in a week or less and chill out and realize I'm PMSing instead of having real feelings.[76]

The sentiments expressed by participants are common ways individuals understand and speak about their menstrual experience, particularly emotional and physical symptoms that are framed as deviant. As in the second example, these justifications often serve as a way to ascribe negative emotions to an individual's uncontrollable cycle phases. Through self-tracking, participants were able to attribute their experience to the phases of the menstrual cycle, using this information as a way to justify and even dismiss their feelings or behaviors.[77] While the study is ultimately critical of these apps, it emphasizes how the algorithms and structures of the app can be improved to support this structure of knowledge production, reinforcing the menstrual cycle as a central cause of emotional and physical experiences.[78]

Thus, any atypical behaviors or reactions risk becoming pathologized or interpreted as indicators of an underlying health problem. While individuals are advised to use the "vital sign" understanding of menstruation to monitor overall health, the testimony above shows how individuals are more likely to understand any change as a product of unseen and uncontrollable shifts in their hormones or cycle. This perspective does not encourage individuals to see themselves as "sick" or "unwell," but it does create the sense that the "true self" is distinct from the hormonal body, subject to fluctuations caused by the menstrual cycle. In other words, despite efforts to reunite body and mind, the biomedical cycle-awareness perspective that underlies menstrual-tracking apps risks encouraging bodily alienation by promoting the perception that individuals are powerless against the hormonal body.

Historically, the uncontrollable hormonal body has been used to reinforce standards of femininity[79] and suppress women's role in society.[80]

Shortly after the discovery of hormones, researchers became focused on chemicals linked to sex-specific reproductive systems, leading to the development of the field of endocrinology and sex-based hormone research. This turn marked a shift away from psychological or neurological interpretations of many diseases toward biochemical processes. Most notably, the discovery of hormones helped undermine nineteenth-century pathologies of hysteria, which often located the condition in the nervous system or psychology. However, as scholars have noted, the discovery of hormones didn't lead to the rejection of hysteria; instead, many of the physical and emotional symptoms associated with the condition were explained through biochemical processes that eventually became attached to symptoms associated with PMS. In 1931, Dr. Robert Frank published the first known article describing "premenstrual tension," which links emotional and physical distress before menstruation to the buildup of female sex hormones.[81] His early work laid the foundation for linking sex hormones to emotional and physiological distress associated with the menstrual cycle, which would later be reinforced and expanded through the work of Dr. Katherina Dalton. Dalton is credited with establishing the term "premenstrual syndrome" in the 1950s, which she attached to the deficiency of the progesterone hormone before menstruation.[82] The shift from "tension" to "syndrome" was a critical "step forward in the medicalization of women's menstrual cycles," framing the physiological and emotional responses to sex hormones as a problem (to be fixed by medicine).[83]

Frank and Dalton's theories of hormones and PMS have since been dismissed, but their work helped establish a biomedical framework for the uncontrollable menstruating body. Deviations from "normal" behaviors or emotional states become attributed to unseen and uncontrollable chemical processes supposedly unique to the female body. This led Dalton and Frank to argue that their work provided scientific evidence that women should remain out of the workforce.[84] Subject to the hormonal body, they claimed that women are not in control of their emotional or physical reactions and therefore should face restricted access to society. Though hormone theories of PMS often worked to justify gendered exclusion, they were also used as evidence for the absolution of guilt. Dalton's work, in particular, shifted toward the legal implications of the biomedical model, going as far as to argue that hormones could turn women into criminals. Throughout the 1960s, her publications were used to support numerous legal cases in the UK, including, most famously, a trial where PMS was successfully argued as a defense for murder.[85] By the 1970s and '80s, scholars and scientists increasingly dismissed this highly gendered understanding of PMS and the hormonal body more generally. However, much of the damage had already been done: PMS as a condition had been firmly established in popular discourse through popular magazines, self-help, and pharmaceuticals designed to treat the condition.[86]

Dalton and Frank's hormonal body is often invoked when people who menstruate turn to biomedical models of the menstrual cycle to absolve personal guilt. The statements from the Epstein and colleagues study illustrate how the logic of the unruly hormonal body has been internalized, functioning as a way for people who menstruate to justify any "atypical" or "abnormal" behaviors, reactions, and emotions. Indeed, since the 1950s, biomedical models of the menstrual cycle have been framed in positive terms, offering an explanation—a hormonal cause—for any behaviors that violate personal or social norms. Unlike Dalton's legal defenses, which suggested women were entirely out of control of their bodies, the popular application of the biomedical model is invoked to shift focus away from the menstruating person, to the unruly menstrual body. In her history of dysmenorrhea research (menstrual cramps), Louise Lander details how the biomedicalization of cramps not only helped enfold menstrual research into the "doctrine of medicine," but shifted the perception of accountability. Popular medical texts on cramp prevention promised to help women "realize that it's not your fault if you suffer from menstrual pain. There is a chemical basis for menstrual pain and women who suffer from it are neither neurotic nor weak."[87] Sociological studies on women's experiences of PMS have shown how this rhetoric of blame, responsibility, and guilt has become incorporated into the way individuals understand their bodies and behaviors. This most often emerges when women use PMS as an "excuse" to violate feminine social norms and to avoid forms of domestic labor.[88] But as a result, these feelings and behaviors are often invalidated, seen as simply products of hormones, rather than legitimate experiences generated from a range of intersecting social, cultural, *and* biochemical factors.

By locating the source of physical and emotional disruptions, the biomedical model is sometimes framed as resistant or empowering because it gives women license to express themselves outside of the social codes of femininity. Elizabeth Kissling describes PMS as a kind of "safety valve" that allows women to "reject" the demands of femininity, labor, and motherhood. It offers a socially acceptable and medically "approved way for women to temporarily escape their responsibilities."[89] Indeed, in their analysis of studies on PMS, Joan C. Chrisler and Paula Caplan note that PMS may be the "only time that some women 'allow' themselves to be angry . . . because they can attribute their anger to their hormones rather than to any of the many things that could legitimately anger them"[90] Thus, popular discourses often frame the biomedical model in positive terms because it seemingly allows individuals to preserve a sense of their "normal self" against the deviant emotions and behaviors that result from uncontrollable biochemical processes.[91] Likewise, menstrual-tracking apps couch this biomedical understanding of the body and self in the language of empowerment: once an individual sees the relationship between their cycle, behaviors, and emotions, they can "better prepare for them and better manage them."[92] For example, Della Bianca's study recounts how one participant used the fertility app as a lens through which to understand her day:

> The very first thing you do in the morning sets a tone for the day. . . . [The measure] helped me to get to a better question faster. So, if I feel irritated . . . it helped me to get to "OK, why am I feeling this?" faster, so I can avoid being a big jerk. And accusing others of being a big jerk . . . I'm going to adjust the day today. Or I'm just not going to talk to these people today because I'm not going to be nice [laughs]. (Robin, age 42, US)[93]

Like sociological studies of PMS, this testimony speaks to how cycle awareness can function as a way for individuals to navigate the pressures and stresses that contribute to distress. Here, cycle awareness is framed as a potential source for not only self-knowledge (or policing), but also as a resource for communicating with others—a tool for negotiating the relationship between the reproductive body, the self, and others.[94]

Ultimately, a focus on management within the biomedical model risks reinforcing the perception that the hormonal, reproductive body is "disordered, unruly, and deviant, [and] the outcome of . . . self-policing is a direct assault on the woman's corporeality."[95] The hormonal body is framed as the enemy of social order[96] and even of the "true self," as individuals understand the body as something to monitor and manage.[97] Menstrual-tracking apps risk extending the scientific logic of the hormonal premenstrual body to include all stages of the menstrual cycle. Today, people who menstruate often blame their feelings on PMS, on an unruly body they can't control at particular times of the month. Rather than contextualizing their experiences in terms of social standards of femininity, stress triggers, or a range of other factors, menstrual experiences are reduced to "markers of pathology."[98] Neatly organized alongside my cycle timeline, Clue's interface encourages such logic. With a glance, I'm inclined to correlate my social, physical, and emotional experiences with the phases of my menstrual cycle: to see my stress as a product of ovulation, a biochemical process I cannot necessarily feel, access, or control. In their current design, the aesthetics of menstrual-tracking apps encourage individuals to see their lives through their menstrual cycles—to reduce feelings, physiological conditions, and behaviors to unseen biological processes.

Indeed, the Eve app takes this logic a step further, offering daily "cyclescopes" that people can use to explain away or anticipate feelings and behaviors through their menstrual cycle phases (Fig. 8). Every day, they can open the app and learn about the biological stage of their cycle and its influence on their emotional and physical well-being. The app uses gendered language, often addressing the user as "Girl," and couples the cyclescope with a funny pop-culture gif. Many of these "scopes" draw upon menstrual stereotypes, including the emotionally unstable, chocolate-obsessed PMSing woman. Likewise, the hormone-centric MyFlo Period Tracker fully embraces a biomedical understanding of life by asking individuals to use their cycle and hormone fluctuations to determine how they go about their days. Through self-tracking, users are meant to "get in sync" with their cycle by coordinating all of their habits, behaviors, and choices according to their cycle phases: "use your cycle to choose what's easiest for you at the ideal, the most optimal time for your brain and body."[99] The app helps determine how the user should live their life by giving recommendations about whether they should "go out or stay in," eat raw versus cooked food, or whether it's "mommy time vs. playing with the kids." By organizing your life around the biomedical body, MyFlo claims, you can be "symptom-free."[100] MyFlo and Eve are perhaps the most extreme and gendered versions of the menstrual tracking and fertility apps, but the cyclescopes and recommendation systems perfectly distill the vision of self-knowledge offered across menstrual-tracking technologies: if I track my cycles long enough, I can discern a direct cause-effect relationship between my bodily and emotional experiences and my cycle. With this information, I can perhaps anticipate disruptions to social order, but ultimately, I'm at the disposal of my hormonal body, which remains out of my control. Propped up by the authority of biomedicine and big data, this image of self-knowledge offered by menstrual-tracking apps risks promoting a biologically deterministic understanding of the self, body, and health.

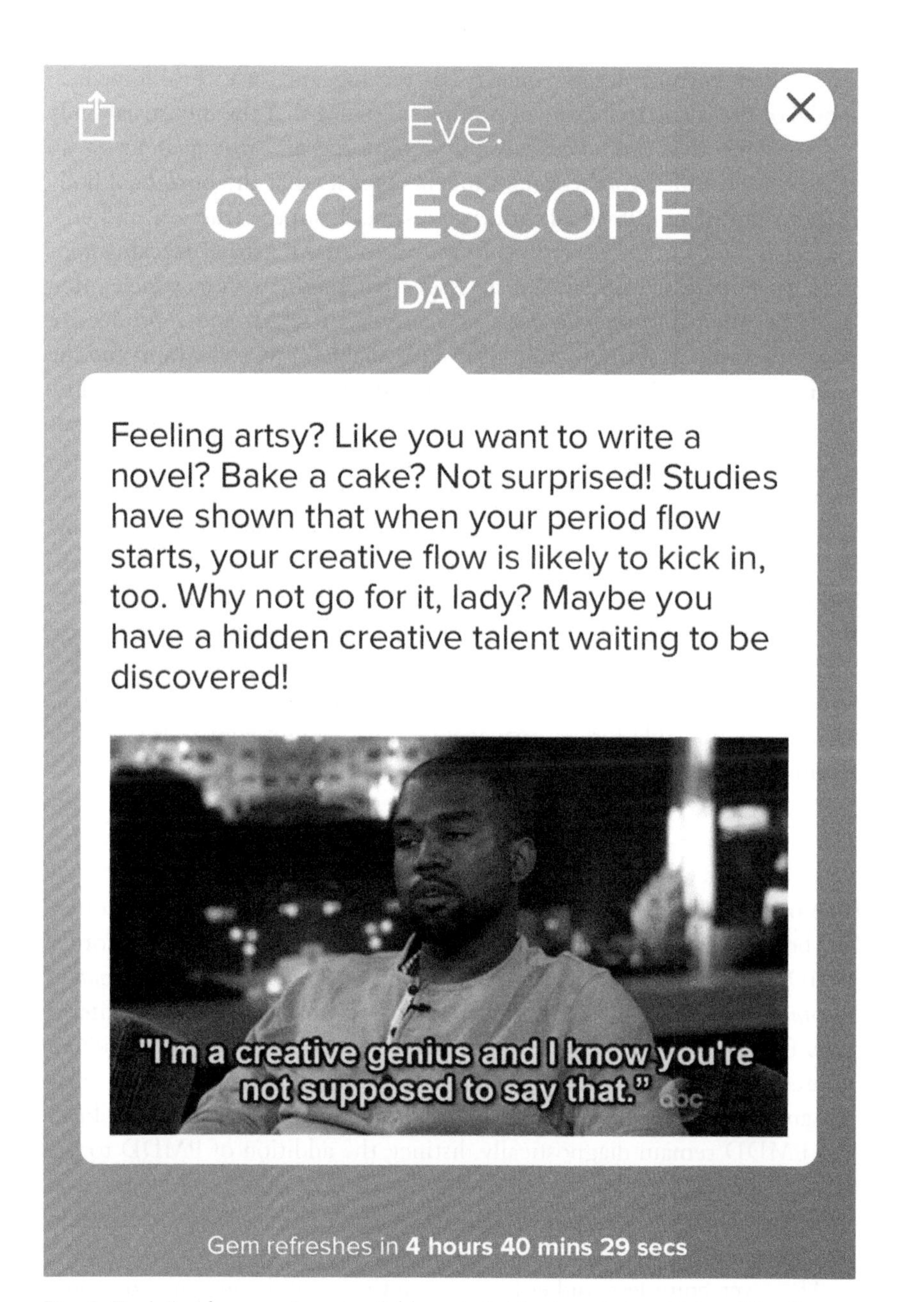

Fig. 8. Eve's "cyclescopes" are available to individuals each day. (Glow, "Eve," vers. 2.15.5., accessed November 2019.)

In their current design, menstrual-tracking apps use the biomedical model of the menstrual cycle to promote the idea that the menstrual body is something that should be carefully monitored and managed across all phases, at all times. At the same time, it suggests that the hormonal body remains out of an individual's control, distinct from the true self, and ultimately at fault for any deviations from the norm. Menstrual-tracking apps thus participate in the "mixed messages" of menstruation, which often move between framing the cycle as a source of sexual and reproductive power (a sign that the body is healthy and capable of reproduction) and the linguistic and symbolic promotion of menstrual concealment.[101] Aided by self-tracking technologies and supported by statistical analysis, individuals find themselves in an impossible position: caught up in the need to monitor and suppress traces of menstruation while their body and emotions are still continually driven and determined by their uncontrollable menstrual cycle. As a result, these apps continually oscillate between two poles: seeking to empower individuals through self-knowledge while still reinforcing the perception that menstruation is an uncontrollable abject process that should be managed and suppressed. In this sense, menstrual-tracking apps reinforce a central contradiction of femininity, in which individuals are both responsible for self-management, yet cannot control the deviant feminine body.[102]

Rethinking Menstrual Management

The power of the biomedical model of menstruation and PMS discourse has been solidified by the inclusion of premenstrual dysphoric disorder (PMDD) in the fourth edition of the *Diagnostic and Statistical Manual of Mental Disorders* (*DSM-4*).[103] Often conflated with PMS in popular literature, PMDD includes a huge range of symptoms but requires individuals to present specific psychological symptoms, including depression or anxiety, and places greater emphasis on severity and intensity. Though PMS and PMDD remain diagnostically distinct, the addition of PMDD to the *DSM-4* helped increase the credibility of PMS in popular discourses on menstrual health.[104] In other words, PMS, by proximity, took on the aura of medical authority established by the *DSM-4* edition.

However, countless studies have shown there is ultimately no hormonal or physiological basis for PMS.[105] Researchers continue to struggle to understand the direct cause of monthly emotional and physical distress, while the list of symptoms associated with these conditions continues to expand, now surpassing 100 behavioral and emotional markers. To meet the basic diagnostic criteria, these symptoms simply need to "occur i*n any combination at any time* during the second half of the menstrual cycle."[106] By these standards, nearly every person who menstruates meets the criteria for diagnosis, reinforcing the perception that they "suffer" from a reproductive health condition. Thus, some scholars argue that "PMS is a form of social control and victim blame that masks itself as value-free."[107] The lack of empirical evidence and the vague list of symptoms have led scholars to argue that PMS is essentially a social construct[108] or "culture-bound syndrome . . . a constellation of signs, symptoms, and/or experiences that have been categorized as a dysfunction or disease in some societies and not in others."[109] But labeling PMS, or any forms of menstrual distress, as a product of culture risks undermining the very real forms of discomfort and emotional shifts experienced throughout the menstrual cycle, as well as the role of medical diagnosis in how individuals understand their bodies, emotions, and behaviors.[110]

While it's easy to attribute the self-alienating, negative perceptions of menstruation to biomedical models of reproductive health, numerous studies on the experience of PMS, PMDD, and menopause have shown how medical definitions and data tracking can function as essential forms of validation.[111] Likewise, more recent work in human-computer interaction (HCI) design has examined how menstrual-tracking apps can participate in ongoing processes of "sense-making" of the menstrual experience. With these considerations in mind, I end by offering two ways to think productively about the future of menstrual-tracking technologies: as a personal tool for menstrual reflexivity that can potentially push back on biomedical understandings of the body and health, and as a resource to aid underexplored areas of reproductive health research.

Recent work by Jane Perz, Jane Ussher, and colleagues has sought to complicate constructivist readings of PMS by taking a "critical realist epistemological standpoint," which aims to "recognize the materiality of the body, and other aspects of experience, but conceptualizes this materiality as always mediated by culture, language, and politics."[112] Their methodology takes experience seriously while still always acknowledging that experience exists in a specific cultural and historical context. Examining women's accounts of PMS and the menstrual experience, Ussher and Perz argue that individuals do not necessarily experience PMS as a "fixed illness," "but rather an ongoing process of negotiation with levels of distress." Part of this negotiation is facing the cultural pressures to suppress the menstrual body and maintain standards of the feminine body. However, this does not necessarily lead directly to pathologization or self-alienation; instead, it may often create forms of self-awareness that can encourage negative interpretations of the body and self but also can allow women to acknowledge and cope with real physical and emotional distress.[113] Rather than critiquing women's PMS self-diagnosis, Ussher and Perz advocate for acknowledging women as "PMS sufferers,"[114] which "*both* evokes connotations of the monstrous feminine and makes meaning of women's distress through legitimizing their experiences as 'real' and something that may require support."[115] In other words, the language of "sufferer" shows how PMS through cultural and biomedical models of menstruation can encourage instances of bodily alienation and self-condemnation, but also acknowledges the range of menstrual experiences and takes seriously the lived distress of people who menstruate. For Ussher and Perz the multiple and often contradictory ways women understand PMS and their menstruating body open up the space for "Western women [to] . . . resist cultural discourse associated with PMS, reject self-pathologization, and avoid or ameliorate premenstrual distress."[116]

Through an emphasis on data tracking and analytics, menstrual-tracking apps can similarly create complex structures of self-alienation and self-reflection. After several years of menstrual tracking, I've found myself slipping into a biomedical way of thinking about my body promoted by the app's aesthetics, but these moments do not necessarily slip into self-alienation or menstrual suppression. While I would not identify myself as a "PMS sufferer," I have found that I experience some pressure and light cramping just before the start of menstruation. There will be moments when I feel my pelvis tighten, as though filled with air, or feel a pulsing pressure just below my navel. This isn't necessarily painful—it's more discomfort I'd liken to feeling too full, but displaced toward my lower abdomen. Initially when I experienced these pressures, because they did not correspond to menstruation I assumed they were gastrointestinal disruptions. Their arrival may prompt me to think about what I've eaten and when, in an attempt to understand my body's reaction to particular foods. But through menstrual tracking, I've come to associate these bodily sensations with the impending arrival of menstruation, indicators that my body may be preparing to shed the uterine lining. By reading these bodily sensations through my menstrual cycle, I am ostensibly operating through the logic of the biomedical model as I attribute my body's behaviors to internal processes out of my control. But in these moments of discomfort, my inclination isn't to explain away or blame my body; it's more of a noticing of my menstruating body, a novel way I'm paying attention to how my menstrual cycle prompts attention to my body.

These moments of bodily self-reflexivity can be quickly undermined by situations in which I use the app to justify or explain my emotional reactions. There have been times when I find myself "overreacting" to a film or television show and have an inclination to turn toward my menstrual tracking app for an "answer." I'm not someone who often cries while watching media or reading, so when I find my eyes welling up and sense a pressure in my chest as my heart speeds up, I pause to deepen my breathing to slow it down. As I feel the pressure of my eyes as tears risk pooling over, I'll shift into a reflexive mode that questions the relationship between my bodily reactions and the content I'm seeing on the screen. These moments can create frustrations with my body, which feels somewhat out of control, uncontained by logic telling me the images on the screen aren't all that sad. Opening up my Clue app, if I see that I'm ovulating or close to menstruating, my reaction will feel "justified," explained through shifting levels of hormones as my body prepares for a physiological process of release. As someone who studies technology and gender, I'm fully aware of the dangers of seeing my emotions through this biomedical lens. I'm also conscious of how my frustration with my bodily reactions is probably the product of other stresses in my professional and social life, as well as my relationship to norms of femininity. But in these moments, there is simultaneously comfort in the biomedical explanation as a way to maintain my sense of self.

Menstrual-tracking apps can often prompt bodily reflexivity, but that reflexivity doesn't necessarily lead directly to biomedical resistance or subjugation. It's often an oscillation between both relationships to the body, resulting in feelings of ambivalence, blame, satisfaction, and empowerment. The range of bodily sensations, reactions, and feelings about the body cannot be reduced to specific formal properties or the goal of the app, nor to the "authority" the app wields over the user. Indeed, most menstrual-tracking users do not see the app as a source of authority capable of explaining their bodies or health: any sense of "self-knowledge" or power the app has is relative, shaped by "multiple elements, through which users themselves produce 'serviceable truths.' The data operate as an active mediator between the body and the embodied self."[117] My use of Clue to explain diversions from what I consider "normal" behavior or a "typical" bodily sensation is a negotiation between the information provided by the app, and my bodily sensations, social pressures, and my sense of myself. The biomedical model, as well as the app, function as tools for self-reflexive practices, but do not necessarily determine my interpretations or understandings of my body.

In her phenomenologically informed study of fertility trackers, Della Bianca argues that the use of the biomedical model of menstruation and "the role of Biology (as the biomedical system of reference) and biologies (as experienced bodies) is ambivalent, potentially acting as both validating as well as invalidating entities."[118] To truly understand the role of biology and work to counteract the possibility of self-alienation, researchers must first acknowledge the "dual tension" between these two roles. This tension extends to the relationship between the function of the biomedical model in the design and interactive features of the apps, and their role in the perception of menstrual health and the future of menstrual health research. As I have argued, current designs do not necessarily acknowledge the diversity of menstrual experiences or frame physical and emotional changes as "natural" or "normal" parts of menstrual embodiment. However, by transforming self-reported experiences into data points, menstrual-tracking apps can help translate these experiences into a form of scientific evidence that has epistemological authority and cultural value in our society. Medical diagnoses and scientific explanations for physical and emotional symptoms can often function as an essential form of recognition for individuals, particularly those whose experiences have historically been dismissed due to gender, class, and racial bias.[119] While the datafied structures of menstrual-tracking apps should not provide diagnoses, they can provide visual and informational records—forms of acknowledgment—of an individual's menstrual experiences. Thus, the biomedical model continues as a troublesome mediator, capable of translating bodily experiences into powerful forms of evidence, and also into abstract processes that remain out of an individual's control.

As with PMS, the key will be avoiding negative and medicalized *interpretations* of menstrual experiences via the biomedical model. In other words, menstrual-tracking apps should seek to cultivate awareness and acknowledgment, and avoid diagnostic frameworks that reinforce norms, standards, and the homeostatic model of reproductive health. Fox and Epstein have sought to explore forms of menstrual self-tracking that encourage bodily reflection and trouble the biomedical models of the body as "wholly knowable and controllable."[120] Through interviews, they found that predictive algorithms and data structures did not always impose statistical norms on the body but could provide ways for individuals to cope and prepare for emotional and physical shifts. For example, in their study, Robert, a transgender man, describes how the prediction features of the menstrual-tracking apps often allowed him to mentally prepare for menstruation, which ultimately helped him resist the anxiety and self-rejection that typically accompanied his menstrual experience.[121] Fox and Epstein note, however, that the current structures of menstrual-tracking apps could not account for the changes in Robert's menstrual cycle once he began to take testosterone supplements, and consequently advocate for technologies that can be adapted and personalized to account for a variety of uses, gender identities, and menstrual experiences.[122]

In addition to creating more modular and adaptable technologies, menstrual-tracking apps could ideally support increased attunement to sensorial and emotional shifts that occur during the menstrual cycle. Rather than seeking to draw correlations between particular phases and logged symptoms, the act of self-tracking could be used as a way for individuals to recognize the small shifts in the embodied sensations that occur throughout the cycle, which may or may not be attributed to a specific phase, hormone fluctuation, or physiological process. There should be a way to incorporate the forms of noticing and attunement, such as the instance of cramping I described above, that don't automatically attempt to explain those sensations exclusively through my menstrual cycle. Ideally, an app could prompt reflexivity and allow me to reflect on the potential contributing factors, and to assess how these sensations affect my body as it moves through the world. Ultimately, my abdominal pressure is not disruptive, and therefore should not be pathologized or interpreted as an example of the discomforts of menstruation. It's merely an example of how my body shifts throughout a cycle.

Ussher and Perz found that participants who focused on "understanding" their menstrual distress, by becoming more aware and tracking patterns, were "less likely to self-pathologize," instead they simply recognized these shifts and cultivated strategies of "tolerance of negative premenstrual change, which was recognized to be temporary."[123] Menstrual-tracking apps could be used to support these forms of understanding by offering a tracking system that encourages individuals to "sense-make" bodily experiences by acknowledging change, distress, and small shifts in the body. By de-emphasizing the four-phase visualizations of the cycle, and encouraging strategies for self-reflexivity, these apps could help destabilize the perception of the homeostatic healthy body. Placing greater emphasis on embodiment, by encouraging individuals to reflect on precise bodily sensations, can help cultivate a bodily awareness that pushes back against the dominant, biomedical understanding of the reproductive body.

At the same time that cultural understandings of menstruation need to shift away from preventative, biomedical models, countless menstrual experiences remain unexplained by modern science and medicine, including the prevalence of heavy flows for particular racial groups, extended amenorrhea, and even the exact cause of endometriosis. These conditions have received less attention and funding from the scientific and medical community because research often relies on subjective, reported experiences. Women's experiences, in particular, have historically been overlooked or dismissed due to gendered stereotypes that figure them as overly emotional. This stereotype is further influenced by other markers of identity, such as race and class.[124] While datafication can function as a way for individuals to feel that their menstrual experiences are valid and legitimate, it likewise situates these experiences within the biomedical paradigm. Datafication currently aims to convince individuals of the authority of the patterns and correlations that emerge through analytics. However, shifting focus to the use of this self-reported data in ongoing scientific and medical research can ideally help reduce the sense that these apps are transparent forms of medical or scientific authority. Instead, I would suggest framing individuals as collaborators, stressing the possibilities for participating in large-scale data analysis on menstruation. Current design practices frame the log and analytics sections as transparent sources of self-knowledge, but by foregrounding the act of participation in research, individuals may come to understand that the algorithm and insight features are still works in progress: tools that can be developed through active engagement in data science projects. A focus on collaboration could hopefully also work toward undoing the emphasis on individual management, and by extension, concealment. Framing engagement with the app through research collaboration would ideally help break down some of the barriers of expertise in a way that avoids placing responsibility in the hands of individuals and open up conversation between patients, researchers, and practitioners. For individuals, this could promote the perception that their experiences are significant contributions to emerging health research, and, it is hoped, reduce the shame and stigma surrounding discussions of menstruation.

Of course, this would require a dramatic rethinking of the way data sharing currently operates in most of these apps. Flo, for example, was recently outed for selling user data to Facebook, and indeed many of these apps currently monetize through data mining and advertising.[125] The personal nature of this information necessitates better anonymization and new security protocols.[126] Moreover, clear definitions of privacy would have to be established to ensure that individuals are protected from healthcare or health insurance discrimination and legal ramifications, particularly in the US with the recent overturning of *Roe v. Wade*.[127] Through partnerships between app developers and research institutions, privacy and data-sharing policies could be developed to facilitate research efforts without violating medical privacy rights. For example, Clue currently partners with several universities, including Stanford and Oxford, sharing its data to promote menstrual health research. Through collaboration with Oxford, the research found no evidence for the myth of period syncing, which is often used to support highly gendered stereotypes about cohabitation among women and female friendship.[128]

With greater attention to individual privacy, these apps can begin to collect demographic information to help target specific populations and potentially reveal patterns and correlations related to factors such as behavior, geography, and family medical history. Currently, none of these apps solicit demographic information beyond age and sometimes location. Allowing individuals to provide information on race, ethnicity, dietary practices, family medical histories, and existing afflictions such as endometriosis could offer insights into specific menstrual health conditions.

The sheer scale of menstrual-health data archived by menstrual-tracking apps means that it could be used for future analysis. But to pursue these possibilities, major revisions must be made to the current design and data-collection features of these apps. While Clue's platform still requires adjustment, its work with universities offers a model for future research. Moreover, the emphasis on inclusive data science and academic research has made it the most highly recommend app by the American College of Gynecologists and Obstetricians.[129] As the second-most-downloaded menstrual-tracker in the Apple app store (as of September 2019), Clue suggests there is a financial and social incentive for companies to change the way these apps frame menstrual experiences.[130] Descriptions of the aesthetic experiences of menstrual-tracking apps can serve as a useful tool for interrogating the impact of these technologies, but true revision and change will require collaborations across individuals and researchers, health scientists, designers, and scholars.

CHAPTER 2

Pleasure Points

Sextech and Measuring Sexual Wellness

> It's like a Fitbit for your sexual pleasure and health!
> —Lioness[1]

> One day soon, buying a vibrator will be viewed like buying a yoga mat.
> —Andrea Barrica, *SexTech Revolution*[2]

In a 2019 interview on *This American Life*, Lora Haddock DiCarlo, CEO of the Lora DiCarlo sextech brand, pushed back on the criticism that her products do not qualify as health and wellness devices:

> REPORTER LINA MISITZIS: When I think of, like, the sex toys that I have been aware of in my lifetime, the point, as I understand it, is pleasure. And I think it's OK for products to be marketed to women simply for the fact that they create pleasure. And I actually just—I wonder why Health and Wellness. I wonder why it couldn't just be in a category called Pleasure. Why isn't pleasure just good enough?
>
> DICARLO: It is pleasure, but as far as I read it, pleasure is also a part of health and wellness.[3]

DiCarlo is specifically referring to how her products (and erotic technologies more generally) should be categorized and marketed at the annual Consumer Electronics Showcase (CES). In 2018, DiCarlo's company was the center of a controversy at CES: after receiving the prestigious innovation award for her sex robot, the Consumer Technology Association (CTA), which runs the annual showcase, revoked the title and banned the company from attending, stating that the device was "immoral, obscene, indecent, profane, or not in keeping with the CTA's image."[4] DiCarlo criticized the decision publicly, sparking a media outcry against sexist and discriminatory practices at the CES. Eventually, the award was reinstated and DiCarlo was asked to consult on how to navigate the inclusion of sex toys in future showcases. Following her recommendation, sex toys and other devices can now be displayed prominently under the category "Health and Wellness."

The movement of sex toys to "Health and Wellness" is, in part, related to CES's complicated history with the adult entertainment industry. Situating the DiCarlo incident in the history of CES, Li Cornfeld describes how the annual conference has had to contend with the fact that erotic markets are often central to the development and economic success of emerging technology. For example, CES's choice to shift its marketing language from "pornography" to "adult entertainment" is related to an attempt to legitimize the erotic industry, which was directly responsible for the popularization of home video systems (VHS). Cornfeld argues that the move toward entertainment frames pornography as "a legitimate business sector, and supplies categorical justification for porn's inclusion in a field devoted to bringing commercial entertainment into the home."[5] Likewise, categorizing sextech as "Health and Wellness" products aims to legitimize the sex toy industry.[6] As health and wellness devices, sex toys can be featured in the main showcase space, so long as they avoid describing or depicting sex acts, or demonstrating how to use the device. In other words, the "Health and Wellness" category functions as a smart business decision: as a way to increase the visibility and economic viability of the products. Indeed, at the end of the *This American Life* segment, Misitzis concedes that DiCarlo's view is largely motivated by business: "she wants to sell to everybody on the main floor with the mainstream products. And if calling her sex robot a health and wellness product gets it out of the lab and into the world, she's fine with that. It's still hidden, just in a different way."[7]

Through a focus on the economic and industrial motivations for the "Health and Wellness" categorization, Cornfeld argues the DiCarlo controversy returns sex toys to the early history of the vibrator, which was first marketed as a device for health.[8] Like the sexual health and wellness toys on the floor of the CES showcase, early commercial vibrators drew on the language of health to sell their products and mask any direct connection to sex. Historical ads for the vibrator in the early twentieth century avoided any explicit references to sex, instead marketing them as tools to treat a host of conditions, ranging from dysmenorrhea (the absence of menstruation), constipation, uterine prolapse, and hemorrhoids.[9] However, by the 1920s and '30s, the prevalence of vibrators in pornography provided an explicit visual link between the device and sex, and public marketing campaigns became increasingly infrequent as products shifted into the adult entertainment industry.[10]

The recent reemergence of the vibrator as a "sexual wellness technology" or "sextech" device is related not only to the commercial and industrial history of sex toys, but to how the science of sex and pleasure has been incorporated into definitions of health, and how these discourses have, in turn, been mobilized by feminist movements in the last half-century. DiCarlo's insistence that pleasure is part of a definition of health suggests that this is not simply a return to the vibrator's commercial origins. Like early ads for vibrators, sextech is increasingly marketed as a tool for self-care. But the recent, explicit emphasis on sexual pleasure as a feminist form of self-care has only emerged in the last half-century, due in no small part to scientific research on sex and health, which helped push back on psychoanalytic theories that reinforced gendered conceptions of sex and the female body. Drawing on this body of work, many second-wave feminists considered the orgasm as both a symbol of women's oppression and as an act of liberation. To understand the emergence of sextech and the rise of sexual wellness, this chapter situates the recent boom of sextech in the intersecting and entangled histories of midcentury sexology, feminist sex shops, and postfeminism. This history reveals how the quantification of sexual pleasure has been mobilized to support shifting feminist agendas and emerging health and wellness discourse.

For pleasure to be included in definitions of health, it must be defined through biomedical frameworks. Once pleasure is measured—quantified—it can be inscribed into the systems through which biomedicine understands health: pleasure can be linked to other biological systems, compared across population groups, and normed according to statistical data. But like pain, pleasure is a deeply subjective experience that is difficult to identify, measure, and track according to scientific and medical standards. Over the last half-century, scientists have used MRI, EKGS, heart rate, vaginal and anal contractions, and qualitative pleasure scales to visualize, track, and measure sexual pleasure. However, across these studies, pleasure is almost always conflated with the presence of orgasm, and consequently the "health benefits" are often attributed to quantitative measurements, including the total number and frequency of orgasmic events. To examine the biomedicalization of sexual pleasure, I begin by tracing how midcentury sexology helped establish the orgasm-as-pleasure paradigm. Founded in biological, naturalist understandings of sexuality, Alfred Kinsey's sociological studies used the orgasm as an indicator of sexual activity. While this helped move away from penetrative models of sex, it simultaneously framed normal sexual behavior through the quantifiable accumulation of orgasms. This framework continues to support how normal sexual behavior, sexual health, and sexual equality are defined, particularly through the rhetoric of the "orgasm gap," wherein sexual satisfaction and equality are measured by the discrepancy in the number of orgasms between men and women. I show how this quantitative model creates a system where pleasure is understood through the logic of "more"—more orgasms, more pleasure—which effaces questions of the multifaceted experience of sexual pleasure itself.

The second section explores how the scientific and health-based models of sexuality that emerged from midcentury sexology have informed the aesthetics of feminist sex shops and contemporary postfeminist sextech. Through quantification, Kinsey aimed to undermine moral and psychoanalytic understandings of sexuality that emphasized prohibition and sexual difference, and instead to promote the idea that sexuality is a natural and normal expression of human biology, regardless of gender or sexual preference. This scientific approach to sexuality provided a foundation for second-wave feminism and the rise of feminist sex shops in the 1970s. Like Kinsey, these early sex shops used science and health to distance sexual pleasure from moralizing discourses on sex and from any association with pornography. I draw on histories of feminist sex shops to explore how the aesthetics and rhetoric of health were used to "naturalize" women's sexuality. However, these new aesthetics of sexual health promoted a highly gendered and classed model of feminist sexuality that continues to inform feminist sex retail today.[11] Through descriptions of the websites and designs of contemporary sextech companies, I show how the aesthetics of sexual health have been extended and revised through postfeminism. Through feminized aesthetics and health rhetoric, these companies aim to "normalize" sexual pleasure and distance sextech from pornography and the adult entertainment industry. In doing so, sexual pleasure becomes reframed as "sexual wellness."

As I discussed in the introduction, within contemporary definitions of health and wellness, health is often *performed* through knowing and training the body. This logic has been extended to sex and sexual pleasure, which are increasingly understood as critical elements of holistic health.[12] Sexual wellness discourse frames sexual pleasure through positive health or health-promotion models: sexual pleasure, orgasms, and sexual activity are all framed as "normal" and indeed *necessary* for maintaining good health. Yet when biomedical models of quantification and tracking become central to maintaining and supporting sexual wellness, this limits the questions that can be posed concerning health maintenance: how many times do you have sex, how frequently, and how many orgasms? In the third section, I show how this logic is tied to the work of William Masters and Virginia Johnson, who helped establish a physiological model for sexual pleasure. This framework, like Kinsey's, operates under the assumption that orgasms and sexual pleasure are the natural product of physiological processes and that any disturbances to or diversions from this norm can be "fixed" through increased knowledge and skill. Second-wave feminists mobilized this scientific model, framing self-knowledge and the cultivation of skill as political tools to fight the patriarchy. Sexual pleasure thus became a symbol of women's liberation from the social systems that inhibit women's sexuality. Through descriptions of the app interface and tracking features of Lioness, a smart vibrator designed to measure and track orgasms, I show how feminist messages about pleasure and orgasm have since been adopted and depoliticized by postfeminist sextech through an emphasis on quantification and sexual wellness. Lioness measures vaginal contraction and temperature data to encourage individuals to locate, track, analyze, and ideally improve their orgasms. This model reinforces the conflation of orgasmic presence and sexual pleasure and inscribes neoliberal values of accumulation and improvement. Individuals are encouraged to use self-tracking to have more frequent, more intense, and longer orgasms. Rather than framing sexual pleasure as a tool for liberation, this postfeminist, quantified model focuses on individual improvement in pursuit of sexual wellness.

While the Lioness app and tracking features perpetuate a biomedical model that conflates orgasm and pleasure, I end by briefly considering how quantification and sextech could be used to help expand definitions of sexual pleasure. Through phenomenological descriptions of my experience using the Lioness platform, I show how the data and tracking features the app provides are almost entirely illegible and unusable: improving one's pleasure or increasing the number of orgasms based on this data feels impossible. The interface and data-visualization features are so abstract and divorced from my experience of sexual pleasure that they have little bearing on my perception of my body or health. Yet rather than dismissing this product as another failed digital health device, I end by considering what Lioness's data-tracking features may be able to tell individuals about their bodies and offer up ways to think about how sextech may be able to encourage a more embodied, sensorial understanding of sexual pleasure.

Numerous sociological studies of masturbation have shown that especially cisgender, heterosexual women continue to feel shame about masturbating or see solo stimulation as a "less satisfying" form of sexual pleasure.[13] This is due in part to cultural norms that continue to privilege partnered sex and stigmatize women's sexuality. The push toward understanding masturbation through the lens of self-care has helped destigmatize and normalize women's sexual pleasure. But because it remains tied to the conflation of orgasm with sexual pleasure, it continues to reinforce the idea that orgasm determines sexual satisfaction, a model of sexual pleasure that has been derived from male-centric sex research. A phenomenological account of the embodied experience of sextech and sexual pleasure can help expand how individuals understand their pleasure and satisfaction, and indeed may offer an example of the experience of health itself. Sexual pleasure often emerges from a hyper-attuned relationship to the body; it requires a great deal of attention to the minute changes in sensations, subtle acts of stimulation, and shifts in feeling. Through recent work on pleasure, orgasms, and embodiment, I suggest possible ways in which technologies may be taken up to help support sensuous attention to the embodied experience of sexual stimulation, which can help expand how pleasure and health are measured, understood, and defined by medical practitioners, app designers, and individual users alike.

Quantifying Sex and Pleasure

While sex and health have been linked through the study of sexually transmitted infections (STIs) since the eighteenth century, the configuration of gender, orgasms, and health is a relatively novel concept that only began to receive scientific and medical attention at the turn of the twentieth century.[14] In his detailed study of the female orgasm, Thomas Lacquer describes how by the end of the eighteenth century the orgasm's presence or absence had come to be associated with sexual difference. Before this era, orgasms were largely understood as sensations and feeling with little consideration of their relationship to reproductive functioning or differences among genders. But the eighteenth-century "discovery" that women did not often experience orgasm during sex helped establish a "biological signpost for sexual difference" and a physiological foundation for "female passivity" and "frigidity."[15] The association of biological difference with the presence or absence of an orgasm was linked explicitly to pathology and health in the work of Sigmund Freud. Most famous in this context for distinguishing between vaginal and clitoral orgasms, Freud extended the sexual difference model to suggest that orgasms not only mark gender but can be used to detect underlying pathology. Freud argued that the clitoral orgasm was a "less mature" form of sexuality, and that a fixation on the "erotogenic zones" unrelated to reproduction was an indication of underlying psychosexual problems.[16] While Freud's work was not based on biology, it helped establish the connection between orgasms and health norms.

In the 1930s, psychoanalyst Wilhelm Reich helped inscribe the psychosexual model of the orgasm into scientific frameworks. He opposed Freud's theory of the clitoral orgasm, pushing back against gender difference theories through his theory of sexual energy and the body. Reich theorized that the orgasm helped bridge the gap between the mind and body.[17] He posited that sexual energy could be charted and that orgasms were, in part, related to the flow of biological energy. Through the language of electricity, Reich described the process of arousal and orgasm as a wave, current, and charge. Sexual organs possessed an "underlying current"[18] that could be activated through psychological and physical stimuli that built up and resulted in the release of tension through orgasm or "bioelectric discharge."[19] This energy model of the orgasm helped support his theory that the intensity of an orgasm was an indicator of psychological and biological functioning. In other words, sexual *satisfaction* and *pleasure* were indicators of health (not simply the presence or absence of an orgasm). Reich built on Freud's model of sexual tension and release, suggesting that arousal and orgasms could not simply be reduced to psychology, but instead are part of a psychophysiological system. Thus, orgasm was not simply an indicator of psychological health, but also functioned as a "yardstick of psychophysical functioning, because the function of biological energy is expressed in it."[20] While Reich's charting of arousal and orgasm would be extended in the work of Masters and Johnson in the 1960s, the connection between intensity and satisfaction and psychological factors would be lost as sex research migrated toward biomedical and quantitative methodologies.

The major shift toward quantified models of sexuality is attributed to the sociological work of Alfred Kinsey. His research conducted throughout the 1950s aimed to legitimize the scientific study of sex through empirical methods and biological essentialism. As a trained biologist, Kinsey claimed to approach sex objectively by focusing on physiological rather than psychological conditions of sexuality. He positioned himself in opposition to Freud and psychoanalysis, which he claimed mystified sexuality, instead offering science as a means to objectively establish norms of sexual behavior. For Kinsey, sex was a "material phenomenon," a physiological response, as opposed to an expression of psychology or psychosexual development. Scholars have critiqued Kinsey's attachment to the scientific method and empiricism, claiming it was a way for him to avoid issues of race and class. For example, though Kinsey's surveys included Black men and women, he did not believe his sample size was large enough to make scientific claims. Consequently, any consideration of the specificity of sexual experience for Black men and women was excluded from the data analysis.[21] Moreover, his definition of the orgasm drew directly from reproductive models of sex and men's experiences,[22] as "the moment of sudden release."[23] This "release" was not tied to the satisfaction of any psychic processes related to the unconscious, but instead to underlying biological systems. The "capacity" to experience orgasm was not the product of sexual maturity, but instead

> depends upon the existence of end organs, of touch in the body surfaces, nerves connecting these organs with the spinal cord and brain, nerves that extend from the cord to various muscles in the body, and the atomic nervous system through which still other parts of the body are brought into action.[24]

In her analysis of Kinsey's research, Janet Irvine claims that the quantification of orgasms supported his insistence that sexuality was simply an extension of the "natural" processes shared by humans and animals.[25] The orgasm serves as an "accessible and quantifiable unit of measurement"[26] that was understood as an expression of the underlying biological system.

Framing the orgasm as the definitive marker of sexual behavior for both men and women, Kinsey helped redefine the presence of an orgasm as the new sexual norm. In her study of the meaning of the orgasm, Hannah Frith describes how Kinsey's quantitative system framed the orgasmic presence as "normal," where its absence denoted dissatisfaction and even dysfunction. This in turn shapes the assumption that normal sexual behavior *should* be accompanied by orgasm.[27] The orgasm as a sexual norm was further reinforced by Kinsey's claims that metrics were a direct reflection of "sexual function." While Kinsey never explicitly defines his theory of "sexual function," Irvine argues that his belief in sexuality as an expression of natural biological processes led him to equate frequency with "capacity." In other words, "those with a low sexual capacity had sex less often than those with a higher capacity."[28] He compared "low capacity" to other physical conditions such as blindness or deafness, which he likewise saw as "sublimation of those capacities."[29] Thus the presence of the orgasm was understood to be a marker of the functioning of an individual's underlying biology, and any diversions from the norm would indicate inhibited functioning.

While Kinsey did not directly connect sexual frequency to health, this quantitative understanding of sexual functioning has been central to the definition of sexual norms and dysfunction. With the presence of an orgasm as the new bar for normal sexual response, "counting the frequency or consistency with which the individual experiences orgasm, enables the identification of gaps and absences which are taken as indicative of problematic or dysfunctional sexual responses."[30] Kinsey's quantitative work and the physiological models provided by William Masters and Virginia Johnson have helped establish the frequency of orgasm and its absence or presence as the defining features of sexual disorder diagnoses in both men and women. Though the field of sexology has attempted to move away from Kinsey's biological model of sexuality, the *Diagnostic and Statistical Manual of Mental Disorders* (*DSM-5*) continues to rely on the logic of frequency as a marker of normal sexual function. For example, "female orgasmic disorder" is defined as "when an individual consistently or repeatedly is unable to have an orgasm after she has been sexually stimulated or aroused."[31] While the latest edition acknowledges that orgasmic absence should be accompanied by "distress,"[32] absence remains central to the definition of "disorder," which the manual claims may be caused by a variety of factors, ranging from stress or abuse to underlying health conditions.[33] As a result, orgasms become an indicator of health, a vital sign for monitoring social, psychological, or physiological functioning.

The movement toward a physiological understanding of sexuality was also directly tied to Kinsey's attempts to undermine theories of sexual difference and an exclusively reproductive model of sex. Kinsey counted any form of sexual behavior that resulted in orgasm as a form of sexual activity in an attempt to separate sex from social norms and moral frameworks. This framework allowed him to include both men and women in the same data set and incorporate a range of sexual behaviors. Kinsey developed a taxonomy of sexual behavior that broke down the activity into specific types, including nocturnal emission, masturbation, heterosexual petting, heterosexual intercourse, homosexual sex, and bestiality. Participants would add up their orgasmic totals to calculate their "sexual outlet."[34] Through a focus on the number of orgasms, homosexuality, masturbation, and bestiality were rendered equivalent to heterosexual sex. Irvine links this methodology to his training in biology: in reducing sexual acts to numbers, he was able to suggest that all forms of sexual behavior were indeed normal and "natural."[35]

Applied to women, Kinsey's methods marked a radical shift in discourses around women's sexuality and pleasure. As Irvine notes, the "use of orgasm as a unit for women's sexuality was progressive" and helped establish a model of sexuality that undermined popular impressions that orgasms and sexual pleasure were less important for women.[36] Historically, the focus on reproduction, rather than pleasure, rendered the female orgasm irrelevant. Unlike the male orgasm, which has a direct relationship to procreation, the female orgasm does not appear to have an evolutionary function. While Freud attempted to link female orgasms to reproduction by distinguishing between vaginal and clitoral orgasms, scientists to this day have not come to a consensus on whether the female orgasm aids conception. Biological anthropologists have offered several theories linking orgasm to reproduction, ranging from mate-bonding hypotheses to the contraction of the vaginal walls during orgasm as a way to aid the suction of sperm into the uterus.[37] However, all of these theories remain speculative due to the variety of ways the female orgasm is induced and expressed, leading some scientists to concede, "we may never be able to definitively state the female orgasm is an adaptation."[38] Kinsey was able to avoid the question of evolution by instead focusing on the "release" of an orgasm as a natural biological instinct. From this perspective, he did not have to question the function of the orgasm; instead, he merely documented that function's existence. He argued, "there is no scientific reason for considering particular types of sexual activity as intrinsically, in their biological origins, normal or abnormal," any interpretations of "abnormality" are the product of culture, not biology.[39]

Despite the progressive stakes of Kinsey's work, he repeatedly insisted he was merely presenting data, not providing interpretations of behavior or reflections on social and cultural norms. He begins *Sexual Behavior in the Human Male* by stating that the work aims to "accumulate an objectively determined body of fact about sex which strictly avoids social or moral interpretations of the fact."[40] Any judgments or interpretations that may emerge are the product of the reader, not the science: "scientists have no special capacities for making such evaluations."[41] However, by reducing sexual behavior to orgasmic quantities, Kinsey also helped produce a system through which different populations can easily be compared and contrasted—a framework that today is still used to measure and interpret normal and healthy sexual behavior.

Indeed, Irvine notes that Kinsey's entire quantitative methodology supported his philosophy of sexuality, which implied "that what is 'natural' is right, that sex is good and more is better."[42] With orgasms linked to natural sexual functioning, and quantity associated with "goodness," a higher "sexual outlet" number is often interpreted as a positive reflection of attitudes toward sexuality and healthy sexual behavior. In other words, a higher number of orgasms indicates higher sexual functioning and a better attitude toward sex. For example, Kinsey's data showed that men and women engaged in sexual activity at relatively similar rates. This statistic is then interpreted as evidence that women are not inherently less desirous than men (e.g., they have equivalent sexual functioning to men), and suggested that many women did not adhere to social standards that condemned and shamed female sexuality.[43] Thus, Kinsey's "more is better" model of orgasms functions to measure not only health but also attitudes toward sex: more orgasms is better, better is healthier, healthier is happier.

This quantitative logic continues to inform claims about sexual norms, attitudes, discrepancies, gaps, and inequity between population groups, such as men and women, and heterosexual and queer populations. Most famously, Kinsey's work helped "reveal" the "orgasm gap" ("pleasure gap"), the discrepancy in the frequency of orgasm between men and women. Over the last century, studies and surveys that borrow from the logic of Kinsey's research have shown a 20 to 30 percent difference in orgasm frequency between heterosexual men and women. Follow-up research has examined social context (e.g., long-term partner versus a single encounter, or college students versus older adults), or solo versus partnered sex, and compared these results to studies of gay and lesbian populations.[44] Across this body of work, the results are most often read as indicating and being caused by the inequity of heteropatriarchal models of sexual behavior. Circulated through popular articles, interviews, and marketing campaigns, the orgasm gap has become the emblem of gender inequality, touted as evidence that heterosexual women repeatedly engage in unsatisfying sex based on social expectations, and as proof of the sexual dissatisfaction widely experienced by heterosexual women everywhere.[45]

These interpretations of the orgasm gap draw on and reinforce the logic of Kinsey's methods and statistical research. By framing the absence of an orgasm as a problem, the orgasm gap promotes orgasmic presence as the sexual norm. In her cultural analysis of the pleasure gap, journalist Katherine Rowland points out that the data illustrate that orgasmic absence in women is statistically normal.[46] To frame the gap as a problem is to assume that orgasmic presence and the accumulation of orgasms is the sexual norm by which women's pleasure should be judged, but data show that a large percentage of heterosexual women do not experience orgasm during penetrative sex. In other words, absence is the norm. It also assumes that orgasmic presence is synonymous with pleasure and satisfaction, and that this pleasure reflects an individual's relationship to sex and their partner.[47] In this model (and Kinsey's research), "equality" is framed entirely through accumulation, obscuring any underlying experiential, cultural, or social conditions that may inform how an individual perceives sex or pleasure. While the discourse around the orgasm gap aims to make claims about social behaviors and attitudes, the data it presents ultimately obscures questions about how pleasure and satisfaction are defined, and how those experiences are inextricable from social and cultural contexts. Irvine describes how Kinsey aimed to remain entirely separate from sexual politics in favor of focusing on the "facts." His dedication to objectivity and science led him to ignore and willingly obscure the impact of culture.[48] While this allowed him to offer a more comprehensive and inclusive account of sexual behavior, it promotes a model of sexuality and pleasure that obscures key questions about how pleasure is experienced. With an emphasis on biology and physiology, it makes pleasure appear self-evident and attached to a quantifiable sexual event—an idea that continues to support cultural discourses of sexual pleasure, politics, and health.

Selling Sexual Wellness

As inheritors of Kinsey's quantifiable model of pleasure, contemporary sextech companies often frame their politics in terms of the orgasm gap. Dame, Lora DiCarlo, and Lioness all sell their devices as tools to achieve sexual equality by explicitly citing orgasm-gap statistics, or using the language of quantity or improvement.[49] Under Dame's "About Us" section, they offer a visualization of a 2005 study that showed that 91 percent of cis heterosexual men experienced an orgasm during sex, while cis heterosexual women only reported orgasm 39 percent of the time (Fig. 9). Next to their minimalist data visualization, they proclaim, "We began our mission to close the Pleasure Gap—the disparity in the satisfaction that people with

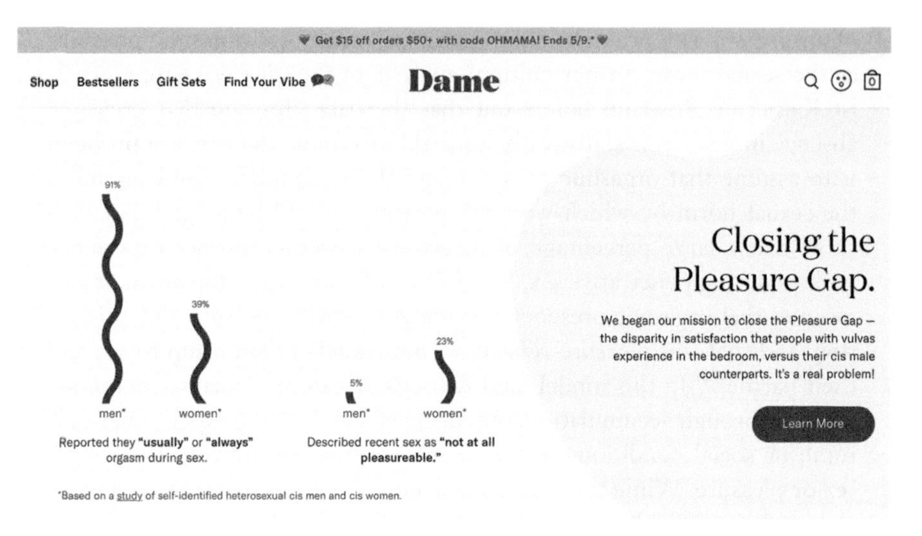

Fig. 9. Dame's "About Us" foregrounds the pleasure gap to sell their products. ("About Us," Dame, accessed May 2020, https://www.dameproducts.com/pages/about-us.)

vulvas experience in the bedroom, versus their cis male counterparts. It's a real problem!" Their supplemental blog post on the pleasure gap argues that lack of knowledge about the clitoris has been central to the discrepancy and that through a greater focus on clitoral stimulation (using their products), "we can help everyone have immensely pleasurable sexual experiences that are fulfilling, empowering, and equitable."[50] As in Kinsey, the implicit logic of this statement is that an equal number of orgasms results in an equal experience of pleasure.[51]

However, operating within postfeminist discourse, Dame and other sextech companies use the population-scale model for orgasmic equality to promote individual actions through the language of self-care and wellness. Dame's homepage declares: "You deserve pleasure. Upgrade your self-care with toys, for sex." Deservingness and equality become attached to individual actions and products: people with vulvas deserve to take care of themselves by having more orgasms using Dame's technologies. The "more is better" logic of orgasm quantification shifts from population-scale models of pleasure equality, to care of the self, the implicit message being that *individuals* can help close the orgasm gap by engaging in *self*-pleasure.

Dame's website is an example of a new aesthetics of sexual wellness that combines the language of postfeminist empowerment with the visual rhetoric of wellness and technology. The goals of health and wellness have become essential in efforts to integrate pleasure and politics and to distance sexual pleasure from the adult entertainment industry. Like Dame's website, self-care rhetoric helps rebrand sexual pleasure as a tool for liberation and wellness. This message is reinforced through the website design, which draws heavily from tech aesthetics and foregrounds the language, iconography, and values of health. Today, if you browse online for a vibrator, you're likely to encounter a site that closely resembles the Apple Store or a boutique health-and-wellness clinic. For example, Lora DiCarlo's website features carefully lit images of their vibrators displayed like sculptural artworks. Devoid of any images of sex, the website's homepage features pictures of diverse women smiling and relaxed, alongside buzzwords such as "empowerment" and "wellness." They refer to their products as tools for "self-love," rather than vibrators, and use nonerotic names, such as "Baci" and "Filare." All of their devices are proudly displayed, but few resemble explicitly sexual iconography. The smooth, round, and oblong devices come in a pleasing range of colors typically used to address millennial consumers, including dusty pink and saturated turquoise. Next to an image of what appears to be a lesbian, interracial couple, the company states its philosophy: "We're determined to continue speaking up for everyone's right to explore their pleasure, and to embrace the idea that sexual wellness is wellness."[52] Lora DiCarlo, like many other sextech companies, uses design to situate their products within the wellness industry. Their websites and marketing campaigns resemble other popular niche companies marketed toward millennials with an eye for design. But by foregrounding politics they simultaneously offer a visual culture of pleasure that emphasizes health, wellness, self-exploration, and empowerment.

This aesthetics and ideology sextech have evolved from second-wave feminism and early feminist sex-toy retailing. During the mid-twentieth century, the United States saw a major shift from reproductive models of sex toward the rhetoric of reciprocity and pleasure.[53] Over two decades, Kinsey's sex studies were published, the contraceptive pill became widely available, and in 1966, Masters and Johnson published their landmark scientific text, *Human Sexual Development*. These key scientific and medical developments all helped change the definition of sex and reframed pleasure as an equal-opportunity experience that should be available to all. For second-wave feminism, sexual pleasure became an essential symbol and tool to fight against patriarchy and dominant models of sexuality that privilege men's sexual pleasure over women's. In response to pornography's phallocentric depiction of sex, many second-wave feminists advocated for a "woman's right to pleasure," framing masturbation or prioritizing pleasure as an inherently political act.[54] For example, in her highly influential article, "Myth of the Vaginal Orgasm," published in 1968, Anne Koedt directly critiques the psychoanalytic interpretations of the vaginal orgasm and calls for a redefinition of sexual pleasure based on orgasmic equality.[55] In response to the historical emphasis on penetrative sex, other sexual practices, including masturbation, oral sex, and lesbianism, became ways to resist patriarchal models of pleasure—the orgasm outside of the context of heterosexual intercourse became a symbol of the "political power of women's self-determination."[56]

During this period, sexology research was used to undermine preexisting, patriarchal assumptions and myths about sex and sexual pleasure, which had historically obscured the female body or supported the myth of feminine mystery. Drawing on the scientific work of Kinsey and Masters and Johnson, sexual pleasure was framed as a way to combat this mythology through self-knowledge.[57] Koedt turns to midcentury sexology because it presents a "neutral" account of sexuality that resists Freudian interpretations of femininity.[58] Sexology offered a medical model of female pleasure centered around the clitoris, citing physiological data on the lack of nerves located in the vaginal canal.[59] Additionally, Masters and Johnson's research promoted the idea that women were multiorgasmic, and therefore superior to men. Following Kinsey's logic that quantity is a reflection of capacity, Masters and Johnson claimed that their work revealed that women "actually had a physiologic capacity *greater* than [that] of men . . . authoritatively deflating the myth of male sexual superiority."[60] Thus, for Koedt and other second-wave feminists, physiology confirmed that practices such as masturbation were expressions of women's power.[61]

For many second-wave feminists, heterosexual intercourse was an institution of patriarchy, a system that was never designed for women's pleasure and functioned as a way to uphold men's power.[62] The clitoris became the symbol of this resistance: the most efficient way to achieve orgasm, and physically distinct from a model of sexual pleasure reliant on the phallus. To embrace clitoral orgasms was to take control of sexual pleasure. Koedt placed responsibility in the hands of women to create their pleasure: "we must discard 'normal' concepts of sex and create new guidelines which take into account mutual sexual enjoyment."[63] This dismantling of the sexual norm was largely the responsibility of women, who were encouraged to demand pleasure from their partners or to masturbate as a way to remain free from the oppressive structures of heterosexuality.

Second-wave discourses around masturbation, liberation, and responsibility helped create a market for feminist sex toys and sex retail. While vibrators were openly sold as sex toys by the 1960s, feminists claimed the device was a tool for sexual liberation.[64] By the early 1970s, feminist sex retailers opened catalog services and storefronts in New York City and San Francisco. In her history of feminist sex shops, Lynn Comella details how these early retailers provided a space for women to learn about feminism and sexual pleasure, and to access technologies outside of traditional, male-dominated sex shops. Beyond simply selling vibrators, feminist sex retailers gave women access to a huge range of political and medical materials and resources. For example, Del Williams, founder of Eve's Garden, which opened in New York in 1974, connected women with therapists and distributed sex education materials.[65]

From the very outset, feminist sex retailers used the rhetoric of health, science, and wellness to distinguish their businesses from traditionally "seedy" sex shops. Indeed, Williams envisioned "Eve's Garden as both a feminist outpost for sexual consciousness-raising and a health shop specializing in sex."[66] By creating connections with sex therapists and educators and using expert testimony to promote the use of vibrators, Williams aimed to destigmatize discussions of sexual pleasure and the sale of sexual technologies. Heavily influenced by Reich's energy theories of the orgasm, Williams believed women could channel their "erotic energy" to become more productive and creative and "be free sexually and responsible for their own bodies."[67] Framing the business as a "health shop," Eve's Garden created an early model for health-driven feminist sex retail that has been expanded through wellness discourse today.

The emphasis on health and the destigmatization of sex was communicated through an aesthetics of hygiene and femininity. Early feminist sex shops selected decor, displays, and devices designed to make sex more "approachable," "clean," and "safe." To further distinguish themselves from the stereotypical sex shop and the porn industry, stores like Good Vibrations tried to make their shops as "unerotic as possible." Comella describes how this often played directly into femininity and class by constructing a dichotomy between the "low" model of the phallocentric sex shop and the middle-class, respectable feminist retailer.[68] Hygiene and safety were communicated via stereotypical codes of white, middle-class femininity. Through "homey" aesthetics including warm lighting, colorful signs, "tasteful" displays, and "painting the walls lavender,"[69] these stores helped craft an "alternative sexual vernacular"—a different way of representing sex and organizing sexual knowledge that pivoted on highly gendered appeals to what women supposedly wanted when it came to sex, and by extension, sex-toy stores.[70]

Over the last forty years, this sexual vernacular has evolved and been fortified through the development of the sexual wellness industry. While feminist sex shops no longer stage their stores to resemble domestic spaces and have moved toward more inclusive models of sexuality, sexual wellness extends the health-focused logic and classed models of hygiene to an entire industry focused on respectable models of sex and sexual pleasure.[71] The sexual wellness industry pairs postfeminist empowerment with wellness rhetoric to promote sex-positive messages and expand the definition of health. In postfeminist models of health, sex is framed as a necessary component of health with the (multi)orgasmic women as the model of liberated, healthy femininity.[72] For example, in *SexTech Revolution*, entrepreneur Andrea Barrica argues, "sexual wellness companies understand sex as a source of energy, power, and self-care. A sexual wellness company incorporates sexual health, mental health, and general wellness to help someone feel at home in their body, free of psychological and physiological issues around sexuality."[73] Combining second-wave rhetoric of pleasure and liberation with the ideology of wellness, sexual wellness frames the orgasm as a form of liberation and a way to maintain health. Unlike second-wave discourses that saw masturbation as a political act because it resisted phallocentric models of sexuality, the emphasis on wellness suggests that sexual pleasure and orgasms are a necessary part of basic health maintenance. This implies that to be a liberated woman is to be a healthy woman, with the presence of an orgasm as the marker of both qualities. Thus, sexual wellness ostensibly extends Kinsey's quantified model of the orgasm, where orgasmic presence not only comes to mark normalcy (or health) but also signals "a particular relationship with the body (how 'in touch' with the body you are)."[74]

Notably, sexual wellness often excludes the language of desire and satisfaction in favor of an emphasis on holistic health. As Barrica proclaims, "sexual wellness is not sexy," it is a legitimate, science-backed sector focused on inclusive pleasure and "closing the orgasm gap."[75] This push toward science is likewise echoed in the shift from "sex toys" and "sex shops" toward "sextech." Moving away from the frivolous connotations of "toys" and the "sexiness" of adult entertainment, "sextech" helps signal a company's connection to the burgeoning sexual wellness industry and endows their products with the aura of technoscientific authority. Indeed, technology has been a key way to integrate discourses of pleasure and liberation with health and wellness. Coined in 2009 by Cindy Gallop, CEO of MakeLoveNotPorn, "sextech" includes technology designed to promote sex positivity and "enhance, innovate and disrupt . . . human sexual experience."[76] Rather than foregrounding pleasure, desire, or sex itself, Gallop sees technology as a tool for sex-positive liberation, which can educate the masses about the relationship between sex and happiness. While sextech may draw on second-wave discourses that framed pleasure as a key to promoting a holistic understanding of the mind-body, it primarily foregrounds products and technologies (consumer objects) as the source of liberation through ties to medical institutions and technological expertise. Operating within the logic of postfeminism, "liberation" is expressed through consumption and the further biomedicalization of sexuality in pursuit of wellness. Barrica, for example, advocates for including sexual wellness in our medical systems, and sex-toy historian Hallie Libermann argues that vibrators should be covered by medical insurance.[77] Thus, in postfeminism, "sextech" expands the strain of feminist entrepreneurship that emerged from early feminist sex retail to push toward an "empowered consumer" model, using institutionalization and expertise as a way to sell products.

The rhetorical and aesthetic shift toward health and wellness has become an essential way for companies to distinguish themselves from pornography and adult entertainment.[78] Indeed, leading figures in sextech such as Gallop and Barrica have no ties to the adult entertainment industry. Creators and CEOs increasingly come from backgrounds in industrial design, computer science, and robotics, and often include a consultant or lead engineer with a background in health science or medicine. For example, Lioness's website describes their products as "meticulously made by badass women engineers, designers, health care experts, and dreamers. Lioness brings patented technology never before seen outside of research labs."[79] The creators of Dame come from backgrounds in sexology and engineering and describe their employees as "engineers for sexual wellness."[80] The websites for Dame, Lioness, and Lora DiCarlo prominently feature awards for technology and wellness from major technology shows such as CES, or from health and wellness publications. In their ethnographic study of the emerging sextech industry, Jeffrey Bardzell and Shaowen Bardzell describe how all participants viewed their devices not as toys, but as "consumer electronics," akin to the ordinary technologies that populate our day-to-day lives: "more and more people are coming from industrial design backgrounds going, 'I don't want to design a new watch, I want to design a sex toy.'"[81]

The move away from sexiness toward wellness has been incorporated into the aesthetics of these technologies. Sextech is rarely sexually explicit in its design or marketing. Like Lora DiCarlo's "tools for self love" or Dame's emphasis on "self-care," maude [*sic*], Lioness, and other online sextech retailers often avoid words such as "masturbation" and "vibrator" in favor of the language of "self-pleasure." This is reinforced by the devices themselves, which avoid phallic iconography or realistic representations of genitalia. iroha [*sic*] by Tenga, for example, offers a range of vibrating, handheld silicon devices with gentle dips and grooves that resemble abstract cute animals such as a bird, hedgehog, or whale. The cream-colored "kushi" features a teardrop shape with rubber ridges that slope down the sides and intersect at the tip, while the "iroha stick" is designed to resemble lipstick for discrete portable pleasure.[82] iroha's website manages to avoid the word "sex" entirely, and instead draws on the naturalist language of Kinsey to sell tools for pleasure: "We believe that the pleasure our bodies seek is something to be valued as a key element of self-care. iroha is a series of self-pleasure items designed to respond to these natural needs."[83] Kushi and irona's philosophy speak to how sextech aims to make these technologies more approachable, less intimidating, and higher quality than the devices associated with pornography and lurid sex shops.[84] By using coded language (the only reference to masturbation on the irona site appears to be "insertable pleasure"), and foregrounding sleek, tech-inspired designs, sextech companies have rebranded vibrators as "tools for self-care."[85]

The push toward emphasizing pleasure as self-care has simultaneously supported efforts to mask any connections to sexuality. Despite the language of empowerment and sex-positivity, the design and marketing of these devices often place a great deal of emphasis on disguise. Like the kushi, many sextech devices avoid colors, shapes, and sounds explicitly associated with sex or the human body. The maude vibe, for example, is shaped like a simple, rounded cone and comes in a sleek cream or olive green; further, the company says, "Our packaging is purposely very discreet. Products in pouches will arrive in a neutral-toned bubble mailer with the maude [*sic*] company name on it and the words 'A better morning is coming' faintly printed on one side."[86] Across all of these major companies, the websites stress the beauty, simplicity, and discretion of their products and shipping procedures: users can be empowered to take control of their pleasure using high-end products, but also keep it private. While the design and shipping practices of online retailers may make vibrators for masturbation more accessible, the emphasis on privacy and discretion does little to increase visible and open conversations around masturbation. By using design to mask the purpose of these products, companies perpetuate the "relative *invisibility* of women's masturbation[, which] infects women's consciousness about how they *talk about, think about* and *engage in* masturbation."[87] In other words, following postfeminist emphasis on individuality, the empowerment and destigmatization offered by these companies appear to be entirely personal and something that should remain private. Sexual wellness seems to be less concerned with making sexual pleasure more visible or changing the public perception of sexual pleasure; rather, wellness provides a new way to mask ties to sexuality. Like Misitzi's claim that DiCarlo was using the rhetoric of health and wellness to hide her vibrator "in a different way," many of these companies use the aesthetics of tech and the rhetoric of health to suppress ties to sex.

Moreover, this shift toward wellness, empowerment, and technology comes at a cost. The sexual wellness industry thrives on the fact that women are likely to pay more for higher-quality, expert-designed products.[88] Framed as sexual wellness tools, and designed to be beautiful, discrete objects, these devices (or "personal massagers") are sold at price points akin to those of tech accessories, with costs ranging from $50to upward of $400 for "tech-centric" products such as Lora DiCarlo's robotic vibrator, the Osé, or Lioness's smart vibrator. These prices are meant to serve as a direct reflection of quality, but they simultaneously further emphasize the difference between sextech and sex toys: as legitimate, health tools, they "should" cost more than your cheap, plastic vibrator at the local sex shop.[89] Despite sextech's shift toward more inclusive audiences and attempts to move away from biologically essentialist language,[90] the form of sexual wellness offered by these companies remains targeted toward the postfeminist ideal of upwardly mobile, middle-class women with extra capital to spend on health and wellness products.[91]

In other words, through the combination of postfeminist empowerment rhetoric, health, and technology, a new aesthetics of "respectable" sex retail has emerged, which intensifies the classed image of sexual liberation that developed in second-wave feminism through an emphasis on health and wellness. This is not unique to sexual wellness or sextech: as I discuss throughout this book, the preventative health model of the wellness industry continually offers new ways (products) for individuals to work at their bodies and health. Wellness increasingly becomes performed by purchasing the "right" products,[92] eating the "right" diet, and using the "right" technologies in pursuit of a "better, healthier, you." Sextech and sexual wellness follow this logic, offering individuals new ways to improve their pleasure and engage in forms of self-care to be more "liberated," and "healthy" users. While these companies may indeed help expand and normalize sex technologies and self-pleasure, they simultaneously reinforce a model of sexuality performed by purchasing the right devices and accumulating more orgasms. The ideal buyer is presented as an upwardly mobile, sex-positive woman who has the income to "invest" in her pleasure and self-care by pursuing the latest technologies and continually seeking out more and better orgasms.[93]

In this sense, sextech adapts a postfeminist sensibility in which the language of sexual liberation and agency continually works to inscribe women into traditional gender roles and social frameworks. Within postfeminism, women are "characterized as actively desiring sexual subjects who are adventurous, knowledgeable, empowered and who choose to engage in sexual activities and interactions to please *themselves*."[94] But as numerous scholars have shown, these depictions of empowered sexuality in pop culture and self-help often reinforce gendered forms of self-surveillance and maintenance. This is often illustrated through an emphasis on "sexiness," where women can have a lot of sex with several partners, and "choose" to express their power and freedom by dressing in tight clothing, showing off their bodies, and wearing makeup.[95] But this image of the empowered woman simultaneously reinforces a model of liberation attached to commodity choices (clothing) and increased bodily maintenance (makeup and working out to maintain a sexy figure). Through wellness, sextech moves away from this feminized model of sexiness, adamantly rejecting any overt ties to sex in favor of more "legitimate" health concerns. But by rebranding masturbation as "self-pleasure" and suppressing references to sex, these companies participate in the contradictory messages of postfeminism. As a form of self-care, masturbation is rendered ordinary, a basic ritual for health maintenance, but the emphasis on disguise and discretion projects the idea that these practices (and conversations) should remain private, and individual practices and products should be hidden away from the public eye. That is, despite shifting away from an aesthetic of sexiness and employing the rhetoric of freedom, liberation, equality, and subversion, these companies ultimately reinforce postfeminism's individualized, classed model of sexuality that fails to intervene in public perceptions and conversations about sex and sexual pleasure.

Optimizing Pleasure

Sextech's rhetoric of empowerment is strongly attached to the values of self-knowledge and control associated with neoliberalism and postfeminism. Within this framework, sexual pleasure is understood as the product of increased knowledge of the self and thereby control over the body. Knowledge is constructed as open-ended and infinite: individuals can always learn more about themselves and therefore improve their sexual pleasure.[96] The homepage for Lioness, a smart vibrator designed to track orgasms, proclaims "practice makes pleasure." Next to an example of an orgasm visualization, the company promotes the ideology that increased knowledge equals increased pleasure, which for Lioness is directly related to the collection of data: "We know. Numbers, data, and charts sound like the least sexy way to explore your sexuality, ever. But we've found that removing some of the sexiness from sex can help people learn about, understand, and communicate their own sexuality."[97] Like many sextech companies, Lioness suppresses connections to sex or sexiness by turning toward science and health. In the case of the smart vibrator, self-quantification becomes a way not only to distance the product from traditional sex toys and sex shops, but to produce knowledge to achieve "better, smarter orgasms."[98]

Lioness's understanding of sexual pleasure follows postfeminism's "requirement to develop a 'technology of sexiness,'" or the continuous cultivation of knowledge and expertise necessary to "secure sexual power."[99] Postfeminism and sextech suggest that power and pleasure are directly related to an individual's capacity to learn and control the self and the body. However, like the aesthetics of sexual wellness, this often promotes contradictory messages that inscribe women into traditional gender roles. Frith argues that the postfeminist logic of sexual expertise simultaneously promotes individual empowerment and encourages women to understand the orgasmic absence as a personal failure that threatens their partner's masculinity. The resulting image of empowerment encourages women "to work on their sexual confidence and free themselves from the last glimmer of sexual repression in order to transform themselves into 'up for it' sexual beings, yet they are simultaneously held responsible for maintaining relationships, protecting their male partners and pleasing themselves in ways which also please men."[100] Lioness and other sextech companies extend to health the double bind of the empowered cultivation of the self within postfeminism. Sextech promotes the idea that to be healthy is to be powerful and liberated, and vice versa: striving to improve health (via wellness products and practices) is framed as an inherently political act.

This logic is not unique to sextech or postfeminism, but emerges from the science of sexual pleasure and discourses of masturbation from midcentury sexology described throughout this chapter. This body of research in many ways provided a foundation for the contemporary emphasis on knowledge and improvement. Kinsey's attachment to naturalist theories of sexuality led him to argue that women were inherently capable of orgasm and that any restriction of sexual desire was the product of culture and socialization.[101] While this emphasis on social conditioning avoids pathologizing orgasmic absence, like medical definitions of orgasmic disorders it suggests the problem is *fixable*. In other words, it borrows the logic of biomedicine and suggests that there are strategies, treatments, and skills one can develop to help the body return to a "natural" state capable of orgasm.

For Kinsey, scientific data was a way to fix this problem by revealing fallacies of gender difference and promoting equity and understanding across all groups.[102] This project was taken up a decade later by Masters and Johnson, who furthered the ideology of naturalness and "sameness" by developing the "sexual response cycle," a physiological model of pleasure that resisted discourses of sexual difference. By tracking a range of vitals and physical measurements, including heart rate, breathing rate, vaginal contractions, and ejaculatory pacing, they argued that all healthy men and women were physically capable of achieving orgasm.[103] While they acknowledged that orgasms were "psychophysiologic experiences" shaped in part by social influences, their model of the human sexual response aimed to set a "nonsubjective . . . [and] recognizable baseline."[104] They repeatedly proclaimed "sex is natural," and it was their goal to put "sex back into its natural context," free of the social influences that inhibit basic physiological processes.[105] Their turn toward physiology was directly tied to addressing "sexual inadequacy," which they believed could only be treated by understanding the most basic physical reactions and responses.[106] The biological models of pleasure from Kinsey and Masters and Johnson argue that every person has the innate *capacity* to orgasm; it is just a matter of developing the proper *technique*.

Indeed, placed within this medical framework, Masters and Johnson were able to monetize their research by opening a sex-counseling business. Following the success of *Human Sexual Response*, they used their expertise to establish a counseling and treatment service designed to help train couples struggling to achieve orgasm during sex. While Masters and Johnson's research can be used to support second-wave feminist causes, their clinical work remained largely conservative and focused on supporting the institution of marriage. Irvine argues that Masters and Johnson, and sexology more generally, "have an investment in the maintenance of dominant ideology," which creates their market of individuals in need of sex advice and expertise.[107] By focusing exclusively on the physiological functions of the body, they were able to create a business "with the promise of simple and effective techniques and commodities that will ameliorate, if not solve, the presenting dilemma."[108]

Though second-wave feminists did not adhere to this market-driven model of sexual improvement, they nonetheless adopted the logic of self-knowledge, training, and practice that emerges from scientific models of sexual pleasure. During this period, women's collectives, activists, and institutions published guides, held workshops, and distributed information about female sexual pleasure, with a particular emphasis on masturbation. In 1968, the National Sex Forum was established to centralize and distribute education and training materials for counselors, and in 1972, they published *Masturbation Techniques for Women*. The guide was meant to "assist you in learning to masturbate and come by yourself. This is a natural desire and you have a right to enjoy your own body, all of it, from head to toe."[109] The 1970 publication of *Our Bodies, Ourselves* dedicated an entire chapter to sexuality and masturbation, and in 1974, sex educator and activist Betty Dodson published *Liberating Masturbation: A Meditation on Self Love*, a memoir on rediscovering herself through self-pleasure. Following second-wave consciousness-raising models, Dodson developed her famous "bodysex" workshops, where women could collectively explore their vulvas and learn the "rock and roll orgasm technique."[110] Comella describes how feminists like Dodson aimed to bridge the gap between the science of sex and sexual liberation by translating the research into self-exploration and pleasure exercises.[111]

For many second-wave feminists, orgasmic absence was a reflection of how women were socialized within patriarchal systems. They adopted the logic of self-knowledge of midcentury sexology to argue that it was up to women to liberate themselves through education and practice. For example, Dodson advocated for masturbation and sexual pleasure as a way for women to "take control of their lives." But in contrast to the language of "naturalness" central to Kinsey's and Masters and Johnson's work, Dodson claimed the patriarchal structures—the "norm"—in which women are socialized prohibit the expression of sexual pleasure:

> Sexual skill and the ability to respond are not "natural" in our society. Doing what "comes naturally" for us is to be sexually inhibited. Sex is like any other skill—it has to be learned and placed. When a woman masturbates, she learns to like her own genitals, to enjoy sex and orgasm, and furthermore, to become proficient and independent about it.[112]

While all women may have the physiological capacity to orgasm or experience sexual pleasure, Dodson emphasizes that cultural norms fundamentally shape the expression and understanding of those capacities, and that combating the social and cultural systems that inhibit women's pleasure requires practice.

Across second-wave sex-positive feminism and midcentury sexology, the orgasm is paradoxically framed as the "natural" and inevitable product of bodily stimulation, but also one that requires great skill and concentration.[113] Self-knowledge becomes the key to navigating this contradiction: it is simply a matter of learning how to take advantage of existing physiological processes and response systems. While second-wave feminism connected knowledge to combatting patriarchy—the cultivation of sexual skill symbolized independence from men as the gatekeepers of pleasure—postfeminism repackages and depoliticizes this ideology through an emphasis on health.

The language of "empowerment" and "equality" continues to circulate through sextech marketing, but the expression of that "power" is largely attributed to the cultivation of individual skills, through practice in pursuit of self-pleasure as a form of care. Frith describes the cultivation of skill as a "performance imperative," aimed to increase an individual's appeal in the sexual marketplace. Practicing in pursuit of improvement functions as "a form of 'sexual entrepreneurship' in which men and women are encouraged to 'invest' in sexual selves and to develop their 'sexual capital,' guided by the advice of 'experts.'"[114] With sextech, sexual capital is not necessarily associated with attracting partners or improving one's sexual appeal, but instead is related to the individual imperative to liberate the self and improve health through sexual pleasure. Skill and practice become pathways—investments—in the pursuit of the healthy, progressive, sexual self.

Contemporary sextech companies operate through and reinforce the ideology of skill and training as a way to perform sexual pleasure and health. Most sextech companies supplement their products with instructional articles, videos, and sexual-wellness coaching services designed to help individuals learn more about their bodies to experience more and better orgasms. Dame and Lora DiCarlo have blogs that supply countless articles detailing how individuals can improve their solo and partnered sessions, posts dedicated to "debunking" common myths of sexual pleasure and orgasms by drawing on scientific studies or health research, and anatomy lessons on how to identify different parts of genitalia. All of this content is framed as "sex education," or tools to help develop self-knowledge through the science of sexual health and wellness. Companies are also beginning to expand this emphasis on training and knowledge through supplementary coaching and classes. Lora DiCarlo offers complimentary "wellness coaching," which they describe "as like sex ed, but way more empowering."[115] Lioness advertises masturbation classes in addition to their archive of instructional materials,[116] and Dame offers an expansive selection of wellness workshops ranging from "Mindful Sex" to "Pelvic Floor Pilates."[117]

However, Lioness has taken the emphasis on practice a step further, by incorporating quantification and biofeedback models common to digital health technologies. As the "first and only smart vibrator and app that lets you see & improve your orgasms," Lioness tracks masturbation sessions and provides data analysis and tracking features to help "improve" pleasure over time.[118] The device measures vaginal contractions and body temperature during masturbation or partnered use. The data is fed into a corresponding app, where individuals can access an image of their session and add supplementary data, including tags (e.g., "workout day," "alcohol," or" period"), ratings, and notes. After each session, users are meant to open up the app, where they will encounter a graphical visualization that maps vaginal contractions over time. They can also choose to include temperature data and vibration levels to "better locate" periods of arousal and pleasure.[119] Examining the graph, they are supposed to make a "clip" of their orgasm by comparing their chart to three "orgasm patterns": volcano, ocean wave, or avalanche. To decode the data, the app provides an information section that shows sample graphs for each pattern, along with brief first-person descriptions of the experience: "it feels like I'm in the ocean, with waves of pleasure washing over me" (Fig. 10). After selecting

10:57
◂ App Store
VOLCANO
"Almost every muscle in my body tenses up as the pleasure greatly intensifies, then there's a huge release. It's over when I can relax."
orgasm
OCEAN WAVE
"It feels like I'm in the ocean, with waves of pleasure washing over me."
orgasm
AVALANCHE
"It's like I rocket up to this huge peak in pleasure, and then free fall my way down until finally my body relaxes."
orgasm
BACK TO MY DATA

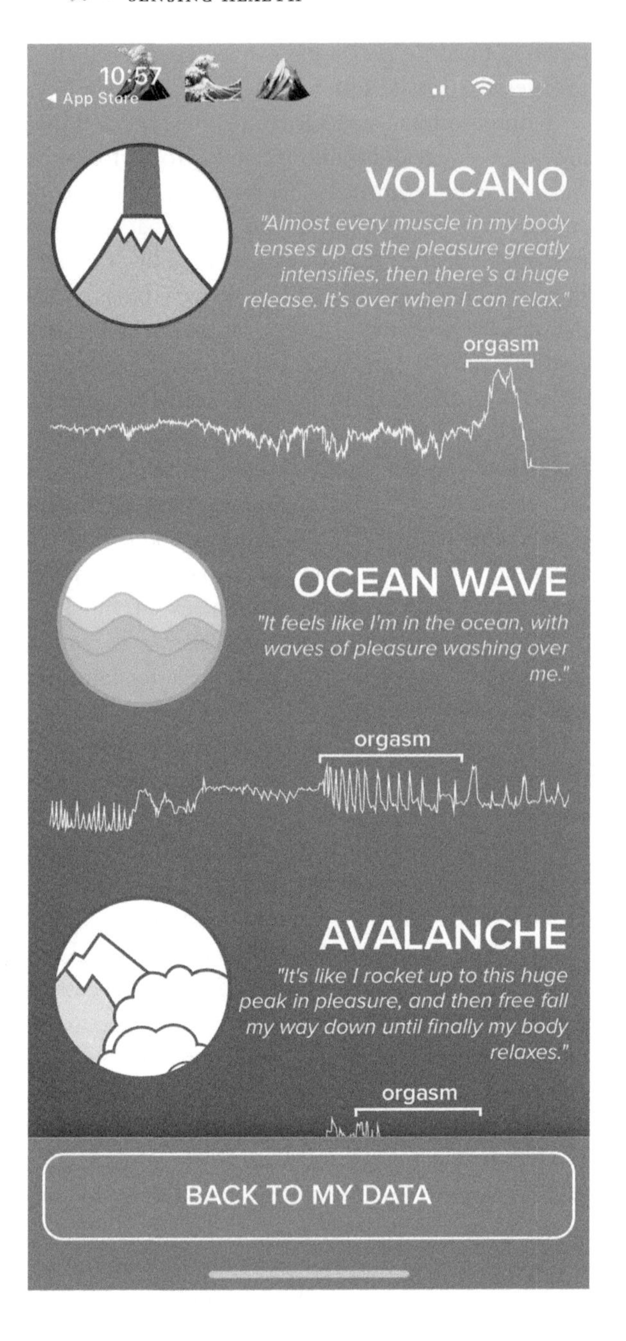

Fig. 10. Lioness offers descriptions and sample graphs for the three "orgasm patterns." (Lioness, "Lioness Health and Sex Tracker," vers. 2.0.07, accessed June 2021.)

the section of a graph as their orgasm, they use one to five stars to rate their session and provide any additional notes for future reference.

"Improvement" using Lioness is figured as in many other self-tracking technologies, where the collection of data is meant to help identify patterns that can be applied to future experiences. Juxtaposing qualitative and social data against the measurement of an orgasm is meant to help individuals locate certain contexts and mediating factors that may contribute to the strength and satisfaction of their orgasms. Ideally, this allows them to identify positive factors that can be applied to create optimal conditions for orgasm and arousal. Lioness invokes the language of science by framing this process as a form of "self-experimentation," suggesting that the device functions as an instrument that can measure the success or failure of a test session. "Improvement" is specifically tied to increased intensity and duration, with "intensity" translated as the strength of vaginal contractions.[120] By framing orgasms as data points measurable via the device, Lioness can thus determine whether the orgasmic experience was "better" than previous sessions. Indeed, each entry in the app includes statistical data comparing the length of the orgasm and overall session to the data archive: "orgasm was *longer* than the average by 1 s."[121]

Lioness's measurement model borrows directly from quantitative methods developed in Masters and Johnson's physiological research, which examines vitals and physical reactions to determine orgasmic presence or absence. While Masters and Johnson were not the first to turn to vital signs, such as heart and breathing rates or vaginal contractions, to detect and measure orgasms, their research collected and combined multiple forms of measurement and provided a public-facing model for the scientific measures of sexual pleasure that have since helped inform both scientific and popular understandings of the orgasm.[122] The graphical representations created by Masters and Johnson continue to provide a basic model or structure for understanding bodily responses. Their sexual response graph maps an upward trajectory through the first three stages of sexual response—excitement, plateau, and orgasm—and a sharp downward turn in the final "resolution phase." This visualization shows how the sexual response cycle involves an intensification of physiological responses that eventually may "reach the extreme level from which the individuals ultimately move to orgasm."[123] Though Masters and Johnson discuss how individual responses to stimulation may influence the duration of each phase, there is the sense that the successful completion of the sexual response cycle is tied to physiological intensity—*increases* in blood flow, heart rate—that culminate in an involuntary orgasmic reaction and the experience of pleasure.[124] Their definition of the phase supports the idea that *accumulation* and *escalation* are directly related to the experience of sexual pleasure.

The attachment of sexual pleasure to escalation is further reinforced by comparing different types of quantified physiological data sets. *Human Sexual Response* includes several graphical representations of their data, including mapping EKG readings alongside "orgasmic platform readings" or vaginal contraction measurements.[125] The juxtapositions show not only how sexual response affects the body as a whole, but show a correlation between specific phases of the cycle and increases in vitals. In the case of the EKG and vaginal contraction graphs, they show a correlation between peak heart rate and the strongest vaginal contractions. The peaks of both graphs align to suggest that orgasmic presence could be detected by examining the maximum heart rate data set. This combination of data creates an image of sexual pleasure directly tied to escalation, with the highest number framed as evidence of orgasm.

While Masters and Johnson's research (as well as contemporary physiological sex research) attempts to "demystify" the orgasm, there is currently no consensus on a definitive physiological marker of orgasmic presence.[126] Nonetheless, Lioness's data-analysis features rely on locating orgasmic presence, and ultimately extend models of quantification and comparative analysis to foreground the orgasm as the primary source of self-knowledge. By combining temperature data and vaginal contraction measurements, individuals are encouraged to locate "hot spots" and graphical peaks to determine where their orgasm is located in their data set (Fig. 11). If they choose to include temperature data, their graph will be colored in varying shades of red; where increased saturation of the hue is meant to correlate with higher temperatures, and therefore indicates "where you're more aroused."[127] Examining the temperature data alongside the vaginal contraction graph hypothetically allows individuals to track a correlation between increased arousal (temperature) and specific types of orgasm, or to track increases in duration or intensity (strength of the contraction). This comparative model encourages individuals to look for points of escalation and to understand their orgasms through the visual rhetoric of intensity, accumulation, and increase.

By drawing on Masters and Johnson's quantitative models of orgasms, Lioness depoliticizes sexual pleasure as a source of liberation in favor of an ideology of sexual pleasure directly attached to neoliberal values of improvement and accumulation. The graphical representations and the

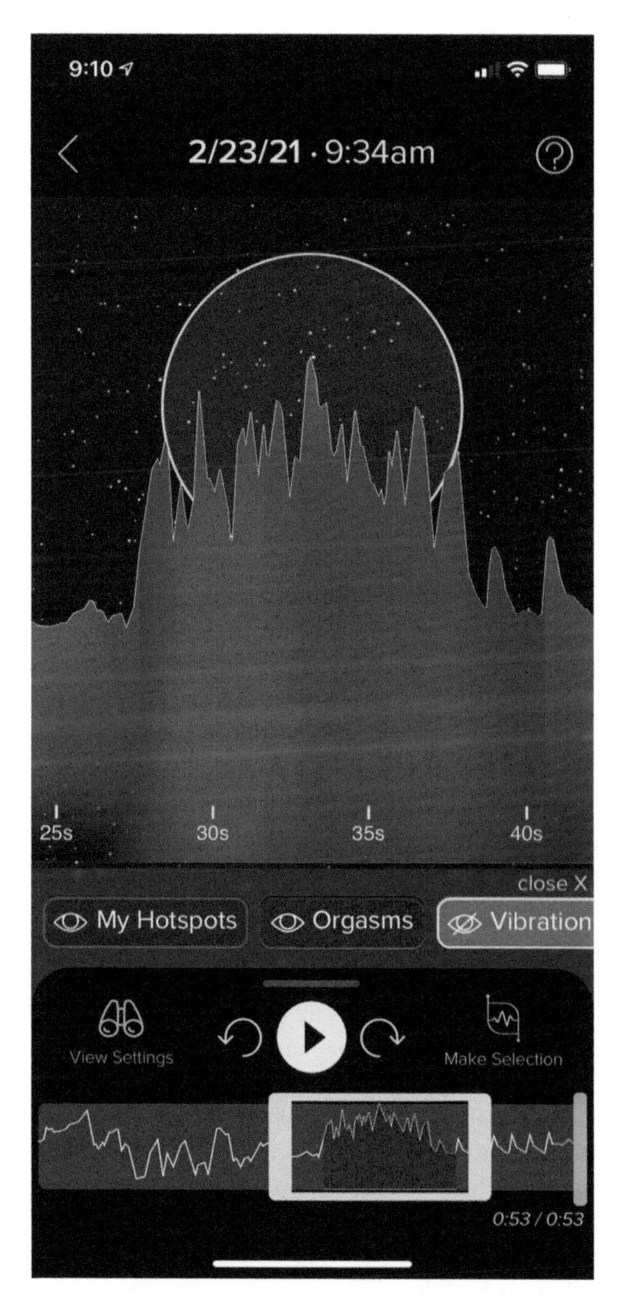

Fig. 11. A sample data set highlighting the "orgasm" section of the graph that includes temperature tracking. (Lioness, "Lioness Health and Sex Tracker," vers. 2.0.07, accessed June 2021.)

orgasm selection process encourage individuals to understand sexual pleasure through identifying an orgasm, which can in turn serve as a baseline for improvement. The tracking features that monitor length and intensity encourage individuals to improve their numbers, seeking higher peaks in their graphs and darker reds. As a result, pleasure is based on the logic of "more is better," "bigger is better," and "stronger is better." While Kinsey's quantitative strategies suggested that more sex is better, Masters and Johnson's physiological models extend this logic to the orgasmic experience itself by suggesting "stronger is better." Lioness borrows from both discourses to locate the value of sexual experience in the strength, quantity, and frequency of orgasms. Pleasure, in this context, is not understood through bodily sensations, but through indirect physiological measures of orgasmic presence.

Indeed, the Lioness app is designed to focus "analysis" on the orgasm phase itself and consequently encourages individuals to frame their entire experience with the device through a small section of data. The information section of the app features "how to interpret your data," but the article focuses exclusively on locating an orgasm based on the contraction and temperature data. There is no indication of how individuals should understand the rest of their graphs; instead, they are instructed to collect more data to help them recognize their orgasm patterns: "After a few recorded orgasms you will likely be able to understand what your orgasm looks like." Consequently, all of the "additional questions and concerns" are framed through the norm of orgasmic presence: "What should I look for if I'm not sure I had an orgasm?" "My pattern doesn't look like any of those"; "Sometimes it doesn't look like anything happened."[128] The tone of these questions is telling. It points directly to how focusing attention exclusively on orgasmic presence and absence can create doubt and anxiety around the experience of sexual pleasure. While Lioness stresses that sometimes the "data isn't always as beautiful as we want it to be" and that you should "trust yourself," the app's design and analytical structures suggest that orgasms are central to understanding and interpreting sexual pleasure.[129] The tracking features and the possibility of "improving" sexual pleasure rely almost entirely on locating and analyzing the orgasm data. Without orgasmic presence, the promise of the app breaks down: one can no longer "keep track of what made your orgasms better, worse, or different to understand your body better and feel more confident."[130]

Quantification and data visualization reduces sexual pleasure to the metric intensity of an orgasm, reinforcing the idea that the orgasm is a "requirement which individuals have an obligation or responsibility to deliver."[131] Despite the wide variety of reasons why people masturbate—from relaxation to a simple element of routine—an emphasis on the presence of an orgasm continues to shape the perception and understanding of sexual pleasure and masturbation. In other words, though studies have shown women often acknowledge the pleasures of finding the time and space to simply explore and stimulate their bodies, the pressure to orgasm haunts these experiences. Sociological accounts of masturbation and experiences of orgasms counter the narrative that orgasms are the sole purpose and goal of sexual stimulation and behavior. In their study of adult cis women, Breanne Fahs and Elena Frank describe how orgasmic labor was central to the meaning and purpose of masturbation: women sometimes found it

> frustrating as they "quested" after orgasm. . . . women may masturbate to avoid the labor they invest with partners to visibly, audibly, and tangibly have pleasure; in other words, masturbation provides a space where women can orgasm without any associated forms of labor (e.g., moaning, groaning, mutual "getting off"), shame, or guilt about their pace and speed of orgasm.[132]

Across accounts from participants is a sense that a focus on orgasms—the presence or provocation of them—encourages women to understand their sexual experiences as work toward the goal of orgasm.

Lioness expands this ideology by suggesting that one must *see* an orgasm to understand and verify its presence. In other words, it's not simply enough to think one has had an orgasm, individuals also must be able to verify its presence and analyze it to improve. The emphasis on data and visualization is part of a broader discourse of orgasm science, which has continually tried to map and analyze orgasms by technologically tracking physiological changes. As in Lioness and Masters and Johnson, orgasm is often located based on correlating indirect data sets. Moreover, many studies that track physiological data alongside firsthand accounts of the orgasmic experience show that participants (primarily women) often fail to locate their orgasm in accordance with the data.[133] This discrepancy is often translated as evidence for how "little" women know about their bodies, but it likewise may point to the limitations of a datafied account of pleasure.[134]

By foregrounding physiological data as proof of an orgasm over individual experiences, these scientific studies, and indeed Lioness, illustrate the gap between two ideologies: pleasure for health versus pleasure for pleasure's sake. On the one hand, a physiological account of pleasure focused on orgasms has aided the scientific study of the health benefits of sexual pleasure. Researchers have examined how orgasms influence a range of other bodily processes, from the release of dopamine in the brain to positive impacts on the body's stress-response system.[135] By focusing on a correlation between indirect physiological markers of orgasm and other data sets, scientists have argued that orgasms have health benefits.[136] But on the other hand, they simultaneously risk effacing the experience of sexual pleasure itself. Once orgasmic presence and the subsequent effects are prioritized over bodily experience, the idea of pleasure begins to lose meaning, or at the very least become displaced. The emphasis on verifying the presence of an orgasm can, as suggested in the FAQ section of the Lioness app, actually encourage individuals to doubt their own experiences of pleasure and their perception of bodily sensations. Thus, despite drawing on second-wave discourses of pleasure and liberation that aim to reconnect body and mind, Lioness's design can effectively remystify the orgasm and reinforce the idea that bodies remain inaccessible to us via ordinary sensations.[137] While the framework of quantification and tracking may suggest knowledge production and control, this tension between data and experience can instead potentially perpetuate and expand the historical idea that certain individuals (particularly women) can't trust their perceptions of their bodily sensations.

The Purpose of Pleasure?

While Lioness draws attention away from bodily experiences of pleasure, the device continues to collect positive ratings, and many articles have stated that the tracking and visualization features have helped some learn about their bodies and improve their experiences of solo and partnered pleasure. But this self-knowledge is largely the result of comparing exterior social conditions to statistical information such as duration and star rating. For example, some have described finding correlation between the intensity of their orgasm and menstruation or ovulation, or between orgasm and the consumption of particular substances, such as alcohol or marijuana.[138] Lioness's website also includes an entire "research" section where individuals who have coding skills can share their data analysis and findings. Similar to "quantified self" online forums that allow individuals to post personal data-analysis projects, the Lioness website encourages sharing analysis conducted using the Lioness device and platform.[139] These at-home experiments have examined different masturbation techniques and the effect of various stimulants, compared Lioness to other sex toys, and even used the data to make data-visualization art. Unfortunately, this approach is only accessible to those who have substantial programming and data-analysis skills. Though this section of the site illustrates the ways that this data can be used to explore sexual experiences, it remains divorced from the core features of the app.

The online forum gestures toward how the device could be used to examine and explore bodies, technologies, and habits, but it remains largely divorced from the experience or perception of pleasure. I end by turning to phenomenological descriptions of my own experience using the Lioness app to show how the app's aesthetics currently obscure and abstract the experience of sexual pleasure. Lioness's primary goal is to help individuals achieve stronger, longer, and more frequent orgasms. But for me, someone without coding or data-analytic skills, the interface design and orgasm visualization features remain so obscure, strange, and utterly divorced from my body that I have little sense that the data or statistics have any bearing on my health or pleasure. However, rather than simply dismissing the device, I turn to sociological and experiential accounts of women's sexual pleasure and masturbation to question whether Lioness and other forms of quantification technologies can be redesigned to encourage a more attuned relationship to the body.

When I open the Lioness app, the graphs are almost entirely illegible to me—I cannot see my body, experience, or pleasure in any of the numbers, lines, or animations. Unlike data collected through other wearables such as my Apple Watch, Lioness's data has not been translated into discernable visualizations that appear to reflect my actions or health. For example, in contrast to the circles that track my progress toward my "move goal" that I described in the introduction, Lioness's interface does not allow me to connect my actions or bodily sensations to the numbers or graphs on the screen. An abstract jagged line with veritable peaks and valleys is mapped alongside seconds on the x-axis: there does not appear to be any identifiable pattern, repetition, or logic to this data. Encouraged to locate my orgasm, I search for the highest peaks, the darkest red, and rapid descents, or any clue to help me locate the orgasmic phase that will allow me to use the app's tracking features. This visualization appears totally incongruous with my bodily experience. The sheer amount of data and the way it is visualized inhibit any possibility of locating any "resemblance" between the graph and the physical sensations I've just experienced. The app does not encourage me to reflect on my experiences using the device or to think back to the unfolding of pleasures and bodily sensations. I'm left scrolling across the erratic peaks and valleys, trying to find a pattern that may coincide with when I think my orgasm occurred.

The search is further impeded by the app's "replay" feature, which is automatically triggered when I select a data set. On opening, the app "replays" the session in real time: the graph moves laterally, gradually revealing sections of the vaginal contractions and temperature data. A large, pulsating circle overlays the ticking graph, which is meant to animate the vaginal contractions. Strangely, rather than displaying the contraction of the vaginal canal, the circle expands as the force of the vaginal contractions increases and contracts as the graph dips and exertion decreases. The combination of real-time playback, vaginal contraction animation, and temperature data is meant to help me "see" my orgasm and "understand" my pleasure. But collectively, these features work to abstract my experience. As it plays in real time, I do my best to locate the orgasmic phase on the graph, "rate" the session, add supplemental information through tags such as "workout day," and write a couple of notes to provide some context for future reference, but it remains unclear to me how the jagged graph and pulsating circle could help me better understand my pleasure, let alone improve it.

Instead, I end up slightly frustrated and utterly baffled by the strange visualization and tracking features. I find myself contemplating what a "star rating" of an orgasm may mean, and whether it would be of any use to me in the future: What's the difference between three and four stars? Am I supposed to develop a system of measurement based on the duration or height of the graph peaks to distinguish between these ratings? Do I look at the pulsating circle and use the rhythm of the contraction to determine pleasure? While I can treat the app as a kind of "sex diary," the data and animations make it difficult to reflect on my experience of bodily pleasure. Indeed, turning to the journal feature of the app often draws attention to the fact that there are too many exterior conditions of experience to determine whether a workout, dietary choices, or sleep may have any impact. Though I may be able to control some elements, such as whether or not I work out, and I can be mindful of where I am in my menstrual cycle, the fact remains that factors such as stress or work fluctuate all the time and remain largely out of my control. Thus, the structure of the app often risks reinforcing a sense that all of these exterior social pressures and environmental factors that I cannot control are negatively impacting my orgasms, and by extension reflect declining health.

This perception emerges in part from a sole focus on orgasmic intensity. Lioness's focus on the orgasm phase effaces any pleasures that may emerge throughout my experience; instead, stimulation, feeling, and sensation are rendered as tools to develop "better" orgasms, rather than understanding these experiences as pleasurable and satisfying in themselves. It also suggests that the only "purpose" of sexual stimulation—partnered or solo—is higher chart peaks and deeper reds. If orgasm becomes the metric through which sexual pleasure is understood, there is no space for accounts of sexual pleasure that are not directly related to this outcome. In contrast to the orgasm-centric model, experiential and sociological studies of cis women's accounts of masturbation and orgasms have shown that definitions of sexual pleasure and the purpose of self-stimulation are highly variable. Women often describe how sexual pleasure and masturbation create an intense attunement to their bodies, a feeling of "presence"—of being "in" their bodies—that is distinct from their everyday experiences in the world.[140] This is echoed by accounts of masturbation that frame it as an "escape" or resource for relaxation and respite from day-to-day life.[141] Rather than helping individuals get closer to this experience, datafication through Lioness only further abstracts the body and sexual pleasure.

At the same time, moving away from an orgasm-based model of pleasure risks reviving the idea that women do not "need" sexual pleasure or have the same libido as men. It may also work to support the gendered stereotype that women prefer intimacy to sex, whereas men only desire sex without intimacy. To be sure, these ideas lurk beneath the experiential accounts above and may very well shape women's perceptions of their sexual encounters. But rather than assuming that orgasmic absence or a relatively low level of orgasmic intensity is emblematic of the sexual repression of women (or of poor health), embodied accounts that describe sexual stimulation as "presentness" and "escape" can help expand definitions of sexual pleasure beyond orgasm. A phenomenological account of sexual pleasure more generally shows how bodily attunement can provide pleasure, and that physical stimulation offers a sense of satisfaction that should not be dismissed or understood as "lesser" forms of sexual gratification.

The current structure of Lioness foregrounds orgasms as the source of self-knowledge and liberation, and thus extends the orgasmic imperative. However, it should be asked whether it's possible to design a technology that could encourage an expanded definition of pleasure beyond the orgasmic event. Studies of women's experience of masturbation have shown positive correlations between regular masturbation and a sense of their bodies, agency, and sexuality. While these benefits are ultimately shaped by racial, socioeconomic, and cultural contexts, they suggest that sexual pleasure continues to be a key place for women to become more attuned to themselves and their bodies.[142] The question is whether technology can be developed to support, rather than abstract or exploit, the bodily attunement afforded by sexual pleasure.

One possible solution would be to use the technology to specifically support medical treatment and scientific research on the pelvic floor.[143] In blog posts and reviews of Lioness, some women have described how they have used the device to strengthen their pelvic floor muscles following major medical procedures or having children. For example, following surgery for ovarian and uterine cancer, Karen Holly described using Lioness to regain the strength of her pelvic floor and increase the experience of sexual pleasure. Rather than relying exclusively on the orgasm phase, Holly was more interested in tracking the overall strength of her vaginal contractions. Over time, she describes moving away from data in favor of simply using the device for self-pleasure: "I just enjoyed and let the data collection and my journal expand so that I could compare at some later date in time. . . . I didn't let the data or science interrupt my pleasure."[144] While there are currently a handful of smart Kegel exercise devices on the market, including Elvie and Perifit, these are largely designed to aid in pelvic floor disorders, particularly following a pregnancy. In other words, the devices are situated within biomedical frameworks of disorder, promoting a sense that the body is abnormal, broken, or divergent and requires fixing. Holly's account suggests the possibility of not only supporting treatment but of using the device to become more aware of the body, which can support the pursuit of sexual pleasure.

However, as long as the device focuses exclusively on the orgasmic phase, escalation, and accumulation, it will continue to promote a narrow definition of pleasure and the orgasmic imperative. Pleasure, like pain, is deeply subjective, inaccessible, and exceptionally difficult to describe, let alone quantify. Likewise, the sensation of pleasure draws a great deal of attention to the body, but unlike pain, pleasure does not draw attention to the surface of the body or the body's interior mechanics; rather, as Drew Leder describes, pleasure creates a kind of "opening," an "expansive" experience that pushes one out toward the world and possibly toward others.[145] In describing the difference between pain and pleasure, Leder uses the example of the pleasure of eating: "I find myself enjoying the taste *of the food*, not that of my own tastebuds."[146] Likewise, the pleasure of an orgasm or sexual stimulation is often not experienced as the physiological mechanics of the body—the contraction of the vaginal walls or the release of dopamine—but rather as the physical sensations of touch and stimulation that result from working with the body. This experience is likewise not necessarily confined to the orgasm itself, but to the entire process of directing attention to specific parts of the body, following sensorial feedback, and feeling the small shifts in temperature, pulse, and breath.

By removing the orgasm phase focus of the app, Lioness could help support an expanded understanding of sexual pleasure as a combination of sensations across the body. Contemporaneous to Kinsey's research, Simone de Beauvoir pushed back on an orgasm-centric definition of pleasure, describing the experience as

> enjoyment [that] radiates out throughout the whole body; it is not always located in the genital organs; even when it is, the vaginal contractions constitute, rather than a true orgasm, a system of waves that rhythmically arise, disappear, and re-form, attain from time to time a paroxysmal condition, become vague, and sink down without ever quite dying out. Because no definite term is set, woman's sex feeling extends toward infinity.[147]

While de Beauvoir's account reinforces a theory of sexual pleasure associated with gender difference, her description illustrates a phenomenology that pushes back on understanding the orgasm as the main event and purpose of sexual experiences.[148] Rather, she illustrates how the fluctuation of sensation and dispersal of feeling across the body undermine the sense that pleasure is located in a particular place or confined to a temporal event. Lioness's graphs showing veritable peaks and valleys in fact illustrate that physiological reactions shift during sexual stimulation to suggest that there is not necessarily a linear, upward trajectory toward an orgasm. However, this suggestion is undermined by the app's focus on the isolation of the orgasmic phase and emphasis placed on the orgasmic event. By eliminating the orgasmic isolation and creating a biofeedback structure that attunes individuals to the shifts in sensation (with audio feedback, for example) or modules that emphasize description and self-narrative to track the varying degrees of pleasure they may feel over the course of using the device, Lioness can help expand definitions of sexual pleasure. Ideally, this would also be extended to devices designed to track physiological responses outside a genital framework to create systems of biofeedback for those who do not have a vagina or prefer a nonpenetrative form of sexual stimulation.

In-the-moment feedback or tracking (also see chapter 5), or postsession personal narration where individuals could provide their phenomenological accounts of their experiences, would ideally promote greater attention to specific sensations, feelings, and even distractions that may arise over the course of sexual stimulation. As a result, they may help promote the sense of "presentness" described by some women, and greater attention to the immediate state of the body. Unlike postfeminist models of sexual wellness, a phenomenological approach to tracking sexual pleasure highlights how it creates hyperawareness of the body. Sexual stimulation is one of the rare moments when bodily sensations are the center of attention. Pursuing pleasure becomes a process of attending to the body: the sense of touch, sounds, and other forms of stimulation that create novel and enjoyable feelings across the body. In other words, it requires a sense of feeling "at home" in the body; one must be curious and comfortable enough to work with the body to generate feelings of satisfaction and pleasure. As part of the legacy of midcentury sexology, second-wave feminism, feminist sex retail, and postfeminist sextech, my call for a more phenomenological approach is yet another attempt to understand the difficult concept of pleasure. But it is one that ideally places technology in conversation with the body, encouraging a return to the sensations, feelings, and pleasures of being a body in the world.

CHAPTER 3

Every Step Counts

Analyzing Fitness-Tracking Technologies

On the walk to the weight room or in the last mile.
Somewhere between first tries and finish lines. Pillow fights and pushing limits. That's where you find fitness.
Every moment matters and every bit makes a big impact. Because fitness is the sum of your life. That's the idea that Fitbit was built on—that fitness is not just about gym time. It's all the time.
How you spend your day determines when you reach your goals. And seeing your progress helps you see what's possible.
Seek it, crave it, live it.
—Fitbit[1]

The above manifesto, which was once proudly displayed in the "Why Fitbit" section of Fitbit's website, articulates how the booming fitness-tracking industry is redefining "fitness." Fitness, as Fitbit states, is no longer an isolated activity—a run, swim, or bike ride—but the "sum of your life": every action, every step, every movement that occurs during the day "counts" toward "fitness." Underlying the logic of this statement is the idea that "life" can be counted—datafied—thereby transforming "pillow fights" and "finish lines" into fitness. In other words, fitness, according to Fitbit, is anything that can be quantified, tracked, and accumulated via their products. Only by purchasing their devices, which can transform "life" into data, can individuals "see" their fitness.

On the one hand, Fitbit's fitness philosophy appears to be a continuation of shifting definitions of health that promote a holistic approach to well-being. Fitness is framed through the rhetoric of lifestyle, which includes all the ways individuals care for themselves that collectively define an individual's health and well-being. On the other hand, Fitbit's manifesto marks a movement away from fitness' association with leisure time. Rather than understanding fitness as a discrete workout or activity completed for relaxation or as a hobby outside of work, Fitbit breaks down these categorical and temporal barriers to render all elements of life "fitness."[2]

In a sense, Fitbit's vision of fitness marks a return to pre-nineteenth-century assessments of "fitness" (or lack thereof), which largely concerned individuals' ability to carry out physical labor.[3] By the nineteenth century, modernity and changing labor practices led many Western countries to turn to fitness as a way to counteract the effects of the increasingly sedentary jobs of adult men.[4] Physical activity, sport, and exercise all became separate activities outside of work associated with attempts to reclaim the masculinity, morality, and productivity lost to urbanization and the "brain work" of a rapidly modernizing society.[5] Fitbit appears to recall an earlier, more holistic understanding of the term, directly associated with carrying out the actions and labors of everyday life.

However, Fitbit incorporates a key modern revision of this approach to fitness: quantification. The emphasis on goals and "seeing progress" suggests that fitness is not confined to an individual's lifestyle, but an active pursuit that requires measurement, monitoring, and improvement. This is precisely why many scholars have argued that fitness-tracking technologies promote a neoliberal understanding of fitness (and the body). By quantifying everyday life, Fitbit and other trackers create a "subject that is, on the one hand, the object of surveillance him/herself and, on the other, becomes a responsible citizen who is expected to construct a healthy self and prove so through constant and continuous measurement."[6] Datafication functions to make the body and behaviors (the user's lifestyle) an object of surveillance that can be assessed at all times in pursuit of "health and fitness." Thus, through quantification, fitness is framed in the same terms as contemporary biomedical definitions of health, as an active, ever-receding pursuit rather than a static state of the body. By extension, scholars argue that fitness tracking, and self-quantification more generally, marks a dangerous turn in the assessment and understanding of health and fitness. By defining what bodies and activities "count," these technologies establish health and fitness norms that can shape human behaviors and habits. In comparing themselves to the datafied norms set by the device or platform, users may self-objectify in an unending pursuit of "more" data, higher numbers, "improvement," and "optimization."[7]

Counter to these arguments, many scientists, physicians, and researchers celebrate the possibility of fitness tracking to motivate and hold individuals accountable for their physical activities and pursuit of health.[8] Despite countless public health campaigns in the last half-century to educate and encourage individuals to exercise in pursuit of health, statistics continue to show overall poor national health, including low rates of physical activity and rising rates of what the medical industry calls "lifestyle diseases"[9]—a term that in itself suggests the source of illness is rooted in the choices of individuals, rather than environmental or genetic factors. For some, fitness trackers serve as a useful tool to monitor and improve these harmful practices. The technology's use of quantification offers a way for individuals to see, track, and improve their daily behaviors and ideally develop positive, lifelong fitness and health habits.

While seemingly opposed, these two interpretations operate through the assumption that there is a direct relationship between the desires of the company or the intended function of the technology and the actions and understanding of the users. In other words, they assume that the design of the technology determines the user's beliefs and behaviors. However, as I discussed in the introduction, fitness trackers and other digital health technologies often produce diverse and uneven experiences of the body and health. Both critical and celebratory positions assume that individuals see the data, goal structures, and fitness and health messages as authoritative reflections of their habits, health, or fitness, and that they will correspondingly respond directly to the prescribed framework of the device. But how individuals use, understand, and perceive their data and bodies varies from person to person and does not necessarily align with the goals and functions set by physicians, researchers, or digital health companies.

This chapter foregrounds how aesthetic analysis and phenomenological description can be used to critically examine the relationship between the design and the lived experiences of individuals who use fitness-tracking technologies. This work begins by first situating the aesthetics of fitness-tracking technology in the nineteenth- and twentieth-century histories of American fitness culture. While today fitness is a well-known subset of health (if not a synonym), the incorporation of exercise and physical activity into official definitions of health is relatively new. Over the last 200 years, medical research, economic incentives, and media have helped firmly attach fitness to the performance of health. With the rise of chronic "lifestyle" diseases, public health officials, doctors, and political leaders in the mid-twentieth century turned to exercise as a key resource for preventative care. However, without established intensity levels and duration recommendations, the application of "exercise as medicine" remained ambiguous and difficult to apply to day-to-day life.[10] The publication of Dr. Kenneth Cooper's *Aerobics* in 1968 marked a turn in how individuals were to use fitness in pursuit of health. Cooper, the "grandfather of the fitness movement," extended medical frameworks for fitness by establishing quantified benchmarks for fitness ability and offered structured improvement plans. Individuals could use his self-help book to track distance and time for specific exercises and convert the activities into rate of oxygen intake, VO_2 max. *Aerobics* provided one of the first quantitative guides for how to measure, assess, and improve fitness and thus overall health, and it would go on to sell more than twelve million copies in the United States. Situated at the emergence of neoliberal economic and healthcare policies, self-help guides for health and fitness like *Aerobics*, along with public health campaigns, helped shape contemporary fitness culture, which largely stresses individualized efforts to maintain and monitor exercise habits in pursuit of health. This era also helped fortify the connection between fitness and white, middle-class culture. Much of the medical research and many products and ideologies behind the rise of the American fitness industry and public health campaigns were grounded in middle-class values and lifestyles, which have been inherited and extended by contemporary fitness-tracking technologies.

In the second section, I use descriptions of the aesthetic experience of the most popular commercial fitness trackers, Fitbit and Apple Watch, to analyze how the interface and feedback features use datafication, data visualization, and technological feedback to reinforce and extend the fitness and health-monitoring structures that have developed over the last half-century. While *Aerobics* offered a way to use manual distance and time tracking to calculate vitals, fitness-tracking technologies shift self-tracking from the individual to a technological device that appears to provide automatic and objective information. Moreover, as Fitbit's manifesto suggests, through datafication these devices offer increasingly granular ways to monitor fitness. Fitness trackers take the form of apps, clips, bracelets, or watches, and track a range of vitals, including calories burned, steps walked, distance traveled, exercise minutes, VO_2 max, and heart rate. Most contain an accelerometer and gyroscope that registers and records a change in displacement to track distance and activity. Activity data is processed through algorithms, compared with other data sets such as heart rate, and interpreted as "calories burned," "steps," or specific exercises. For example, my Apple Watch "thinks" that I'm exercising when it registers changes in displacement—which it reads as "steps"—and my heart rate reaches "a brisk walk or above." These two data points are correlated and interpreted as "exercise minutes," counted toward my daily thirty-minute goal. This information is communicated through elegantly designed interfaces that draw on the visual rhetoric of data visualization and are reinforced through push notifications. I argue that the combination of the interface's aesthetics and quantification creates the impression that the information presented is an objective and authoritative reflection of an individual's health and fitness efforts.

Because of the emphasis on data, many scholars argue that fitness-tracking technologies alienate individuals from their bodies.[11] The actual body—the sensations, strains, and affects of fitness and health—appear to be fragmented and obscured by numbers, statistics, graphs, and visualizations. However, in the final section, I complicate the assumption that fitness-tracking technologies objectify the body and lead to self-alienation by turning to my own phenomenological descriptions of Apple Watch, and accounts from former students collected in IRB-approved and exempt studies that I conducted in my courses between 2017 and 2020.[12] These descriptions illustrate the myriad ways that fitness-tracking technologies can both abstract *and* draw attention to the body. Often, self-alienating and reflexive embodied experiences coexist, giving way to a complex and sometimes contradictory understanding of fitness and health that pushes back on a generalizable theory of fitness tracking and self-quantification. Following the goal to move away from generalization, the descriptions from my students are not meant to provide a clear assessment of what health and fitness mean or "feel like" in the digital age, but instead show how phenomenological description and reflective practices can create critical modes of engagement between individuals and technology.

Building on the work of the previous chapters, which emphasize the value of aesthetic analysis, this chapter makes a case for incorporating phenomenological description to understand the impact of design and encourage critical reflective practices. Description reveals the way specific design elements and interactive features shape bodily experiences and perceptions of health, but my work with my students also showcases how the practice of description itself can also serve as a tool for reflection. In describing their experiences with Fitbit, they often found themselves questioning the structures of the device and evaluating the impact it was having on their bodies and behaviors. Through description, they identified how aesthetic features, including interface design, numbers, and feedback structures, were shaping their experiences. Their accounts thus demonstrate how phenomenological description functions not only as a tool for researchers to capture aesthetic experiences, but also as a way for individuals to reflect on how their devices or platforms may be influencing their behaviors, bodies, and perceptions of health. I end by suggesting that incorporating modules and design features that prompt description may encourage critical reflection on the biomedical and quantified definitions of health promoted by existing digital health technologies.

Health as/and Fitness

> [E]xercise is medicine that keeps countless people alive. But like all medicine, it must be taken according to prescription.
>
> —Dr. Kenneth Cooper, *The New Aerobics*, 1970[13]

Scholars have traced the connection between health and exercise to ancient China and the Greeks, most famously citing Hippocrates as a seminal figure in linking poor fitness with poor health.[14] However, most agree that the nineteenth century marks a key shift in the social and cultural value of fitness, where exercise and physical activity began to become increasingly intertwined with morality, virtue, masculinity, and nationalism. The institutionalization and professionalization of fitness during this period helped establish the connection between fitness and a white, middle-class lifestyle—a framework that continues to shape contemporary American fitness culture, industry, and discourse today. Fitness and sport historians Harvey Green, James C. Whorton, and Roy J. Shepard cite Jacksonian America and Victorian England as key places where modern understandings of exercise, sport, and fitness were born. They argue that in this period, exercise and physical activity emerge as antidotes to changing behavioral and environmental conditions of modernity. The rapid pace of urbanization and increasingly sedentary work practices were framed as a threat to the morality, health, and fitness of the nation. In response, "health reformers" in the US and UK developed physical-fitness education programs and established journals, societies, and institutions dedicated to physical education and training. Simultaneously, the fitness industry and exercise culture were cultivated through the rise of sports such as bicycling and gymnastics, and the founding of the Young Men's Christian Association (YMCA), which created a novel commercial space for sport.

Nineteenth-century exercise and fitness cultures were closely associated with moral and religious values. Many scholars point specifically to the YMCA and the broader "Muscular Christian Movement" as a model for the way fitness was framed as a way to cultivate strong, healthy, moral character. Green argues that this early movement helped promote the principle of "perfectionism," still closely associated with American liberal values and fitness culture,[15] or the idea that the body (and soul) should be worked on in pursuit of physical perfection, in the model of God.[16] Fitness is framed as a way to counteract the immoral, impure, and polluting conditions of modern society, anything from the effects of urban life and desk work to the threat of immigrants.[17] For example, President Theodore Roosevelt famously tied the health of the nation to exercise: "A life of slothful ease, a life of that peace which springs merely from lack either of desire or of power to strive after great things, is as little worthy of the nation as of an individual. . . . In the last analysis, a healthy state can only exist when the men and women who make it lead clean, vigorous, healthy lives."[18] Within this ideology, fitness functioned as an extension of middle-class, white, and nationalistic (Protestant) values: exercise, sport, and physical activity became ways to strengthen and cultivate the physical, spiritual, and moral health of the middle class and the nation more broadly.

At the same time, the nineteenth century also included the development of modern theories of biomedicine and secularized discourses of health (including germ theory). While the new paradigm would eventually replace existing theories of medicine that drew from religious and spiritual practices, for decades, biomedicine continued to overlap with existing morally inflected and religious behavioral diagnoses, such as hysteria and neurasthenia. Fitness, as a way to build the strength of body and mind, often traversed both secular and religious treatments. For example, exercise was often prescribed as a treatment for neurasthenia, a catchall term for nervousness or weakness of nerves associated with an urban middle-class lifestyle.[19] Dudley Allen Sargent, who developed one of the first standardized muscular-training programs for fitness educators, claimed his "Sargent System" helped combat neurasthenia and other nervous conditions. Exercise, according to Sargent, could "break up morbid mental tendencies, to dispel the gloomy shadows of despondency, and insure the serenity of spirit."[20] Sargent's claim illustrates how the early iteration of "exercise as medicine" often emphasized the holistic health benefits of fitness through discourses of religion.

By the early twentieth century, fitness was increasingly secularized through the institutionalization of physical fitness and the development of exercise science. In the US, scholars, doctors, and politicians helped establish physical education programs and academic journals dedicated to exercise programs and medical research.[21] This period also saw the rise of research on the physiology of exercise, which became increasingly popular in both the US and Europe with the expansion of eugenics. In his history of fitness culture, Jürgen Markutschat argues that the publication of Charles Darwin's *The Origin of the Species* in 1859 was a key turning point in the study of exercise and health. With the theory of evolution, fitness came to be closely associated with "survival of the fittest," and the cultivation of the ideal physical body produced a strong species.[22] In the early twentieth century, these evolutionary understandings of fitness were adopted by eugenicist efforts to study the ideal physical body, with researchers exploring anything from physiology based on race, to fitness and virility, and blood "impurities" associated with poor fitness.[23]

Despite the popularization and professionalization of fitness and the rise of fitness consumerism, at the beginning of the twentieth century, the public and medical community remained skeptical of a direct connection between fitness and health.[24] However, with the rise of chronic illness, physicians, researchers, and politicians began to explore fitness as a form of preventative medicine (as opposed to a moral and spiritual treatment, or a practice focused on optimal physical performance). Yet it was not until the "cardiac crisis" that arose after World War II that fitness became firmly incorporated into modern definitions of health.[25] Just as nineteenth-century efforts used exercise to combat modern life, the affluence of postwar lifestyles presented dangers to the physical well-being of Americans that exercise could ameliorate. Historian Shelly McKenzie argues that postwar economic transformations not only shifted the work of many American men but supported the growing culture of individualism and responsibility that would shape the explosion of fitness culture in the latter half of the century. In 1952, the National Institutes of Health declared obesity to the be nation's "number one problem," and by 1956, heart disease rose to become the number-one cause of death of men over thirty in the US (and it remains in the top spot today).[26] The sedentary lifestyles of white, middle-class American men were labeled as the source of the problem, and doctors, self-help guides, and government institutions all increasingly turned toward diet and exercise to combat the crisis.

In conjunction, the medical profession shifted toward a focus on preventative care, moving attention away from treating ailments, and toward prescribing behavioral changes to decrease the risk of future illness. "Executive health" briefly emerged as a subspecialty specifically focused on the health conditions of men working in high-stress desk jobs, with physicians often prescribing dietary changes and exercise to decrease the risk of developing heart disease and related conditions. While throughout the 1950s and '60s, studies repeatedly reinforced the connection between exercise and decreased rates of heart disease, professional opinions on fitness and health remained a source of debate. During this period, some doctors argued that exercise could in fact increase the stress on the body created by high-pressure executive work.[27] Without clear, direct correlations between types of exercise, intensity, duration, etc., and specific health benefits, some continued to warn of the dangers of fitness.[28] McKenzie describes how this debate was part of a broader cultural shift in the perception of medical expertise: some even argued that "doctors were only able to treat disease, not promote health."[29] As I discuss in the next chapter, this growing distrust of medical expertise and treatment contributed to the rise of wellness culture in the 1970s, but also created the cultural conditions for popular self-help focused on individual exercise efforts to improve health. Combined with the increased focus on prevention and lifestyle, the early debates among experts and the failure of medical institutions to decisively link the prescription of exercise to positive health benefits during the 1950s and '60s helped cultivate the culture of health that moved expertise away from institutions and toward the efforts of individuals.

Rather than focusing on how exercise could improve the body's physiological functions, early advocates focused on fitness as a way to combat the stress of modern work. Unlike the nineteenth-century exercise movements, fitness was not a means to enhance physical strength or shape the body, but instead served as a source of relaxation. McKenzie argues that the emphasis on stress and diet was largely associated with class and gender. While bodybuilding and sport were popular among working-class men in the early twentieth century, in middle-class culture attention to body shape or figure was largely seen as homosexual and feminine. In the 1950s and '60s, exercise was sold to women as a way to improve appearance, weight, and shape, but for men, the greater focus was on the psychological and sensory benefits of fitness to avoid gendered stereotypes.[30]

The emphasis on relaxation in discourses of health and fitness led to a very broad understanding of "exercise as medicine," offering men a wide variety of activities and intensities to choose from. However, the lack of parameters made it challenging for men to adopt regular fitness habits. Self-help guides from the 1950s and '60s include a wide range of recommendations, including types of exercise (golf, tennis, etc.), and vague suggestions about duration and frequency.[31] Much like the Fitbit manifesto, early self-help guides for men as well as public health efforts attempted to locate exercise in the pre-existing routines of middle-class life. For example, McKenzie describes one guide that recommends "getting an hour of exercise a day, which included stretching in bed after the alarm rang, using one's towel 'vigorously,' bending over 'all the way' to pick up one's socks, and performing isometric buttocks contractions while waiting for the elevator."[32] In 1963, YMCAs across the US, in partnership with Paul Dudley Wright and John F. Kennedy, created the "Measured Mile" program, which provided mile markers on the streets of cities, designed to encourage businessmen to use breaks in their workday to exercise.[33] Both of these efforts illustrate attempts to redefine existing spaces and activities through the framework of health and fitness. The "Measured Mile" program uses quantification as a means to transform a city street into a kind of gym, while the self-help recommendation encourages individuals to see basic movements and habits as forms of exercise. Today, Fitbit has ostensibly combined these ideas, using quantification to help individuals "see" every facet of their lives as a potential site and source of fitness.

While the above accounts offer sporadic examples of the use of quantification and everyday habits to guide early fitness adopters, it was only with the publications of *Jogging* and *Aerobics* in 1967 and 1968, respectively, that exercise programs became increasingly standardized and popularized in middle-class American culture. These two publications mark the rise of popular self-help works penned by professionals from the fitness and medical professions ("fitness crusaders") who used their expertise, scientific research, and health rhetoric to support their arguments and methods. Drawing on the authority of science and medicine, they offered explicit, quantitative guidance on how to execute fitness in pursuit of health. Both of these books received strong recommendations from public health officials and institutions and were celebrated for their use of scientific data and expertise to improve the health of Americans. Coauthored by University of Oregon track coach Bill Bowerman and cardiologist W. E. Harris, *Jogging* adapted the training methods of professional athletes for the masses, promising improvements to the health of the cardiac, respiratory, and circulation systems. Bowerman brought his experience in military training and coaching to Harris's scientific studies of heart health to fashion a system through which individuals could train their bodies and improve their health and fitness.[34] Born out of a series of small experiments Harris and Bowerman conducted on the health of joggers at a range of fitness and age levels, the book offered three different twelve-week training schedules for adults.[35] Unlike performance-based fitness training, their guide was designed to incorporate jogging and exercise in moderation over time, framing both physical fitness and health improvement as a product of sustainably incorporating exercise into one's day-to-day life. Situated within the cardiac crisis of the postwar period and the growing medical and public health interest in fitness, McKenzie argues that *Jogging* helped lay the foundation for the explosion of fitness culture in the 1970s. The book helped launch the "jogging craze" that would spread across middle-class America during the 1970s and 80s, and helped firmly establish "jogger" as a recognizable fitness identity.[36]

Since the 1970s, health has increasingly become something that is *performed* through the purchase of specific goods, the consumption of particular foods, and the execution of specific types of exercise.[37] *Jogging* provided one of the early models of the modern health-conscious identity and helped establish exercise as one of the key ways to pursue and perform "good health." By linking regular exercise to health benefits and encouraging individuals to incorporate jogging into their day-to-day lives, Bowerman and Harris helped support a model of fitness and health based on continuous maintenance and lifestyle: "Exercise should be part of a long-range health program. Regular exercise year in and year out is what counts."[38] Their training systems suggested that efforts and intensity should build over time, as individuals continually strive to improve their physical strength, and by extension, maintain and support good health. This ideology was simultaneously supported by the growing commercial fitness industry, which marketed exercise (and its products) as tools to support health and wellness. Shoes, clothes, and accessories all became additional ways to signal the jogger identity and perform health.[39]

Jogging offered a specific strategy for individuals to maintain and improve their health, but the publication of *Aerobics* helped expand this culture beyond jogging to encompass a range of exercise types, durations, training schedules, and fitness levels. Rather than focusing on a particular type of exercise, training schedule, or health benefit (e.g., weight loss), *Aer-*

obics offered a quantitative system that could be widely applied to a range of activities and adopted by varying levels of fitness capability. Selling over twelve million copies worldwide, the book's highly adaptable system promised a way to assess, measure, and improve fitness and therefore health, over time. Written by Dr. Kenneth Cooper, *Aerobics* measured fitness and health based on the rate of oxygen intake (now referred to as VO_2 max): "Forcing more oxygen through your body with aerobic exercises is what produces these [positive health] effects in your bodily systems, and the total amount of oxygen that your body can process becomes, in turn, a measurement of the health of these systems."[40] VO_2 max continues to serve as a way to assess aerobic fitness, and indeed many wearable fitness trackers provide metrics that allow individuals to track their aerobic capacity. But in 1968, without the technology for at-home vital measurement, Cooper provided a series of fitness tests with corresponding charts to indirectly translate distance and time into VO_2 max. *Aerobics* asks individuals to complete one of two "tests" to set the baseline fitness level: they can walk or run as far as they can in twelve minutes, track the distance, and use a corresponding chart to locate their level, or they can record the time it takes to walk or run 1.5 miles and likewise use a chart to assess oxygen intake levels.[41] Without any technology to automatically track distance, Cooper suggested driving the distance of the planned running course and reading the car's odometer to gauge the mileage. He in fact warns against the use of commercial pedometers: "none are sufficiently accurate."[42] The test results allowed individuals to take advantage of the book's point-based exercise training system. Charts provided conversions for exercise types and duration into points that are meant to reflect the aerobic exertion of each activity. Cooper set the "minimum level of fitness" at thirty points, providing both plans to build up to this baseline, as well as to exceed it in pursuit of better health and fitness.

The health benefits of fitness were located in what Cooper called the "training effect," or "the changes induced by exercise in the various systems and organs of the body."[43] VO_2 max functioned as the indicator of whether the effect was triggered, with the points reflecting "the amount of oxygen required to perform it."[44] The logic of the system is that more points mean greater energy expended, which results in a greater "training effect." Most of the book was composed of charts that translate exercise types and duration into points, and corresponding training schedules designed to increase weekly point levels to improve fitness. Each schedule was modified based on activity level: those with lower aerobic capacity are asked to accumulate fewer points than those with higher aerobic capacity. Ideally, over time, an individual worked through the training schedules, moving up to the next level on completion to improve their health or the "training effect."

By quantifying exercise through VO_2 max and creating a point-based system, Cooper was able to apply his system of measurement and training program to a wide variety of exercises, populations, and fitness levels. *Aerobics* provided charts for running and walking inside and on treadmills, and for racket sports, swimming, and cycling, each converting time and distance into oxygen consumption and points. Individuals had the freedom to select training programs based on a single exercise or to use the charts to set weekly point goals that can be satisfied through a variety of activities. Like *Jogging*, the system encouraged individuals to gradually incorporate exercise into their day-to-day lives over time. The weekly point goals and suggested frequency helped individuals moderate and build these habits to ideally establish fitness not as an isolated activity, but as a component of lifestyle.[45]

Cooper's point system also suggests that fitness can essentially be reduced to a physiological process—oxygen intake—that subsequently affects the functioning (health) of the body as a whole. This biomedical model of exercise that defines fitness based on vital signs and unseen biological processes is the foundation of scientific and medical research on exercise and health. *Aerobics*, and the second edition, *The New Aerobics*, published just two years later, brought this framework to the masses and offered individuals a way to assess, monitor, and improve their well-being like a scientist or medical researcher: "*Aerobics* puts the lab in your pocket."[46] Throughout both editions, Cooper cited research studies and stressed how his methods and training regimes were grounded in scientific methods. *New Aerobics* foregrounds this desire by repeatedly stating that his book attempts to make laboratory methods accessible to the general public: "The beauty of the system is that it allows you to choose your own form of exercise, secure in the knowledge if you do enough exercise—earn enough points—there is a scientific basis for measuring the medical benefits."[47]

While Cooper's biomedical system seemingly breaks down the boundaries between the lab and ordinary life, it likewise muddles the boundaries of fitness itself. Rather than understanding fitness as an isolated activity or sport, Cooper's biomedical system suggests that fitness is defined by physiological processes of exertion, intake, and intensity. Exercise, in these terms, is not a specific type of movement or category of action, but exertion placed on the body. Thus, any action that results in increasing oxygen intake is a potential act of fitness. While *Aerobics* never suggests that "pillow fights" or other everyday activities qualify as fitness, his quantitative system provides a framework that—like Fitbit's manifesto—suggests that fitness is "all the time."

Aerobics helped fortify quantification as a central way to communicate the relationship between fitness and health to the public. In 1978, the American College of Sports Medicine established the official recommendation of exercise three to five times per week to maintain good health.[48] While this number has since been revised and qualified based on developments in health and fitness research, public health and medical recommendations continue to frame health maintenance in terms of the amount and frequency of exercise. *Jogging* and *Aerobics* used quantification and goal-based systems to lay the numerical foundation for the incorporation of fitness into institutional and popular understandings of health—a system that would later be taken up and extended through fitness-tracking technologies.

Measure and Improve

In 1975, the Yellow Pages replaced "gymnasium" with "health club."[49] This marketing shift is emblematic of the emergence of contemporary fitness culture, as discourses of sport and communal spaces of exercise signified by "gymnasium" were replaced by the language of health and wealth. Over the course of the 1970s, the commercial fitness industry and public health campaigns would help solidify the conflation of health and fitness. Fitness companies stressed the importance of exercise (and their products) for maintaining health, and government efforts to reduce healthcare spending promoted exercise as an effective form of preventive health. With these industrial and economic considerations in mind, Jennifer Smith Maguire argues that the American fitness industry coevolved with health-promotion discourse to help shape the contemporary ideology of fitness that is closely aligned with neoliberal values, which stress individual self-management, control, and improvement. In the introduction to the 1979 Surgeon General's Report, "Healthy People," Jimmy Carter argued that a focus on prevention (through activities like exercise), can "substantially reduce both the suffering of our people and the burden on our expensive system of medical care."[50] Insurance companies and businesses alike promoted fitness as a way for individuals to care for their health, but also to drive down their healthcare costs. The 1970s also saw the rise of workplace wellness programs and the expansion of benefits to support gym memberships and fitness efforts.[51] All of these programs and public health campaigns reinforce fitness as a form of health maintenance, an ideology of health that has since become the dominant paradigm in the US and beyond.

While the quantitative recommendations that emerged in the 1970s supposedly offered stable guidelines to maintain health, contemporary understandings of fitness and preventative health are rarely figured in terms of static weekly or daily goals. As in *Jogging* and *Aerobics*, fitness is often framed as a continuous effort where individuals are encouraged to work to perpetually increase their capabilities and decrease the risk of future illness. In other words, improving one's fitness will improve one's health. But as many scholars have pointed out, "fitness [and therefore health] can never be reached, and fitness does not stay."[52] This conception is apparent in the never-ending supply of new fitness products, trends, diets, and technologies that supposedly allow individuals to pursue the ever-retreating ideal of fitness.

With the rise of datafication, the ways in which individuals can monitor their bodies and behaviors in pursuit of health and fitness have expanded and consequently reshaped the way health is assessed and monitored. Datafication and data mining have created new forms of commodification, as the data created by individuals is used to sell more fitness products. Fitness can now be performed not only through the purchase of specific goods, but through the continuous "prosumption" that individuals engage in via the data surveillant structures of the device.[53] Beyond these novel forms of commodification, quantification has also created new ways to reinforce and promote the values of improvement, perfectionism, and self-work.[54] Fitness culture of the 1970s, '80s, and '90s often invoked the rhetoric of improvement and perfection through a focus on appearances: individuals were encouraged to monitor the shape of the body, muscle tone, and other aesthetic traits of the "fit" and "healthy" body.[55] Today, fitness and health remain closely tied to physical appearance, but the rise of datafication technologies has expanded how individuals can now track, monitor, and improve their well-being. *Aerobics* provided an early example of how fitness metrics could be tracked and improved on in pursuit of health, but today's apps and wearables surpass this initial qualification system, collecting metrics on seemingly endless data points and amassing incomprehensible archives of information. A run is no longer simply measured by distance, duration, or even VO_2 max, but also by heart rate, cadence, elevation changes, temperature, and pace. Each activity is broken down into increasingly specific types of data, offering novel places to improve and perfect in pursuit of fitness.

The expanded use of quantification is why many scholars have argued that fitness-tracking technology expands the self-surveillant practices associated with neoliberalism.[56] Datafication creates new sites and ways for individuals to monitor their lives and shift their habits according to the structures of the technology. The most basic example is the 10,000-step daily goal set by many fitness apps and wearables. Without an Apple Watch, Fitbit, or another pedometer, this metric remains inaccessible to human perception. In revealing this data, fitness trackers appear to offer individuals an automated way to strive toward quantifiable measures of health and fitness while simultaneously suggesting that steps can and should be monitored every day. Through my Apple Watch "Activity" app, I can monitor my daily step count, while the iPhone "Health" app will help me track my numbers over time. The inclusion of steps within the fitness and health tracking features of the watch and phone suggests that steps are yet another facet of my life that requires continuous attention if I want to maintain "health." The step surveillance by my watch and other fitness trackers is ultimately used to encourage individuals to meet quantified health norms, thus standardizing and extending the power of the "medical gaze." Drawing on the work of Michel Foucault, many scholars argue that fitness tracking (and digital health, more generally) makes the "medical gaze virtual," breaking down the boundaries between the clinic and everyday life. For example, my Apple Watch's step count creates the technological conditions for self-monitoring, encouraging me to govern my actions and health pursuits according to a statistical norm.[57]

By quantifying daily activities and setting numerical goals, fitness-tracking technologies suggest that fitness, and by extension health, can and should be monitored every day. Fitness-tracking technologies often set default daily goals for distance, calories, or time spent active. Individuals can adjust their numbers, but the baseline metrics provide a basic framework for how they are meant to understand and pursue health and fitness. For example, the Fitbit app's homepage displays metrics including how many calories are burned, exercise minutes, weight, and water and food logs (Fig. 12). Individuals can also choose to include additional health data, such as heart rate and weight, each of which has a new numerical goal. While all of this tracking information can be customized according to an individual's preferences and lifestyle, it collectively suggests that health and fitness can be maintained by meeting a collection of specific daily numerical goals. "Maintaining health" comes to be defined by whether an individual has burned enough calories, consumed the minimum amount of water,

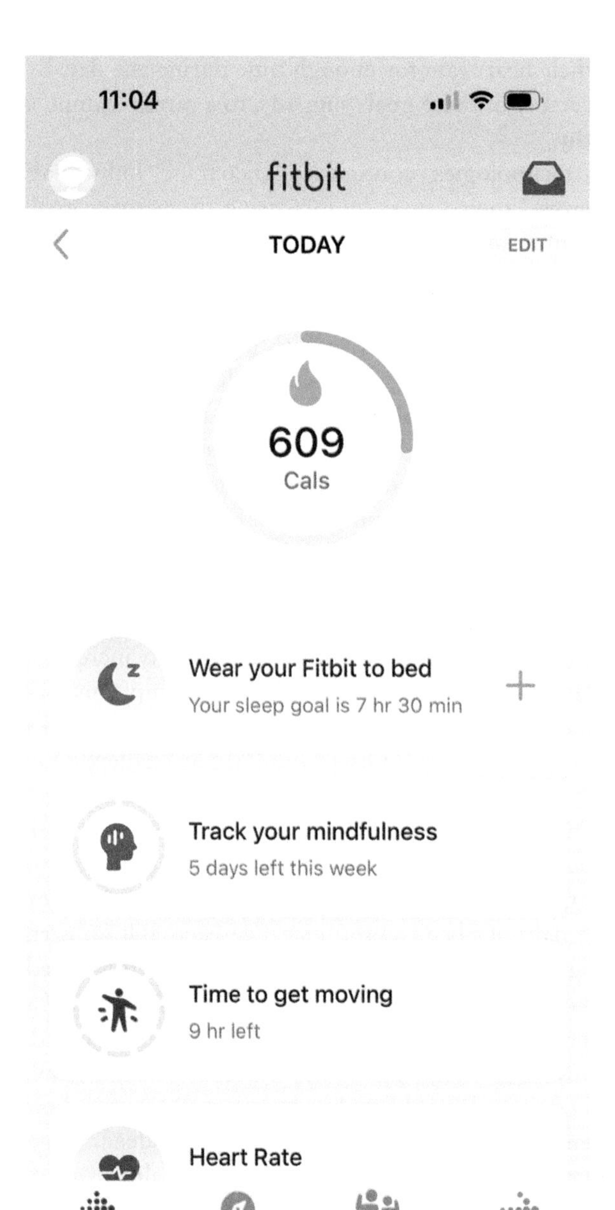

Fig. 12. Fitbit's default home screen offers a circular visualization of calories burned and additional self-reported data portals. (Fitbit, "Fitbit," vers. 3.44, accessed July 2021.)

and managed to raise their heart rate for enough time during the day. By extension, failing to meet any of these goals suggests, to a certain extent, a failure to be fit or healthy.

Additionally, most technologies continually encourage individuals to "progress" and "improve" their fitness by increasing the metrics week after week. Through gamification tactics, such as awards or competitions, fitness-tracking technologies promote health and fitness as an ever-receding, unattainable goal.[58] For example, every Monday morning, my Apple Watch sends me a "weekly summary," which provides an overview of my efforts from the previous week. A bar graph visualizes the number of calories I burned each day, and below the graph I can find statistics on the total steps walked, flights climbed, and hours I've spent active. The notification also includes the average number of calories I've burned per day and then prompts me to set a goal for the coming week. If I have consistently exceeded my daily goal, Apple will suggest a slightly higher number, pushing me to "improve" my health and fitness by burning more calories. This logic is further reinforced through the "awards" I can earn, which include personalized monthly challenges that encourage me to gradually increase a section of my activity data. The "February Challenge," for example, pushes me to spend 3,820 minutes exercising over the month, which breaks down to approximately 136 minutes per day.[59] Other months may challenge me to make my "stand goal" for a certain number of days a month, or to travel a minimum distance. The longer I've used Apple Watch, the harder these monthly goals have become. Due to the magnitude of these numerical goals—I have neither the time nor the physical strength to exercise for more than two hours a day—it's been years since I've been able to earn an activity award through the platform. In addition to these personalized awards, Apple Watch includes badges for "Move Goal 200%" and "300% and 400%," each respectively reflecting whether I've successfully doubled, tripled, or quadrupled my daily calorie goal. Depending on one's baseline, striving to get any of these awards could push someone well beyond their physical limits and even prove dangerous to one's health. Indeed, some doctors and health practitioners have even warned of the health dangers associated with these quantified goals.[60] This illustrates how the ideology of health and fitness-as-improvement often simply stresses accumulation and increase without considering any social or physical restrictions and conditions that may prohibit an individual from pursuing or accomplishing these goals.

This ideology is powerfully communicated through the emphasis on numbers and "raw" data. While critical data studies has repeatedly shown how datafication and quantification are often shaped by the biases of the humans who create the computational algorithms,[61] and studies have questioned the accuracy of commercial fitness-tracking technologies,[62] the numbers, graphics, and statistics feel, to some degree, objective. When I look at my step count, heart rate, or exercise minutes I don't think about the underlying computational systems that have interpreted and processed my behaviors, or potential prejudices underlying the health metrics. Rather, the numbers and graphics I encounter on my watch and smartphone carry a strong epistemological charge—they feel, to some degree, like an authoritative representation of my everyday behaviors. Even as a scholar who is critical of digital health technologies, aware of the problems regarding the accuracy of the technology, resistant to the absurdly high goals it may encourage me to meet, and conscious of the inherent biases underlying the measures of "health and fitness," I cannot help but feel an impression of scientific authority when I look at the numerical interpretation of behavior and activity.

This feeling is indebted not only to the authoritative role of numbers in modern scientific practice, but also to the way these technologies combine the quantification and statistical analysis of big data with the rhetoric of health and fitness. Scholars in critical data studies have argued that big data is not merely a methodology, but a "cultural, technological, and scholarly phenomenon" that operates through the interplay of emerging technologies and algorithmic accuracy to support the "widespread belief that large data sets offer a higher form of intelligence and knowledge that can generate insights that were previously impossible, with the aura of truth, objectivity, and accuracy."[63] In other words, big data support an emerging scientific paradigm in which objectivity is communicated through the combination of technologies capable of quantifying and collecting massive data sets and through the scale of the information archives accumulated via these algorithms.

The big data paradigm marks a shift away from mimetic or indexical understandings of objectivity, in favor of locating authority in the algorithms, computational processes, and analytical protocol that produce and process the data. For example, the steps counted by my Apple Watch are not judged by their indexical relationship to the actual steps I've taken. Rather, their accuracy is determined by the underlying algorithms and hardware that approximate my bodily movements—whether the device's gyroscope is sufficiently sensitive to shifts in displacement and whether the algorithm processing that displacement can accurately translate the minute shifts in space. Historian Orit Halpern argues that this new version of objectivity—what she calls "communicative objectivity"—has emerged with the rise of cybernetics in the second half of the twentieth century, as scientific interests shifted away from "external reality" in favor of increased attention to "purpose" or the revelatory possibilities of processes.[64] In this period, scientists became less concerned with understanding the "essence" of an object or a priori reality, and more concerned with refining the processes of recording, storage, and transmission. Correspondingly, objectivity became associated with the accuracy of the ways information is processed and analyzed.[65] "Communicative objectivity" describes the present epoch, where machines, algorithms, and technologies have become the authorities—the experts—capable of interpreting evidence and information.[66]

Today, "communicative objectivity" is often signified by data visualization, which attempts to transform massive archives of data into legible figures and statistics.[67] Fitness-tracking technologies combine these visualized forms of "communicative objectivity" with the rhetoric of health and fitness to compel individuals to conform to the platform's numerical standards or increase their numbers over time. Because the big data paradigm relies on huge data sets that are impossible for humans to process or analyze, "communicative objectivity" is largely signified through data visualization, statistics, and other numerical outputs. In the case of fitness trackers, wearables and apps generate and produce data about activities and the body at a scale incomprehensible to human perception, forcing individuals to become entirely reliant on the interfaces to translate their behaviors into seemingly legible and objective reflections of their health and fitness. As such, the perception of the fitness tracker's authority cannot be reduced to a naive faith in the algorithms and technology, or even through an understanding of the mechanics of the device. Individuals rely on *aesthetic* modes of communication to derive any information or knowledge from these data sets. The big data presented by these technologies are "both statistical and visual": objectivity is supported and communicated via the diagrams, graphs, and statistics provided by the device or platform.[68]

Fitness-tracking technologies use a common set of aesthetic strategies to signify this authority or "communicative objectivity." Simple graphs and statistics are surrounded by negative space, which places focus on comparing data sets or tracking averages.[69] The data are often presented through visual and numerical comparisons: stats comparing steps to the daily goal of 10,000, or average calories mapped across days of the week. The most

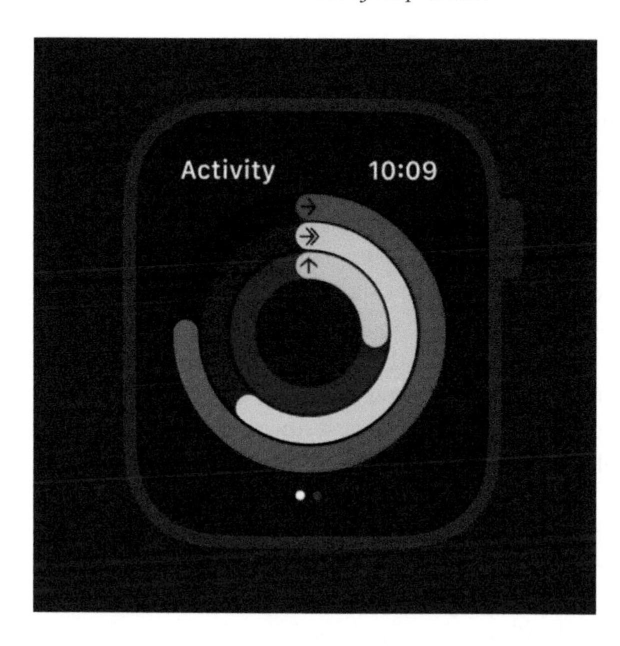

Fig. 13. The three-ring visualization of Apple Watch's "Activity" app. ("Close Your Rings," Apple, accessed February 2023, https://www.apple.com/watch/close-your-rings/.)

common visualizations track progress through circle and bar graphs that either fill in or gain height as the individual works toward their daily goal. Apple Watch uses three concentric rings to visualize the central goals for the day: "move goal," "exercise goal," and "stand goal." As individuals move through the day, the color-coded rings gradually fill in as they stand for an hour, complete thirty minutes of exercise, and burn calories. The simplistic graphics and the layout of the interface are designed to allow individuals to immediately assess their progress toward these goals; with a glance, they can tell if they've moved "enough" to "close" the rings (Fig. 13). If they scroll down, they get additional information, including specific statistics and tiny bar graphs that show activity levels for the day. But ultimately the "rings" provide the most immediate translation of the data, framing their behaviors by completing the circular visualization.

The epistemological power of Apple's visualization is tied to design paradigms in data visualization that link aesthetics and scientific authority. Nearly all fitness-tracking interfaces borrow from the "good design principles" of statistician Edward Tufte, whose theories of data visualization have been adopted by scholars and graphic designers alike. For Tufte, data is inherently truthful, and it is up to the visualization to communicate or reveal this truth through economical and minimalist design strategies.[70]

Minimalist design is not only rhetorically powerful, it communicates logical and clear reasoning. As he describes the issue in terms of negative: "a lack of visual clarity in arranging evidence is a sign of a lack of intellectual clarity in the reasoning of evidence."[71] In other words, there is a direct correlation between the aesthetics of the visualization and the objectivity of the data or analysis itself: "clear and precise seeing becomes one with clear and precise thinking."[72] For Tufte, the "clarity, precision, and efficiency" of ideas are communicated aesthetically through particular representational strategies, and conversely, the presence of these strategies is taken to indicate the clarity of the thought behind them. Recent sociological studies on data visualization have shown a strong correlation between the perception of scientific authority and particular aesthetic strategies, such as two-dimensional graphics, clean layouts, geometric shapes and lines, and labeled data sources.[73] This research and the ideology of design found in Tufte's work attest to how aesthetics convey "communicative objectivity," or to the way particular representational strategies help signify the accuracy and authority of the underlying computational processes, algorithms, and analysis provided by datafication technologies.

Tufte's aesthetic logic is found across fitness-tracking technologies: from Apple's ring interface to the Fitbit app home screen, the simplistic, bold, minimalist design is meant to directly reflect the accuracy and authority of the data it presents. This visual rhetoric is precisely what informs my perception of my behaviors, and by extension, my health. When I open the app on my watch, faint outlines of the circles fill in with red, blue, and green. With a glance, I can immediately compare my activities to the parameters of the technology: my move ring is nearly complete, but I need to stand more today or I won't be able to complete the blue circle. There are no numbers or labels: all of this is conveyed through a simple circular graphic. One might say that Apple Watch's interface "brings absolute attention to the data," creating a strong sense that the visualization is a direct and authoritative representation of my habits, body, or health. Indeed, the ability to immediately assess the data has a powerful effect on my perception of my day and creates the imperative to meet the standards set by the device.[74] The combination of quantification and visualization works hand in hand to suggest that the device reflects my health, while simultaneously suggesting that my health depends on conforming to the measures—biostatistical norms—set by the technology.

The aesthetics of fitness-tracking interfaces directly supports and masks the ideology of improvement promoted by the device. Beyond merely increasing numbers or earning awards, the ring visualization helps inscribe the logic of improvement into everyday habits and behaviors. While my Apple Watch may suggest increasing the number of calories I burn every week, the ring visualization and the task of closing the circles do not change. Rather, filling in my rings just becomes slightly more difficult—I need to walk a bit more, run a bit longer, or push a bit harder during my workout. Trained to glance at my rings to assess my progress, or nudged to meet my daily goals through ephemeral push notifications, I don't consciously aspire to meet a new, bigger number. Instead, I work toward the standard daily goal communicated visually by closing the rings. I may be a bit more tired, or occasionally notice that I need to move just a bit more (Apple will send me a reminder in the evening if this is the case), but the increase in calories burned is relatively small and doesn't necessarily require a dramatic shift in activities or habits.[75] Over time, I may double or triple my daily numerical goals, but caught up in the daily task of filling in rings and moving through the suggested weekly increases, I'm likely to ignore any big-picture trends or achievements.[76]

As a result, neoliberal frameworks for health that stress improvement and accumulation are slowly inscribed into daily habits, behaviors, and activities. The emphasis on small-scale goals and minor increases in data helps support the idea that health and fitness are not states of the body—you cannot "achieve" either—but are instead ever-receding goals that require continuous maintenance. However, fitness-tracking technologies help obscure this idea by focusing on daily tasks and challenges that encourage individuals to improve week after week. For this reason, countless scholars have drawn on theories of governmentality to describe how fitness-tracking technologies frame the body and health to condition ideal neoliberal subjects. The combination of quantification and visualization encourages individuals to slowly shift their habits according to the biomedical structures of the device.[77] Because individuals have control over certain daily goals and must actively work to accumulate higher numbers and more data, this change appears voluntary. As a result, "health" becomes understood as the choice to continually strive toward unending accumulation.[78]

Critiques that draw on theories of governmentality assume that individuals will conform to the structures of the device, thus conditioning them into neoliberal subjects caught up in practices of improvement and accumulation. The combination of quantification and the imperative to fill in a ring, increase the calories burned week after week, or earn an award is enough to fundamentally change an individual's understanding of their health and habits. But the reality is that few manage to become the perfect fitness-tracking subject. Numerous studies have shown that these devices have poor rates of retention as individuals lose interest or grow frustrated with the device,[79] and a wide array of reviews, videos, and blog posts have analyzed the accuracy of the technology or explored ways to hack or game the systems.[80] Indeed, if I pause to consider what underlies the interface, I realize the rings are not an accurate representation of my health, and I don't *have to* close them every day to be a "better," healthier person. While I might feel an initial push to close a ring—feel the epistemological charge of the visualization—I remain conscious of the platform's downfalls. A persistent skepticism surrounds fitness-tracking technologies, and people are aware of their shortcomings. At the same time, the insistence on debating accuracy and objectivity suggests that fitness-tracking technologies do have some authority in society. The information they offer about fitness and health does hold some epistemological power, and as such, individuals—myself included—may continue to use them to explore what kinds of experiences or information they may be able to offer, despite the doubt, hesitancy, and ambivalence.

Feeling Fit?

Tufte's design principles begin to explain how, at a glance, many of these devices can signify authority and encourage individuals to meet quantified fitness goals. However, the use of persuasive aesthetics does not guarantee that individuals will believe that the graphics or statistics are objective facts about their health. Visualizations are powerful not simply because they propose to offer "objective" information, but because they make "it possible to *feel* numbers, metrics, data, and statistics to make sense of the figures in a way that is emotional and affective, not just cognitive and rational."[81] When I look at the unfinished rings on my Apple Watch screen, I have physiological and psychological reactions. I feel the need to complete the circles: my body may tense in anticipation of moving to meet that goal or relax at the realization that I can remain at rest. Moreover, the phenomenological effects of my Apple Watch cannot be reduced to the screen itself: the haptic feedback structures of the device help extend the impact of the visualization to my movements and bodily sensations.

Therefore, to fully understand how these technologies function in individuals' day-to-day lives and shape their perception of health, the embodied experiences of fitness-tracking technologies must be brought into conversation with the aesthetic structures of the devices and platforms. Fitness-tracking technologies reinforce quantified fitness goals through feedback, including push notifications, vibrations, and visual rewards for reaching goals. These mechanisms are designed to draw attention to the data visualizations in the app or on the screen of the wearable device, but they can simultaneously draw attention to the body itself: the point of contact between the device and wrist, the pace of a walk, or the position of the body. Analysis of the visualizations and quantified goals alone cannot account for how individuals interpret, understand, or use this data or the physical sensations and actions that may emerge through interactions with the technology.[82] For example, as I described in the introduction, my Apple Watch will send me a reminder to meet my daily goals each evening. The notification may tell me to go on a walk or attempt to stand up and walk around for the remaining hours of the day. Though my watch suggests I need to complete some task or activity, I rarely follow directions. Rather, I'm likely to reflect on how much longer I'll be wearing the watch and how I plan to fill that time. If I have plans to stand and make dinner, I'll probably settle myself further into the couch, muscles relaxing, confident that I will be able to meet that goal without conscious effort or additional exercise. This certainty comes from a phenomenological awareness I've developed over time. After seven years of experience with wearable fitness trackers, I have gained a sense of how my actions correspond to the numbers on the screen: I can roughly estimate the number of calories I may burn during sections of my day—such as when I make dinner—or sense that my move goal will be a bit further ahead on days when I have to lug my laundry up and down the stairs. This does not necessarily mean I understand these actions or my day solely in terms of numbers, but rather speaks to the way the feedback structures and metrics have become incorporated into my sense of my body and habits.

In their sociological analysis of self-tracking, Gina Neff and Dawn Nafus push back on the claim that self-tracking leads to blind, neoliberal subjugation, arguing that individuals "interact with algorithms not as blind, mindless dupes, but as active participants in a dialogue that moves between data as an externalizing of self and internal, subjective, qualitative understanding of what data means."[83] Sometimes, this may encourage a model of health associated with self-improvement, but at other times, it may produce experiences that lead to interpretations outside of the health and fitness framework the device provided. In other words, it's impossible to offer a generalizable assessment of how these technologies influence the perception of health and fitness, because individuals continue to use, interpret, and make meaning from their devices in a variety of ways and forms. While I may not conform to the suggestions provided by the device, others may immediately head out for a walk or feel mounting anxiety and a sense of dread as their watch reminds them that they must "move more"; some simply ignore the slight pulse to their wrist. All of these reactions illustrate how individuals use, understand, and interpret the aesthetic structures of fitness-tracking technologies and undermine any generalized interpretation of how these devices shape one's understanding of health and fitness.

Thus, rather than attempting to universalize the experience of fitness-tracking technologies, I end by showing how phenomenological description can be deployed as a method for analysis and critical self-reflection for both scholars and everyday users alike. Phenomenological descriptions of my own experiences using these devices, and accounts from former students, reveal the complex range of experiences and relationships to the body, technology, and data that these devices engender. At the same time, such descriptions highlight how this method can be used to encourage individuals who use these devices to perhaps critically reflect on how fitness-tracking technologies may be influencing their understanding of their body and health.

Between 2017 and 2020, I asked students in my courses on health and technology to provide phenomenological accounts of their experiences using Fitbit's Versa and Flex wearables and other free step-counting apps.[84] Their papers highlighted a range of positive and negative affects, bodily sensations, and ways of thinking about technology, their bodies, and fitness. By drawing on this body of work, I am not aiming to provide an empirical or sociological study of fitness-tracking technologies, since their descriptions are undoubtedly influenced by the critical health studies approach I use in my classes. Rather, I offer this assignment and excerpts of their writing to show how phenomenological description can be employed to reveal the variety of ways individuals use, interpret, and understand fitness-tracking technologies. With a focus on bodily sensations and small-scale interactions, a phenomenological account of fitness trackers allows scholars (and perhaps those who use the devices as well) to see both the influence of neoliberal instantiations of health and fitness, and the bodily experiences, sensations, and perceptions that resist, reinforce, or exist alongside forms of subjugation.

At the beginning of the class, students were either given a Fitbit to borrow for the duration of the assignment or asked to download a free step-counting app (or to use an existing app on their smartphone).[85] I provided a lecture on phenomenological description that highlighted the method's focus on a highly located, subjective point of view, through attention to bodily sensations, movements, and perceptions that are commonly overlooked. For their written descriptions, I encouraged students to focus on how to communicate bodily sensations to a reader through careful, creative language. In doing so, they had to both confront their embodied experiences and consider how to translate them to an unfamiliar reader. Their work ranged from accounts of specific workouts, to their attachment to the device, to frustrations or eventual dismissal of the technology entirely. Health and fitness were not necessarily the focus of the reflection, but rather often appear implicitly in the way students discuss the imperative to work out, move "enough," or feel a sense of satisfaction about their day. Across nearly all accounts, there was a sense that the act of description itself resulted in critical reflection on how these technologies affect the perception of the body and health.

Student experiences were also highly influenced by their environment: one class completed their assignment in spring in Chicago, where they were able to take advantage of good weather; another class found themselves highly restricted by the snow of a Michigan winter; the final group had to navigate the restrictions of the COVID-19 lockdown. Despite this diversity, nearly all of the papers showed how the practice of description revealed the ways that self-tracking could reframe their sense of their surrounding environment and how they navigate their day-to-day lives. For example, students described how the metrics transformed how they understand distance or a mundane chore:

> The distance from my apartment to the coffee shop or to class stopped being measured in how many songs I could listen to on the way, but in vague step counts. I would gain two or three thousand steps in the morning walking to class, and an additional two to three thousand walking back in the evening. . . . distances took on new meaning. (Student paper, Chicago, 2017)

> I realized all the steps I took at work with my arms straightened, while vacuuming, running a carpet extracting machine, or other such work was not being counted as steps. I would try to adjust my movements so that my arm was swinging. I ultimately couldn't do

> this while doing certain tasks like carpet extracting, or shoveling when I had gloves on, and I felt like this exorcize [*sic*] didn't count because my step count didn't reflect the work. (Student paper, East Lansing, 2019)

These descriptions highlight how quantification caused students to rethink their relationship to space and actions that were once performed unconsciously, to see their behaviors through the numerical structures of the device. Indeed, this quantified perspective often caused students to make decisions based on the number of steps they may accumulate or "lose." For example, their step count would inform the choice between walking or taking a bus.

At the same time, environmental conditions led other students to question the metrics. Students expressed the difficulty of choosing between a convenient bus ride and the long, cold, snow-covered walk to campus, or the challenge of going for a walk or a run in a neighborhood without sidewalks. Students completing the assignment during COVID-19 found themselves at odds with both the constraints of lockdown and the additional responsibilities of taking courses at home and supporting their families:

> [Fitbit] did make me a bit more insecure on [*sic*] how active I am on a daily basis, but I am doing everything I can to make sure my family and I are safe [during the COVID-19 lockdown]. (Student paper, Los Angeles, 2020)

In describing their experiences of the technology, students encountered the ways that data can change, challenge, and conflict with the environment, illustrating Sarah Pink and Viake Fors's claim that self-tracking produces "data in the environment—with the body" rather than simply producing data "about the body."[86] While datafication may aim to reduce all forms of activity to numbers and extract fitness from social and environmental conditions, the act of quantification itself may draw attention to the way bodies must navigate social and physical spaces in pursuit of "health."

Because phenomenological description emphasizes the locatedness of bodies in the world, many students focused on the relationship between technology and their daily routines. Descriptions often emphasized how fitness-tracking technologies failed to fit in with existing patterns of behavior. Rather than blaming themselves or immediately conforming to the structures of the device, in their papers they emphasized the downfalls and shortcomings of the technology and the quantified measures of fitness and health. Across almost all accounts, students doubted the accuracy and legitimacy of the information. Several questioned whether they should simply shake their phones to increase their step count or fashion some device to game the system. They quickly realized that the device didn't necessarily count every step, or they discovered gaps in their heart rate data that left them questioning how many calories they'd burned for the day. Moments of friction or the discovery of technological deficiency left some disillusioned, and their descriptions addressed the dismay, apathy, and frustration—"[f]umbling with the band, I threw the device on my bed and walked away"[87]—, but most were much more invested in what the device *could* tell them about their habits and behaviors: "At one moment I thought, 'What would happen if I just shook my phone in the air to get more steps?' But that would utterly defeat the purpose of documenting how much I have walked."[88] Like the student above, who learned to swing their arm to log their movements, many descriptions revealed how students adjusted their movements or bodies to work with the technology:

> I realized the Fitbit wasn't counting my steps like I thought it would be able to and any steps I took with the Fitbit in my pocket did not count. I started paying more attention to what was counted and what wasn't. (Student paper, East Lansing, 2019)

> I was extremely conscious of my phone's presence shaking in my jacket pocket, to the point that I was worried they were shaking in the wrong way, and not accurately documenting my every step. (Student paper, Chicago, 2017)

> The weight of the phone in my pocket became reassuring. . . . I became used to having the heavy weight of it grounding me, telling me that I needed to do something. It reminded me to skip taking the bus home and walking instead. (Student paper, Chicago, 2017)

Thus, for some, phenomenological description revealed the subtle shifts in how they sensed their bodies in relation to the technology. Their accounts highlighted how ordinary frictions between the position of a device or the weight of their phone could cause them to adjust their patterns of movement or feel for the way an object moves with the body through space. These descriptions show how technological limitations or deficiencies can create novel forms of attunement to ordinary movements, habits, and behaviors.

In describing these limitations, students discovered how previously passive activities such as sleeping and walking were suddenly felt to be significant once they were registered—quantified—by the technology's feedback structures and visualizations. They described the deep satisfaction they felt as a cause-effect structure was created by the device's tracking and feedback systems:

> As I undergo a routine motion of raising one foot, returning it to the floor, and repeating, the statistics alter. The alignment of the numerical values with the motions of my physical movement creates a feeling of satisfaction. (Student paper, East Lansing, 2019)

> I became aware of each step in the care that I placed in making sure I pressed my foot firmly onto the ground, so carefully and measured so as to create vibrations at the heart of the foot that would echo through the muscles of my legs and, as a confirmation signal, impact the phone in my pocket as it bounces out from my leg and slaps against it again in rhythmic motion. (Student paper, Chicago, 2017)

Phenomenological description provided a way for students to express how the technology changed their perception of their actions: at the same time that steps became meaningful through quantification, stepping itself became sensible. Both of the above accounts articulate how quantification "transforms the taken-for-grantedness of movement by constantly calling attention to actions. . . . It asks us to feel not only the technology on our bodies but also the pace and weight of our own steps."[89]

Students tied novel attunement to the body to the visual and haptic feedback structures: the push notifications, data visualizations, and dynamic statistics. Through the act of description, they found these structures both mentally and physically satisfying as their actions, datafication, and feedback aligned:

> These vibrations are strong enough that they seem to travel up my lower arm, tickling each nerve as it travels up. This is sometimes amplified when I wear my jacket. The sleeve of my jacket covers the device completely, keeping me unaware of my progress. (Student paper, East Lansing 2019)

> The flashing of lights [when I reach 10,000 steps] gives me a sense of pride and satisfaction because I can see a representation of my

> progress being acknowledged and celebrated. (Student paper, East Lansing, 2019)

In trying to describe the moment of meeting 10,000 steps or meeting a daily goal, these two students discovered how the metric structures of the devices were felt through the combination of visual and haptic feedback. The flashing lights on the screen or the buzz of the device against their wrist created the physical and mental feeling of acknowledgment. While for some, this registered as satisfaction, others used description to explore the small frustrations or physical disruptions the device created as it snagged on their clothing or hindered a previously fluid motion:

> Every time I put a shirt with long sleeves on, or when I would wear a hoodie under my coat, and when I wore gloves. When I put my gloves on I could not figure out why one arm felt much more comfortable than the other until I realized it was because of the Fitbit. (Student paper, East Lansing 2019)

> It was intrusive to the point where I would consciously change the way I moved my arms and hands. Every time I reached for a door handle, or any moment when my sleeve rolled back onto my arm and bared that sleek, black, coiling leech around my wrist, I would jerk it back and have to remind myself of its presence. (Student paper, Los Angeles, 2020)

By and large, phenomenological description showed that bodily sensations were never replaced by data. Instead, combined with the reflective act of description, quantification and visual and haptic feedback continually encouraged modes of self-reflexivity. As Deborah Lupton notes, self-tracking can "challenge the non-reflexive, absent body [typically associated with medicine]. The body is hardly able to disappear when its functions, movements, and habits are constantly monitored and the user of digital technologies is continually made aware, via feedback of these depositions."[90] Indeed, bodily attunement often went hand in hand with the sense of validation provided by the technologies. Their descriptions located the feelings of acknowledgment or validation in the combination of quantification that drew attention to the body, and the visualizations and feedback structures revealed by the device or platform. Seeing and feeling their efforts visualized created the sense that their actions mattered or counted toward "something." For some, that "something" was better health or fitness, while others were simply interested in the novelty of seeing their actions quantified. The meaning of their numbers, goals, and bodily experiences seemed to vary widely, from a wholehearted belief in "exercise as medicine" ("[Fitbit] grants me the opportunity to witness incremental personal growth, something that is both very helpful to my self-image and also highly motivating to keep going."), to highly skeptical ("There is something distinctly dystopian and ironic about thinking I've been bitten by an insect only to find that my *health device* is the source of my very slight pain.").[91]

Regardless of students' belief in biomedical definitions of health and fitness that support neoliberal values, the practice of phenomenological description revealed the implicit impact of fitness tracking on their perception of their habits, health, and fitness. For many, describing their bodily experiences illustrated that surveillance and continuous attention to their body and actions created anxiety or resulted in a sense of "failure" when they did not meet the standards set by the device:

> The act of observing myself through a phenomenological lens revealed to me just how much I had normalized the use of the Fitbit that I would have found alarming in anybody else. Through this normalization I allowed the device to affect me deeply. The level to which I allowed my mental state to be determined by the Fitbit was very disturbing and I didn't know how to react to the news that I could be controlled by something so simple. (Student paper, Los Angeles, 2020)

> The Fitbit was meant to help me be a better version of myself, but I felt like a failure for not raising my heart rate enough to meet the app's definition of working out. It made me question if I was actually active or if I should work harder. (Student paper, Los Angeles, 2020)

> Every decision to eschew physical activity—be it taking the bus, skipping a workout, or taking an elevator—evokes a definite feeling of guilt or doubt, as though I can feel the Fitbit grow heavier on my wrist while I am motionless. I am never unaware of the Fitbit's presence on my wrist, but it is never harder to ignore than when I am choosing not to walk. (Student paper, Chicago, 2017)

As students detailed their struggles, description allowed them to critically reflect on how the feeling of being surveilled and the imperative to accumulate and improve at all costs had negative effects on their emotional well-being. In the context of my course, many students were able to tie these experiences to shifting definitions of health, connecting their feelings of "guilt" and "failure" to the rhetoric of personal responsibility and accumulation that often surrounds these devices. The reflective practice of description helped students realize that they began to judge their behaviors and selves based on the numerical and technological structures of the device. Many found the metrics to be a source of surveillant pressure—"an overprotective, helicopter parent"—that had the power to judge the success or failure of their day.

Some students suggested that the negative affects and experiences reinforced the desire to use the technology: in failing to meet the standards of the device, individuals feel bad about their behaviors, and in turn feel compelled to use the device to improve and feel better about their health and fitness. But through reflective description, many students discovered a much more ambivalent relationship to the technology as the feedback structures and goals faded into the background. In detailing how the feedback structures felt, they found that the vibrations and push notifications were just another small interruption like the arrival of a text message or email:

> I am sometimes not consciously aware that I am wearing the device so the sensation [of the vibration] can come as a surprise. The device itself has become an extension of my body. (Student paper, East Lansing, 2019)

> After so many months of wearing it, I now take its work for granted. In fact, I rely on my Fit Bit [*sic*] to remind me not to work for too long and to go outside. (Student paper, Los Angeles, 2020)

> [The] gentle reminders from the Fitbit were as omnipresent as the accessory itself, which I'd grown strangely attached to. For some reason, I particularly enjoyed one feature: raising the Fitbit to my face, and watching as that exact motion caused the time display to light up. Of course, if I checked the time, I couldn't help but also tap to check my step count, regardless of whether I'd even moved in the

> meantime. Combined with the hourly reminders . . . the Fitbit Alta buzzes 10 minutes before the hour when you haven't reached 250 steps in that hour I felt the same disappointment countless times each day. (Student paper, Chicago, 2017)

The above accounts highlight how the mundane interruptions of the device faded into the array of technological signals that make up day-to-day life. But they also highlight how the ordinary feedback structures of push notifications can take on new meaning over time: a signal to take a break or an indicator of time.

By locating the source of these meanings within aesthetic structures, their descriptions also revealed the small ways students pushed back on the quantified imperatives imposed by the device. The three students describe bodily responses to the vibrations, but they did not necessarily conform to the actions suggested by technology. Instead, their phenomenological accounts helped them see how the feedback issued by the device was reinterpreted and decoded according to the flows of their day. The third account details how the vibration structure produced new habits, but rather than encouraging movement or exercise, the notification patterns simply created habitual encounters with the device itself. Through the act of describing, they found that despite repeatedly failing to meet the quantified goals, which resulted in feelings of disappointment, they'd grown attached to the device. The attachment was tied to how the notifications operated as a way to organize time as they learned the cycles of the push notifications, and also gave them a small reminder of their bodily state, which was almost always at rest. While the reminders produced anxiety about their behaviors, they did not result in any behavioral shifts beyond the inclination to check the device. The device simply provided a reminder of the bodily state and provided a small, satisfying physical interaction with the screen.

Indeed, as someone who has used fitness trackers for several years, phenomenological description has served as a way for me to reflect on how the vibration features have become incorporated into my daily habits and movements. Over time, the notifications and reminders have become less and less significant. I no longer need to interact with the screen to decode the vibration patterns: two short pulses after a workout tell me I've met my exercise goal for the day, and the single pulse at around 10 a.m. provides a brief assessment of my progress so far. If I lift my wrist and tilt the screen toward my gaze, a notification pops up on the screen providing an overview of my metrics and either encouraging me to move more or validating my work so far: "you're off to a great start." Toward the end of the day, a pronounced pulse of my wrist may inform me that I've met all three goals for the day. Tilting the screen will trigger a series of continuous vibrations, and three rings of fireworks appear on the screen. While that animation was undoubtedly satisfying at first, today I rarely indulge in the daily firework show. Over time, these reminders and rewards have faded into haptic signs that can be read without the help of my screen: I can now intuit or gauge my progress without them.

At the same time, even after years of using the technology and the persistent awareness of its dangers and downfalls, the absence of these vibrations can still produce anxiety. Through prolonged use of my Apple Watch, I have attached the feedback to a sense of satisfaction with my day. The notifications often function as haptic sources of accomplishment: another checkmark on the list of items to complete. But attempting to meet these goals doesn't alienate me from my body, nor do I simply conform to the structures of the technology. Those pulses draw attention to the relationship between my embodied state and the technology. I feel for that validation as I go about my day: my attention is drawn to my wrist and the feeling of the device against my skin. Without the feedback from the device, I'm abundantly aware of my bodily state: the pinch in my shoulder and stiffness in my lower back that has emerged while I sit for hours in front of my computer. The absence of the haptic feedback can draw attention to the tightness in my joints and tension in my body, as I begin to fidget in anticipation of getting through my work, out of the chair, and moving again. While when I stand, I may attempt to meet my daily "move goal" with a walk or yoga class, these actions are not mindless attempts to discipline my body: they attune me to the fact that I have a body and am a body moving through the world.

Across the short-term accounts provided by my students and my long-term experiences with Apple Watch, description reveals the range of positive and negative affects and the possibility for novel forms of bodily attunement. The act of close, careful description functioned as a critical way for students to reflect on their relationship to technology and simultaneously revealed the way they consciously or unconsciously conformed to or resisted neoliberal instantiations of health and fitness. For some, the description offered a way to link their anxieties and bodily sensations to the imperatives of self-improvement and responsibility, while others focused on novel attunements to the body. What emerges from this collection of experiences is not a portrait of neoliberal subjects, but a complicated, often contradictory account of how datafication technologies can affect what health and fitness mean.

All of the descriptions provided in this chapter are influenced and shaped by my courses on health and technology, but regardless, the act of description itself functioned as a means of self-reflection that can be applied to work beyond the scope of the classroom or this book. Description functioned as an essential way for students to step back and examine their relationship to data, technology, health, and fitness. It revealed a range of experiences, from the feelings of data surveillance and the pressures of quantified health to the sensation of stepping or the body at rest. Whether conscious or not, the practice of phenomenological description helped draw out the embodied experiences that attest to how neoliberal instantiations of health and fitness are navigated and how these imperatives can impact (or fail to impact) individual habits and the perception of the self.

Importantly, phenomenological description locates these structures and imperatives in specific encounters, feedback structures, and design elements. As a practice that focuses on the relationship between bodies and the world, phenomenological description pinpoints how specific features or interactions give rise to bodily sensations and affects. In other words, it identifies moments when technology triggers or provokes a bodily reaction. As such, it could be used more systematically to answer questions about specific aesthetic features. Researchers may use it to ask, "What kinds of reactions—physical and psychological—do hourly reminders provoke?" "How do vibrations impact an individual's day-to-day routine, relationship to the body, or technology?" "What kinds of sensations or affects do data visualizations and statistics create?" Coupled with aesthetic analysis from film and media studies, it's possible to identify how these bodily reactions may be tied to design choices or feedback features that borrow from biomedical frameworks for health and fitness and reinforce neoliberal values such as improvement and optimization.

Combining aesthetic analysis and phenomenological description provides a way to examine how fitness-tracking technologies (and digital health more broadly) are shaping the communication and experience of health. With more and more scientific studies using wearable trackers, like Fitbit, to study disease, fitness, and health,[92] and insurance companies incentivizing individuals to sync their trackers with company websites, there is a need for both scholars and everyday users to critically reflect on how these technologies shape individual experiences.[93] The practice of description offers an accessible way for individuals and researchers to reflect on the impact of fitness-tracking devices and platforms and to identify possible places to resist understanding the body and health through the logic of optimization, improvement, and accumulation. For example, by prompting individuals to perform an embodied description through the app interface, platforms could promote a more critical mode of engagement with quantification. Likewise, researchers could incorporate more descriptive practices into studies to provide a more nuanced account of how quantification and self-tracking practices succeed and fail to reinforce self-improvement ideologies. The incorporation of fitness trackers into insurance policies and workplace wellness programs suggests they have already become firmly situated in health promotion associated with neoliberal economic policies. But the phenomenological accounts of fitness trackers throughout this chapter suggest it's not necessarily so simple: we appear to still be in a period of transition where individuals remain curious, hesitant, frustrated, and questioning regarding datafication and self-tracking. Now is the time to consider how specific aesthetic structures of feedback, design, and biomedical tracking systems affect one's understanding of the body and, ideally, to revise these technologies so they encourage critical reflection and bodily attunement, while still leaving space for individuals to interpret and understand their health beyond the structures promoted by the device. The work of revision can begin through attention to the aesthetic experiences, by identifying the impact of the design and feedback in a way that leaves space for the range of experiences and affects that emerge when bodies engage with digital health devices and platforms.

CHAPTER 4

Meditation and Breathing Technologies and the Biomedicalization of Wellness

I sit hunched over my laptop, head tilted slightly down, eyes fixed on the screen as my fingers press lightly against the keys. The subtle dip at the center of the square key helps me sense when I've met my target. As I press out an email response, I feel a tap-like vibration, as though someone were momentarily pressing their thumb twice against the Reminder. I shift in my top of my wrist. I recognize the vibration pattern as a text message and continue to type away. Lost in the growing list of emails, my attention shifts away from my watch and toward the relationship between my hands and the windows on the screen. My concentration is broken by a rapid series of vibrations, which come in pairs as though someone were impatiently tapping their finger against a surface. I stop my work, lift my hand, and tilt the screen toward my gaze: Medication Reminder. I look out over my computer at the allergy medication on the counter. After a pause, I decide to return to my email: I'll get up and take my medication in just a minute. Moments later, I feel a gentle press, which holds for a moment and retracts. I glance down to my wrist resting on the surface of my keyboard and tilt the screen as a graphic showing overlapping circles that form a flower-like shape appears with the text below: "Even a minute of breathing helps you think clearly."

In the span of a few minutes, my Apple Watch pushes notifications from across my life, reminding me to take my medication, attend to my mental well-being, and communicate with my friends. The success of the Apple Watch's release in 2015 prompted a major transition in the wearable market from primarily fitness-based technology, such as the original Fitbit devices or other pedometers, to smartwatches, or devices that seek to integrate fitness tracking with other personal communication and organization features. Smartwatches imagine an optimized experience of day-to-day life via technology through the centralization of features ranging from electronic payment systems to mobile data chips and geolocation services. Smartwatches aim to not only motivate users to meet their fitness goals, but to help them manage tasks at work, socialize with friends and colleagues, and passively monitor vital signs, including oxygen absorption and heart rate. In other words, they imagine a holistic approach to a user by providing tools to manage the tasks of labor and leisure, from work to social interactions, fitness, and health.

The holistic approach to the smartwatch user extends to the health-monitoring functions of the device, particularly through the integration of meditation and mindfulness features. Apple Watch claims to make users more efficient workers, family members, and friends, but it also reminds them to "stop and take a breath." Apple's Meditation app (formerly the Breathe app) guides users through customizable daily breathing exercises that aim to "calm the mind." With the arrival of the notification I describe above, the user can begin a timed session that uses haptic feedback—gentle vibrations, graphic animations, and heart rate tracking to guide them through deep breathing exercises. Fitbit quickly followed up with the Relax app, which allows users to engage in two- or five-minute breathing exercises. Both companies stress the benefits of breathing and mindfulness to not only improve long-term health but to make you "be a healthier, calmer, more focused you—all from just a few minutes of inhales and exhales each day."[1]

By placing breathing and mindfulness exercises alongside other digital tools used to improve daily organization and communication features, smartwatches implicitly frame these exercises as tools to optimize daily life. Often referred to as "breath work," this ideology of mindfulness understands breath as a tool to improve individual productivity by combatting the long-term and short-term effects of stress. By taking a moment to breathe, Apple Watch users ideally become more focused, "healthier" versions of themselves, capable of taking on the rest of their day. Proponents of breath work and meditation cite the range of studies that have shown it lowers the long-term effects of stress on blood pressure and cardiovascular disease and has short-term benefits for efficiency and productivity[2]: "[breathing can] help centre [*sic*] and focus your body and mind, reducing stress so you are ready to perform at your best."[3] This ideology of breathing and meditation ultimately supports a model of health associated with the neoliberal instantiation of wellness, which promotes health monitoring and maintenance as tools to improve and optimize the self.[4]

Meditation and breathing technologies stand at the intersection of health and wellness. While the terms are often used interchangeably, "health" and "wellness" figure the relationship between body and illness in dramatically different ways. As I described in the introduction, health is often framed through biomedical terms as the body's physiological equilibrium, whereas wellness refers to the active *performance* of health through physical, emotional, and social practices and choices. Importantly, wellness understands health not as a bodily state but as an existential goal. With the vernacular conflation of these two terms, ordinary understandings of health increasingly resemble the active pursuit of an unachievable state of "being well."

Analyzing breathing and meditation technologies reveals how definitions of health have shifted through the incorporation of wellness. The popularization of breathing and meditation as tools to improve health and well-being is the result of a complex history of social, economic, and political changes that emerged after World War II. I begin by tracing this history to show how biomedical methods such as quantification and biofeedback help support the values and economic incentives of wellness, such as the merger of mind and body, and individualized preventative healthcare strategies. To ground this history, I use the highly influential self-help book, *The Relaxation Response*, as a case study of how the quantification of autonomic responses, such as breath and heart rate were used to legitimize holistic approaches to health. Herbert Benson and Miriam Z. Kippler's 1975 publication helped establish a biomedical framework for the study of meditation that continues to inform the study of and promotion of wellness today.

The biomedical studies of meditation and breathing developed in *The Relaxation Response* are in tension with holistic health values and practices. By quantifying breathing and connecting breathing to other biological systems, Benson and Kippler redefine breathing and meditation not as tools for focusing on the holistic connection between mind and body or the present state of the body, but as preventative actions for maintaining and improving overall physiological health. In other words, breathing and meditation are tools to use in the pursuit of wellness. Through the aesthetic analysis of four popular meditation and breathing technologies—Breathesync, Spire, Apple's Meditation app, and the Muse Headband—I show the contradictions between biomedical and holistic models of the body that emerge when quantification is applied to meditation and breathing. By emphasizing numbers and improvement through "exercises" and "training," meditation and breathing technologies appear to undermine the goal of reuniting body and mind, a holistic approach to the body described by medical phenomenologists and wellness supporters alike. Analyzing the design of breathing and meditation technologies reveals how quantification and biofeedback can encourage individuals to self-objectify and reinforce a preventative model of health.

While the aesthetics of many breathing and meditation technologies may encourage self-objectification, I end by asking whether these technologies may be capable of resisting a preventative ideology of health promoted by wellness. Though postwar efforts aimed to incorporate practices and methods that brought the patient and body back into medical practice, definitions of health and wellness fail to articulate how either can be sensed or felt on the level of the body. In both scholarly and popular accounts, health is most often defined in the negative, in opposition to illness, or as a state of physiological equilibrium: the *absence* of pain, physiological disruption, or distress. In other words, health is imperceptible, often hidden until bodily harm or disease upsets this balance:

> [I]n many ways, the phenomenon of illness seems to be far more concrete and easier to grasp than the phenomenon of health. When we are ill, life is often penetrated by feelings of meaninglessness, helplessness, pain, nausea, fear, dizziness, or disability. Health, in contrast, effaces itself in an enigmatic way. [Health] seems to be the absence of every such feeling of illness, the state or process in which we find ourselves when everything is flowing smoothly, running the usual way without hindrance.[5]

Wellness appears to be the opposite of health in that it is framed positively through an emphasis on "feeling good," being happy or content. Early wellness guides frequently stressed how a focus on health can "provide more joy, satisfaction, and zest in living," using vague descriptions to suggest an ascent to an "advanced state of physical and psychological/spiritual health," while more recent discussions focus increasingly on productivity and success.[6] Across historical definitions, wellness is often framed in ambiguous, emotional terms that emphasize possibilities and potential for the future, with little focus on what it means for the body to "feel well" in the present.[7]

One early definition of wellness perhaps gets closer to a description of feeling well. Halbert Dunn, one of the first medical practitioners to lead the wellness movement in the 1960s, described wellness as a "state wherein you are 'alive and clear to the tips of your fingers. You have energy to burn. You tingle with vitality.'"[8] Though Dunn's early account gestures at a sensorial account of wellness, the body is quickly subsumed into the logic of continuous maintenance and improvement: "[an] individual must maintain a continuum of balance and purposeful direction."[9] Like popular accounts of wellness, Dunn's definition remains caught between the holistic impulse to call on the state of the body, and the biomedical logic of prevention and optimization through imagining the future, healthy self. By contrast, recent philosophical work in medical phenomenology has theorized health as an embodied feeling of vitality and possibility. Complicating the claim that health is an imperceptible state, philosophers have argued that health is not passive, but perhaps an encounter with "'being-itself': or the sense that my body is readily able to move in and through the world."[10]

I end by placing phenomenological descriptions of the Muse Meditation Headband and Apple Watch's Meditation app in conversation with the philosophical work of Hans-Georg Gadamer and Fredrik Svenaeus on health and phenomenology to show how these technologies may create encounters with the body in a present state of balancing or an attunement to bodily sensations. Contrary to the biomedical, homeostatic model of health or the preventative structure of wellness, these accounts of bodily attunement offer examples of how technology can prompt reflexive relationships to the body in its present state. By drawing on philosophical discussions of health and attunement, I begin to question whether we might use these experiences as examples for rethinking the feeling of health itself.[11]

From Health to Well-Being

Today, the terms "health" and "wellness" are often used interchangeably. As I discussed in the introduction, the conflation of health and wellness represents a relatively recent shift in the boundaries of medicine. As an "active goal," in wellness discourse health is no longer a biological state but something I can ideally "seek to accomplish" through particular strategies. Thus, health comes to be expressed or performed through *behaviors*: nutrition, exercise, counseling, mindfulness practice, and environmental *choices* made day after day. Individuals are charged with making the "right" decisions about daily habits and long-term healthcare. Determining the boundaries between "healthy" and "unhealthy" behavior, suggesting that certain choices are more "correct" than others, enfolds wellness and health into socially constructed value judgments and power structures that may rearticulate ideological positions.[12] These choices are often determined by the assumption that illness or injury will arise: certain foods *increase the risk of* cancer, moving less *leads* to heart disease, breathing exercises may *ward off* hypertension. Wellness stages itself as a way to intervene in these trajectories: it imagines a patient whose future is laden with illness, offering preventative methods to condition the present to avoid this otherwise inevitable future.

At the same time, wellness is seen as a corrective to the historical approach to the patient as an assemblage of biological parts that work together to produce a functioning whole. In this medical model, the body is understood as a "functioning mechanism," modeled on a "lifeless machine," divorced from the mind or personality.[13] From Michel Foucault's *Birth of a Clinic* to contemporary scholarship in the medical and health humanities, the objectifying gaze of medicine has been linked to dehumanizing structures of power.[14] Scholars and activists alike have pointed to these principles as sources for self-alienation and the policing of bodies through cultural and medical institutions. In contrast, wellness imagines the "whole person" by emphasizing the interconnection of biological, psychological, social, economic, and environmental determinants of "health."[15] Wellness programs and counseling correspondingly advocate for activities and choices that acknowledge the link between mind, body, and society: exercise for mental health, socialization for emotional support, and breathing exercises to reduce stress. The most widely circulated models are authored by clinical psychiatrists and researchers Jane Myers and Thomas Sweeney, whose "wheel of wellness" and "indivisible self model of wellness" have served as central pedagogical tools in counseling programs since the early 1990s.[16] Both these models use circular graphics to visualize the holistic patient whose "self" is composed of concentric and intersecting elements, including but not limited to emotional, social, creative, and economic realms. Across all of these examples, the individual is understood as a network of intersecting elements that operate together to determine well-being.

Wellness thus seemingly functions as a concept that supports preventative models of health and counteracts historically dehumanizing approaches to the patient in medicine. This section traces how this model of wellness emerged in the mid-twentieth century as a way to satisfy critiques of medicine and medical institutions, while still maintaining (and indeed, expanding) the moralizing discourses of health. The wellness model of health has become increasingly institutionalized through governmental, educational, and corporate programs, solidifying the multifaceted and expansive model of health monitoring and performance. In 2013, the RAND Corporation reported that nearly half of US companies included a workplace wellness program.[17] Additionally, most major private and public universities offer students supplementary wellness initiatives in addition to basic student healthcare.[18] Examining the history of wellness in the US demonstrates why this model of health has satisfied stakeholders across the political spectrum, doctors, and activists alike, and has effectively expanded the power of health by locating the monitoring systems, support, and encouragement (or enforcement) in the spheres of labor, education, and beyond.

The emphasis on the treatment of the whole person has been traced back to religious and intellectual healing movements of the nineteenth century, and the concept of wellness has been more broadly associated with a variety of alternative and at-home healing practices throughout history.[19] However, it was only after World War II that the term increasingly became attached to medical understandings of health. The incorporation of wellness into popular and medical discussions of health emerged from a constellation of social, political, and economic forces that brought debates on patient rights, treatment protocol, and healthcare costs to a head in the 1960s and '70s. By the end of this period, wellness principles seemed to offer the ideal tool to appease all parties, from activists and alternative-medicine practitioners to government and medical institutions. With its emphasis on holistic care, prevention, and individual responsibility, wellness became the ideal tool to expand the domain of medicine to include alternative health practices, *and* to support the emergence of the modern "patient-consumer."[20]

The history of wellness is a book in its own right.[21] I offer a brief account here to highlight how this concept is wrapped up in major shifts in patient rights and medical ethics, political regulation of health and safety, and economic reform. In other words, wellness isn't merely a trend or movement, but rather a powerful ideology that incorporates social, political, scientific, and economic values and systems of regulation.[22] Examining this history will illustrate how the biomedicalization of wellness reinforces these values and has given shape to the morally and economically inflected definition of "health and wellness" today.

Modern wellness practices were initially connected to religious and spiritual traditions where treatment of the "whole person" was largely related to belief in the "spirit" or "soul." Christian Science, for example, advocated for the "mind-cure," which considered an individual's mental and spiritual well-being as an indicator of health. Mary Baker Eddy, the founder of Christian Science, employed nontraditional approaches to healing, including mesmerism and other auto-suggestive techniques developed by fringe healers.[23] In his history of wellness, James William Miller argues that early religious adoptions of wellness in the nineteenth century operated under "the basic assumption that a healthy body was the product of a healthy mind and spirit."[24] By the second half of the twentieth century, the alignment of the mind and body would shed its religious affiliations as doctors and alternative health movements and activists increasingly advocated for holistic approaches to patienthood and self-regulated preventative care.

Alongside the secularization of wellness, in the twentieth century, medicine shifted from methods of treatment to prevention. As I discussed in the previous chapter, the rise of chronic or "lifestyle diseases" caused medicine to move from a focus on acute illness to long-term health management. The rising rates of heart disease, particularly in white middle-class men, prompted doctors to become more concerned about long-term habitual shifts in fitness levels, diet, and other behavioral patterns to avoid contracting the illness at a later stage in life. Responses from public health and medicine were largely focused on targeting white, executive men, who were seen as the most "at-risk" group. Consequently, solutions such as diet and exercise directly addressed the behavioral patterns of the postwar white middle class. No longer merely focused on the functioning of the physiological and biological processes of the body-machine, lifestyle diseases required careful attention to working conditions, diet, and exercise habits as a means of prevention.

With the rise of chronic illness came the rise in healthcare costs. By 1970, with the combination of chronic illness and complications in the Medicare and Medicaid billing structures, healthcare expenses for both patients and providers were at an all-time high, and politicians, health insurance agencies, employers, and healthcare providers sought ways to decrease spending.[25] These economic concerns combined with increasing rates of chronic disease led to the rise of "positive health" and health promotion, which moves away from traditional treatment models of health to more inclusive, wellness-driven methods of prevention.[26] Health promotion emphasizes education as a way for individuals to gain control over their health, offering social and environmental strategies for prevention. Advocates such as Dr. Halbert Louis Dunn, considered one of the founders of the wellness movement, aligned health with individual "potential." He developed the term "high-level wellness" to describe an approach to health that aims to "maximize the potential" of individuals within their social and environmental conditions. Dunn suggested that health was a continuum rather than a fixed state: "wellness is about potential—it involves helping the individual move toward the highest state of well-being."[27]

While healthcare professionals like Dunn represented a transition toward wellness practices within existing structures of medical care, the rising cost of care and increasing distrust in medical authority fueled the popularization of alternative healing practices, New Age medicine, and self-care outside of the domain of medical institutions (and coverage of health insurance). In the postwar period, the field of medicine faced a great deal of public scrutiny. Following events such as the thalidomide drug safety scandal[28] and the release of the Surgeon General's report on smoking,[29] the public grew increasingly skeptical about the advice and authority of doctors and medical institutions. At the same time, scholars critiqued the mind-body dualism underlying medical practice, claiming it led to a dehumanized, mechanized vision of the body.[30] By the 1960s and '70s, holistic approaches to health became increasingly accessible and popular among the white middle class. The boom of self-help, in particular, spread alternative and New Age methods across the United States. Books on topics ranging from fitness and diet (*Diet and Disease*, *Fit or Fat*) to meditation and mindfulness (*Mind as Healer*) and opposition to the medical establishment (*End of Medicine*, *Mirage of Health*) were widely disseminated in this period. Individuals who could afford the cost also increasingly sought out treatments from acupuncturists, chiropractors, and those trained in "non-Western" medical traditions.

The rise of alternative and New Age health is likewise indebted to the importation of religious and spiritual wellness practices. Perhaps the longest-lasting and most popular expression of wellness, yoga is emblematic of how religious traditions were incorporated into American wellness culture through a process of secularization and commodification. In the postwar era, yoga studios and ashrams began to emerge on the West Coast, offering retreats and classes dedicated to a holistic approach to the mind, body, and spirit. While yoga had been introduced to the US nearly a century before, the loosening of US immigration policies regarding India in the 1960s allowed more teachers and practitioners to emigrate and establish businesses dedicated to their yoga practices.[31] The influx of immigration helped give rise to "modern yoga," which emphasized the physicalism of the practice over the spiritual or religious benefits. By foregrounding the body, modern yoga was increasingly understood as a practice that could be studied scientifically and empirically as a tool for health and wellness. The focus on muscular movement made it a useful resource for combatting a variety of health concerns ranging from stress to back pain, and framed yoga as a form of exercise, as opposed to foregrounding the mind-body benefits of the practice. As both a wellness practice and a form of exercise, yoga moved into the spaces of commercial gyms and YMCAs, with studios and classes dedicated to fitness and wellness-focused yoga.[32] Wellness practices such as yoga that addressed a wide range of physical and mental health concerns, and existed outside of the boundaries of traditional biomedicine, were able to address a wide variety of audiences, ranging from those interested in novel fitness regimens to those seeking alternatives to the medical establishment.

While the spread of alternative and New Age medicine is in part related to its increasing accessibility, its popularity was simultaneously bolstered through its political affiliations. Activist movements in this period targeted medical institutions and structures of authority as emblematic of the status quo, citing health scandals and scholarly debates as justification for radical political action. For example, health became a central pillar of second-wave feminism, which spoke out against the gendered structures of healthcare funding and medical care.[33] Existing models of healthcare, they argued, reinforced patriarchal or hegemonic structures of power. This was echoed by Black health activists who aimed to fight against the racist institutional practices and structures of medicine and care.[34] Across many health movements in this period, there was a common goal to "obtain rights to health care as well as rights within health care." Thus, for many, taking back power over healthcare was to take back power in our political system at large. Holistic approaches to health, and many of the values associated with wellness, provided a "basis for the development of a coherent oppositional subculture," united in an effort to consider the health and rights of the whole person.[35] Alternative and New Age medicine thus became political statements unto themselves: by seeking out holistic medical treatments and wellness practices, one was asserting one's individual rights and agency.

Indeed, the emphasis placed on individual agency and self-care in wellness discourse made it equally appealing to the political right. With the rise of government spending on healthcare following the establishment of Medicare and Medicaid in 1966, critics advocated for deregulating and defunding government support of healthcare. Health promotion aimed at individually driven, preventative modes of care became an ideal resource to cut down on private and federal spending. By the 1970s, wellness programs were increasingly offered by corporations, including Mobil Oil and General Motors, and also on college campuses.[36] Corporate wellness programs and self-help books during this period (and up to today) suggest that considering an employee's physical and mental health is good for the bottom line: "Rather than throwing money at treating disease, big and little businesses could probably increase productivity, lower absenteeism and improve morale and otherwise decrease the extent of illness by promoting wellness at the company's expense."[37] In 1979, the Surgeon General confirmed and extended such sentiments, claiming that the tenets of wellness offered a pathway to improve the health of America at large:

> Further improvements in the health of American people will be achieved—not just through increased medical care and great health expenditures—but through a national commitment to efforts designed to prevent disease and promote health.[38]

Thus, healthcare emerged as the "centerpiece" of debates across the left and right because it "served well to illustrate the ways the American system had failed key groups of its citizens"; it was an emblem of authoritarian powers responsible for social and economic inequity in the US.[39] In her history of the American healthcare system, Nancy Tomes argues that across party lines there was a shift from the rhetoric of the "patient" to that of the "patient-consumer" as a way to emphasize individual responsibility and choice.[40] "Consumer" signaled individual agency and power in this period, as a modification of the more traditional understanding of patienthood that was "deeply suffused with values of medical paternalism."[41] The growing wellness discourse and industry proved to be a natural expression of this shift in language, creating spaces and social practices where individuals could "choose" to resist the medical status quo and take back "control" over their health and bodies.

However, contrary to the goals of agency and freedom proposed by the rhetorical shift toward consumption, the movement toward wellness has helped extend the boundaries of medical power over the course of the last four decades. Terms such as "patient-consumer" and its emphasis on choice and individual responsibility have helped promote the conflation of health and *lifestyle*. And emerging out of the postwar focus on the health of white men and the expansion of alternative health practices for the middle classes, the model of a "healthy lifestyle" is tied directly to the behaviors and spending practices of the white middle class. By the 1980s, health increasingly connoted "individuality, self-expression, and a stylistic self-consciousness."[42] Scholars have labeled this phenomenon "healthism" to describe how the emphasis on prevention and lifestyle choices has caused everyday life to become increasingly intertwined with the power and structures of medical authority. In line with wellness, healthism proposes lifestyle as the solution to medical problems: "[it] *does not* address the expansion of the jurisdiction of medical professionals or institutions . . . but rather 'the dissemination of medical perception and ideology.'"[43] Healthism encourages individuals to examine their lifestyle through the lens of medicine, defining every action and choice in medical terms and causing individuals to increasingly "internalize and reproduce health awareness spontaneously and without any external coercive force."[44] Wellness functions as the positive expression of these forces. It helps designate the "right" (consumer) lifestyle choices in pursuit of this activated definition of health.

Over this period, wellness emerged as a concept capable of addressing many of the competing political concerns around health and healthcare spending, as well as changing approaches to medical care and patienthood. The postwar period laid the foundation for a definition of wellness (and by extension, health) that was directly related to class. Through an emphasis on lifestyle and choice, wellness has helped reinforce the idea that very specific and costly consumer choices and behaviors are pathways to health—choices and behaviors that remain inaccessible for many who do not fit the profile of the ideal, white middle-class patient-consumer. While wellness is not necessarily a direct product of any specific political action or historical event, its capacity to address a wide array of problems in the American healthcare system has made it an incredibly powerful ideological force today. Wellness practices, as well as breathing and meditation technologies, inherit this collection of political and economic concerns and the classed framework that continues to shape how health is performed, monitored, and evaluated today.

The Relaxation Response and the Rise of Evidence-Based Wellness

In his history of wellness, Miller claims that today wellness often serves simply as an "advertising slogan" used to sell products and services under the guise of health. Profits from lifestyle products ranging from supplements to skincare and other household items are undoubtedly increased through marketing their health benefits. But to reduce wellness to a slogan or marketing scheme overlooks the epistemological power these concepts continue to exert in contemporary culture. While wellness may be focused on individuals and rhetorically oppose itself to the medical institution, health and wellness remain powerful precisely because they remain attached to biomedicine. Since the 1950s, holistic medicine and wellness practices have been explored through scientific and medical research studies, which have supported the public and professional adoption of wellness. For example, Donald B. Ardell, author of *High Level Wellness* (1977) and one of the earliest promoters of wellness, cites evidence-based research on mind-body awareness as a crucial supporter of the wellness movement.[45] He credits the success of wellness to scholarly work that helped suppress some of the religious and spiritual undertones of wellness, in favor of a scientifically informed secular approach to well-being. Ardell and other early supporters invoked the language of science and medicine, claiming that modern wellness advice took a "systematic approach" to self-care through measurement, clearly defined goals, and feedback to promote long-term behavioral changes.[46] These methods were backed by biomedical research, which often used principles of biofeedback and correlations between emotional or physical markers of health and quantifiable vitals such as heart rate and temperature to study an expanded understanding of health and well-being.

The popularization and dissemination of wellness are thus inextricable from the expansion of biomedicine. Indeed, despite activist attempts to dismantle medical institutions, social critiques of healthcare gave way to an emphasis on patient rights and health education: "sweeping critiques of medicine and capitalism gave way to a more domesticated version of medical consumerism . . . providing patients with more information and choice about products and procedures available to them became a means of ensuring greater patient compliance."[47] Underlying this sentiment is the sense that the scientific and medical *methods* were not necessarily the source of doubt; the problem lay in the structures of treatment, information, and financial responsibility for care. Indeed, today, wellness is supported by a variety of scientific studies, expert recommendations from organizations such as the Centers for Disease Control and World Health Organization, and medical practitioners. With support from the government, commercial, and biomedical spheres, Carl Cederström and Andre Spicer argue that wellness has become an ideology: "[wellness] offers a package of ideas and beliefs which people may find seductive and desirable, although, for the most part, these ideas appear natural or even inevitable."[48] That "inevitable" or "natural position, I argue, is tied to the way official discourses of health—reinforced through biomedical standards of evidence—have helped produce this perception of neutrality.

Some of the earliest and most influential examples of this work included research on stress management, meditation, and mindfulness. As a form of care accessible to the general public without the aid of medical practitioners, mindfulness, and meditation give people a relatively simple way to manage emotional and physical health. Like yoga, mindfulness and meditation practices began as religious and spiritual imports into the US from East and Southeast Asia. In the US, modern meditation practices emerged throughout the 1950s and '60s, brought into popular consciousness via figures such as Joseph Goldstein, Sharon Salzber, and Jack Kornfeld, who adapted Theravada meditation practices for Western consumers.[49] In 1975, they founded the Insight Meditation Society (IMS), which acknowledged the ties to Buddhist traditions but largely promoted a psychotherapized version of the teachings.[50] IMS marked the popular turn toward a secular therapeutic version of meditation, and by 1979, meditation was officially incorporated into modern medical training and practice with the establishment of the Mindfulness-Based Stress Reduction (MBSR) program at the University of Massachusetts Medical School. The founder, Dr. Jon Kabat-Zinn, applied his training in biology to the study of his yoga and meditation practices, building out a therapeutic framework for the study and prescription of meditation and other holistic health practices. The MBSR program was "rooted in a scientific and therapeutic framework that seeks to address specific ailments," and established the practice as an evidence-based tool for health treatment and prevention.[51]

The success of the MBSR program and subsequent popularization of medical applications of meditation has been supported by countless scientific studies that used biomedical and quantitative methods to specifically demonstrate how meditation can be used to reduce or combat stress. Perhaps the most publicly influential work was the 1975 publication of *The Relaxation Response*, on the physiological benefits of meditation and breathing. To produce this early example of self-help literature, the authors, Benson and Kippler, drew on studies conducted in the 1960s at the Harvard Medical Center to offer readers a set of meditation practices that used breathing to reduce the harmful effects of stress. Their research offered a complementary physiological reaction to the "flight-or-fight response," or the "inborn" and involuntary reaction to acute or chronic stressors in which blood pressure, heart rate, and rate of breathing increase.[52] As a counterpoint, they offered the "relaxation response," a physiological reaction that combats stress and is capable of reducing heart rate, blood pressure, metabolism, oxygen intake, etc. This response is not manufactured or produced through the introduction of pharmaceuticals, but is rather an "innate and protective mechanism" that helps protect our bodies against the "harmful bodily effects of the flight-or-fight response."[53] Benson and Kippler claim the response can be triggered through meditation strategies that coordinate thought and breath to improve an individual's physical and psychological health. Their biomedical approach laid the foundation for the explosion of scientific work on meditation in recent decades, with hundreds of studies published in academic journals annually.[54]

Benson and Kippler's research marked an important juncture in medical research as one of the earliest studies dedicated to understanding the psychological *and* physiological effects of stress on the human body. While doctors acknowledged the toll stress often takes on a patient's physical and emotional well-being, studies faced the problem of "how to quantify stress" and how to articulate a clear relationship between an individual's psychological state and bodily functions.[55] Drawing on related scientific studies of blood pressure, Benson and Kippler locate stress in four autonomic functions: blood pressure, heart-rate recovery, lactate and hormone levels, and oxygen intake. They argued that meditation practice could systematically reduce all these functions, which are elevated during the flight-or-fight response. Through principles of biofeedback, which uses a reward-based system, they argued, their techniques were capable of "mentally reorganizing a biologic function [so that] you can gain control of that function."[56] However, because Benson and Kippler saw biofeedback as a limited and time-consuming method of treatment, they turned to schools of meditation to research the body's autonomic response.

Through the study of a range of meditative practices, from transcendental meditation to yoga and prayer, Benson and Kippler showed that breathing and meditation practices decrease oxygen use, which in turn lowers metabolism and stress on organs, decreases lactate in blood, and produces positive responses in the sympathetic nervous system.[57] Drawing on historical meditation practices, they conclude, "we offer no innovation but simply a scientific validation of age-old wisdom."[58] The relaxation response

> has always [existed] in the context of religious teachings. Its use has been most widespread in Eastern cultures, where it has been an

> essential part of daily existence. But the physiology has only been recently defined. Religious prayers and related mental techniques have measurable, definable, physiologic effects on the body.[59]

In other words, their research simply legitimizes preexisting methods for combatting stress, offering scientific support for mindfulness and meditation. *The Relaxation Response* provides quantitative evidence of the benefits of meditation, drawing a clear cause-effect relationship between body and mind: thinking "relaxing thoughts" has been scientifically shown to reduce the physiological effects of stress.

The Relaxation Response directly opposed itself to conventional scientific approaches to health, which had tended to uphold the Cartesian separation of body and mind.[60] Benson and Kippler's research instead sought to link psychological state to innate physiological conditions—the flight-or-fight and relaxation response—through "hard, measurable, physiologic data."[61] The goal of their work was to link body and mind through preexisting standards of evidence and to use established biomedical models to connect these two previously independent spheres of medicine. They would go on to reinforce their claims through increasingly technical forms of quantitative analysis, affirming their results through studies using MRI and fMRI to track the aural structures of relaxation and stress, along with genomic research[62] that demonstrated how meditation was capable of producing "enhanced expression of genes associated with energy, metabolism, mitochondria function, insulin secretion, and telepomre maintenance, and reduced expression of genes linked to inflammatory response and stress-related pathways."[63] By providing quantitative grounds for the connections between body and mind, *The Relaxation Response* provided an essential foundation for future research that reinforced the connection between psychology and physiology, and mental and physical health.

The Relaxation Response promoted breathing exercises to unite the body and mind. Individuals were encouraged to sit in a quiet environment for ten to twenty minutes a day and focus on breathing and the repetition of a selected word or phrase. The goal is to use the repetition of breath and thought to "quiet the mind" and bring attention to the body in the present, or what they call "adopt a passive attitude."[64] This "passive attitude," is akin to what today is understood as mindfulness, "a mental state achieved by focusing one's awareness on the present moment, while calmly acknowledging and accepting one's feelings, thoughts, and bodily sensations, used as a therapeutic technique."[65] For Benson and Kippler, "awareness" comes through breathing: "Breathe through your nose. Become aware of your breathing. As you breathe out, say the word 'ONE,' silently to yourself."[66] By bringing attention to breathing—an often-unnoticed autonomic function—one can become aware of one's present mental and physical state.

While Benson and Kippler's research demonstrated the positive effects of breathing and meditation practice, it is ultimately difficult to trace a clear cause-effect relationship between relaxation-response methods and positive physiological changes. Their work is largely reinforced through accounts of meditation from individuals who praise the relaxing and calming effects of their book's meditation methods, leading to questions about whether the benefits of their methods are merely a placebo effect.[67] Benson and Richard Friedman would later go on to endorse the psychosomatic effects of the relaxation response, citing examples of patients who demonstrated no clear cause-effect relationship between meditation and improved physical health. Nonetheless, they claim that this does not disprove the relaxation response or the power of mindfulness; rather, it emphasizes that "for optimal care . . . the placebo effect should be maximized."[68] The relaxation response encourages "positive b liefs and expectations on the part of the patient . . . [and the] healthcare professional . . . and a good relationship between both parties," which is essential for successful patient care.[69] As a way to rebrand the "placebo effect," Benson and Friedman offer "remembered wellness" to describe the psychological and physiological benefits of mindfulness.[70] While the placebo effect is, in part, encouraged by a kind of "positive thinking" or "faith," these beliefs are backed by neural firings in the central nervous system—that is, physiological evidence. Thus, the placebo effect or remembered wellness describes a psychologically motivated expression of cell firings in the brain that "result in feelings of well-being."[71] Breathing in pursuit of mindfulness perhaps does not result in a clear and definite cause-effect relationship, but Benson, Kippler, and Friedman's work exemplifies today's popular understanding of mindfulness, meditation, and indeed, wellness; despite questions about the placebo effect or "remembered wellness," biomedical research has shown that meditation and breathing *improve* health and encourage feelings of well-being.

In 2018, the CDC released a study showing that the practice of meditation and yoga has increased threefold in the US over a period of four years.[72] Meditation and mindfulness are now widely prescribed therapies incorporated into wellness programs and psychological counseling. Ranging from spiritual mindfulness programs to MBSR and mindfulness-based cognitive therapy (MBCT), mindfulness and meditation have become part of popular wellness discourse. Physicians, psychologists, counselors, popular health publications, blogs, and TED Talks, have prescribed breathing exercises for wellness.[73] More than forty years after the publication of *The Relaxation Response*, Benson and Kippler's research continues to provide evidence for many contemporary meditation and mindfulness techniques: they are understood as medically proven strategies to improve health and well-being.[74]

"Making the Intangible Tangible"

In addition to helping popularize wellness, *The Relaxation Response*'s methods continue to underwrite the science of meditation and breathing technologies. Fitbit's Relax app FAQs, for example, cite the flight-or-fight response to support the claim that their product can help reduce its harmful autonomic effects.[75] Contemporary apps and wearables claim to place the quantitative methods of Benson and Kippler's research in the hands of individual users. Apple Watch's Meditation app, Fitbit's Relax app, Spire, Core, and Breathesync couple breathing exercises with quantitative data collection, including heart rate, heart rate variability, and breaths per minute, giving users "direct access" to the autonomic responses that occur during breathing exercises. This data is stored in the app's archive, allowing individuals to track and improve their meditation practice as a metric of their overall well-being.

Meditation and mindfulness technologies go beyond previous meditation programs and use the affordances of mobile technology and quantitative data collection to promote the preventative ideology of wellness discourse. I begin with the analysis of breathing technologies Breathesync and Spire to show how biofeedback operates through quantification and notification features. Rather than providing biomedical evidence for the benefits of mindfulness, biofeedback is instead used to create the *impression* of well-being through the promise of stress prevention, improved productivity, and control over the body. Breathsync and Spire's use of biofeedback to encourage meditation for the sake of productivity contradicts the basic principles of mindfulness. Rather than focusing on the present experience of the body and mind, quantification and tracking shift attention to the future potential benefits of the practice.

While Breathesync and Spire primarily focus on future improvement,

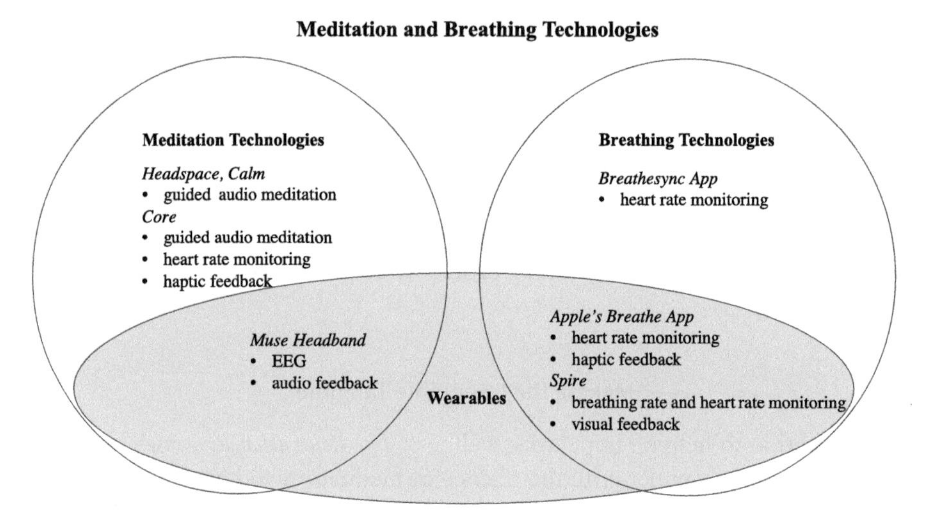

Fig. 14. The diagram offers a way to categorize breathing and meditation technologies based on the design features.

some technologies use real-time feedback in an effort to draw greater attention to present meditation practice (Fig. 14). Both Core and Muse, for example, combine quantification with real-time audio and haptic feedback in an effort to encourage the relaxation response and improve practice over time. In the second half of this section, I turn to descriptions of the Muse Headband interface and phenomenological descriptions of my meditation experiences to examine how real-time biofeedback likewise supports the preventative logic of wellness and can indeed undermine the goal of meditation practices and the supposed health benefits of the relaxation response.

Released in 2013, the Breathesync app for iPhone uses the device's built-in flash to track an individual's pulse during a guided breathing session. On entering the app, individuals are greeted with the company's tagline, "Breathe yourself better," which quickly gives way to a pulsing orb prompting them to place their finger on the surface of the phone camera. A small heart in the upper right corner of the screen pulses until the device registers the presence of a finger and starts the breathing exercise. The one-minute clock at the bottom of the screen begins to count down, and the words "breathe in" appear at the top of the screen (Fig. 15). Concentric blue circles slowly pulse outward from the center of the screen, setting the pace for inhalation. Once the largest blue circle appears, "breathe out" fades in at the top of the screen, and the spherical animation slowly shrinks inward. Individuals repeat this practice seven times, trying to link breath and animation while the phone tracks their pulse using the flashing light.[76] At the end of each session they receive a score, or a "Wellbeing Quotient,®" or "WQ," undoubtedly a pun on IQ. A number between 1 and 100 and a corresponding key (Fig. 16) helps users discern their "wellbeing": under 70: "feeling tired or stressed?"; 70–90: "Feeling ok?"; over 90: "Feeling good?" How these categories are created and quantified remains entirely opaque, but they are meant to provide a consistent and quantitative means for individuals to compare their breathing practices over time. Unlike traditional fitness wearables, Breathesync does not give individuals clearly defined quantitative data; rather, it uses a numerical value and assigned question to create an alignment between a quantitative value and a qualitative feeling.

Through push notifications and quantitative data tracking, Breathesync claims to use the principles of biofeedback to "[directly affect] your autonomic nervous system which helps reduce your stress levels."[77] Biofeedback operates through the principle that knowledge or awareness of automatic bodily functions can lead to greater control over these previously unconscious systems. Over time, this control is conditioned into an unconscious habit, shifting an individuals' autonomic and behavioral patterns. By linking breathing and heart rate, the Breathesync app claims to offer information about "well-being" that ideally can be used to help train individuals to relax. The app proposes that individuals incorporate breathing sessions into pre- and postwork routines and to use the practice in preparation for any task that requires focus: "instantly relax your body and mind."[78] While hypothetically the app tracks long-term data on their breathing and heart rates, the emphasis on instantaneity reveals that it is less interested in the production of awareness than in training users to experience a particular effect. Through repetition, visual and numerical feedback, an animated interface, and the "WQ" score, the app aims to *trigger* relaxation. In other words, by showing users the benefits of breathing through quantified analysis, the app places breathing and relaxation into a numerically supported cause-effect structure—breathing causes relaxation—which over time can be used to automatically produce the positive autonomic benefits of breathing (ideally mediated through the app).

The ubiquity of smartphones and the rise of wearable technologies have made biofeedback increasingly available to scientific research and indeed to individual users. In 1975, Benson and Kippler cited biofeedback research as a critical precursor to their meditation research, one that helped reveal

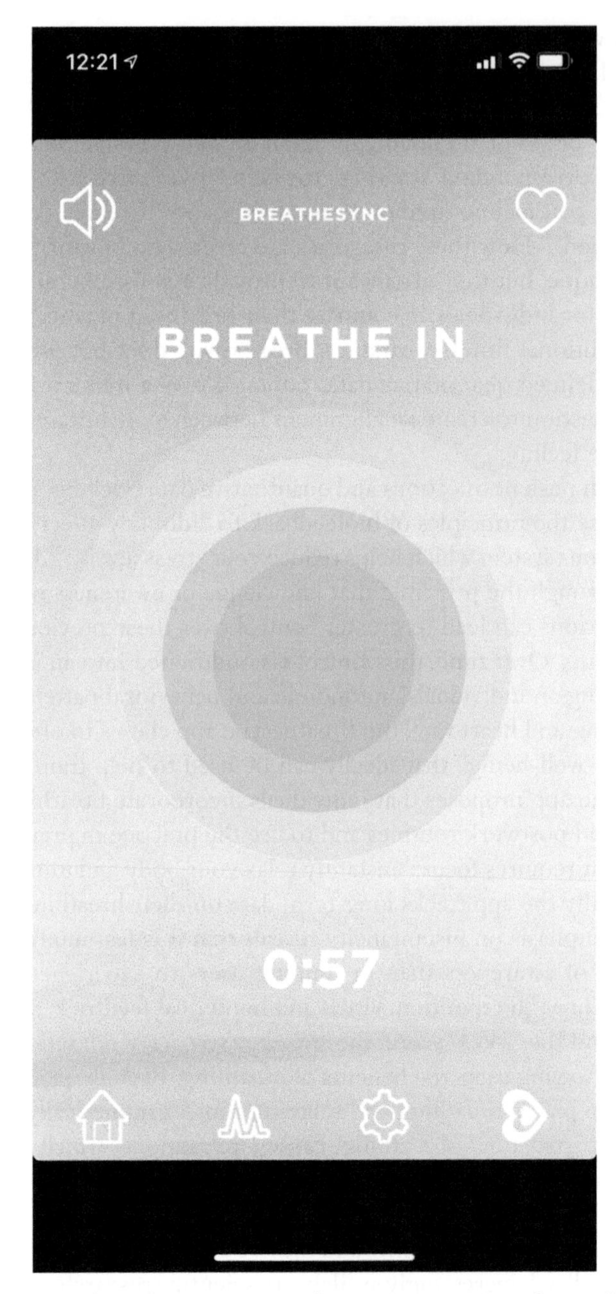

Figs. 15 (*above*) and 16 (*facing page*). Breathesync's exercise interface and "Well-Being Quotient" key. (Breathesync Ltd., "Breathesync," vers. 1.7.0, accessed February 2018.)

12:22

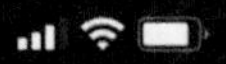

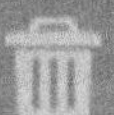

BREATHESYNC

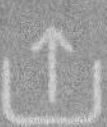

Your WQ

Under 70
Feeling tired or stressed?
Breathe deeply, rest and catch up on sleep when you can.

70–90
Feeling ok?
Slow down and take some more breaks.
Why not go outside for a walk and some fresh air?

Over 90
Feeling good?
You're ready to perform at your best.
Why not take on a new challenge?

WQ (Wellbeing Quotient) is a measure of your wellbeing based on your heart rhythm whilst breathing.

Ok More

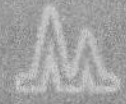

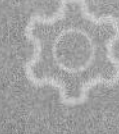

a scientific link between mind and body. At the time, however, biofeedback was incredibly cost-prohibitive, and required highly regulated laboratory settings for proper data collection.[79] Today, however, Apple Watch, Fitbit, Spire, Breathesync, Core, and Muse all integrate the principles of biofeedback in their meditation and breathing programs, offering quantitative strategies to promote the positive physiological effects of breathing and meditation. For example, Spire, the only wearable technology currently designed solely for breathing, tracks breathing and heart rate in real time to visualize a user's "mental state."[80] Information is processed and visualized as a timeline of their mental states, ranging from calm to stressed. Over time, the wearable learns their average breathing and heart rates, provides push notifications when it notices that their vitals are elevated for an extended period, and reminds them to stop and take a moment to engage in a breathing exercise.[81]

Interrupting the individual's stressed state, Spire seeks to use breathing exercises to alter the physiological patterns of stress individuals experience throughout the day to trigger the relaxation response.[82] Biofeedback places awareness of physiological processes into a cause-effect structure, or in the words of Spire, "your state of mind is influenced by how you breathe."[83] The technology suggests that the mind can be controlled through quantified goal markers, including "energize," "calm," and "focus" goals, which are based on breath and heart rate data. "Calm" is measured as 6 to 12 breaths per minute, 18 to 24 breaths is interpreted as "tense," and "focus" is quantified as 16 to 20 breaths over an extended period.[84] Spire supports all of these quantitative categories with the positive and negative physiological effects associated with the corresponding breathing rates. Individuals are thus encouraged to maximize their positive breathing categories to improve mental and physical health.

By quantifying calm, tense, and focus, Spire suggests that one's state of mind, and even mindfulness, is not a "state" one necessarily experiences, but something that can be achieved by simply trying to control one's breathing and heart rate. By examining historical data, the individual can supposedly control their "states of mind and help them anticipate or prevent negative mental states in the future."[85] These training structures are reinforced through principles associated with long-term wearable habits. Through push notification feedback, scheduled breathing exercises, and quantitative analysis, Spire places breathing exercises into the structure: "habit formation, social motivation, and goal reinforcement."[86] To achieve these principles, Spire, and Breathesync, figure breath as the quantifiable cause for positive autonomic bodily responses. Breathing is thus refigured as an exercise not unlike going to the gym—an action that can be counted, controlled, and conditioned to strive for wellness.

Though Spire and Breathesync both claim to encourage mindfulness through breathing exercises, the technologically mediated use of biofeedback places them into the logic of preventive health associated with wellness. The goal-oriented structure assumes that meeting a daily quotient will increase mindfulness and therefore improve physical and mental health, with little regard for what these improvements feel like on the level of the body. The primary concern with both products is the assumption that mindfulness maps directly onto breathing. In other words, Spire and Breathesync take the strategies of the relaxation response as a given: if one engages in a breathing exercise practice, one will achieve mindfulness, and by extension all of its health benefits. Rather than assessing the phenomenological effects of breathing and meditation, these practices are treated like daily tasks one checks off in pursuit of health. The apps do not include any features that encourage individuals to consider whether they feel less stressed or perceive any changes in their physical and mental states. Meditation and breathing are treated like fitness: as a temporal or numerical goal ("exercise thirty minutes per day") that one simply completes to "be well."

By contrast, meditation technologies such as Core and Muse use real-time feedback to focus on the present experience of meditation. While the technologies do foreground improving numbers, the meditation sessions themselves are guided through haptic and audio feedback to hypothetically encourage individuals to focus attention on the present state of the body and mind. For example, Core monitors heart rate as an indirect measurement of brain patterns through small sensors on the surface of the handheld device, and provides biofeedback in the form of vibration to help individuals monitor their state of mind. The corresponding app reveals statistics after the practice, which breaks down the session into periods of "calm" and "focus." At the same time, while Core advertises itself as "meditation you can feel," the device similarly uses heart rate as the metric for the experience of meditation and mindfulness: a slow heart rate becomes the signifier of successful meditation and a calming experience, but this does not necessarily reflect one's mental and bodily state.[87]

Core's vibration feature illustrates how meditation and breathing technologies must provide more than quantified forms of motivation and goal reinforcement through push notifications: users must also *feel* a sense of improvement. Breathing and meditation practices can only be integrated into everyday wellness efforts when "quantitative data and *qualitative experience* mutually reinforce one another."[88] Following the need for qualitative feedback, *The Relaxation Response* reminds readers of the importance of remaining open and responsive to the process. The focus on attitude suggests that the benefits of mindfulness are largely felt due to the placebo effect or "remembered wellness": if one takes a more open and positive attitude toward meditation practice, then one is more likely to see a positive outcome.[89] Benson and Kippler's scientific research and carefully designed protocol for meditation aimed to create a structure that encourages regular practice and a corresponding sense of satisfaction.

To create a sense of satisfaction and real-time feedback, the Muse Headband uses sound to supposedly allow individuals access to the state of their mind during meditation. Muse advertises itself as a research-grade EEG device that can read and collect data on an individual's brainwaves while they meditate.[90] The headband sits just above the brow and features three sensors across the forehead and two behind the ear, which collect brain electrical signals; "machine learning techniques are applied to the brain signal components to control the experience in real time."[91] The Muse 2, released in 2018, added sensors to track heart rate, movement, and breath to give individuals a "holistic view of [their] performance." "Performance" is tracked through the corresponding app where individuals can gain access to the guided meditation options and access their data history.[92]

Muse's EEG sensors read brainwaves that are translated through audio feedback during the mediation practice. To begin a meditation session, individuals set the duration and can select from a range of "exercises" to help set an intention or element of focus for their practice. These exercises, however, merely introduce the session, and are quickly eclipsed by the "soundscape" feature of the app once the clock starts. Biofeedback is provided through fluctuations in the sonic environment provided throughout the meditation session; in Muse's words, the device "translates your brainwaves into the guiding sounds of weather."[93] The app offers a handful of environments, including a rainforest, desert, and city street, and the intensity of the audio weather pattern is meant to reflect the individual's brain activity level. For example, the rainforest soundscape fluctuates between heavy downpours and quiet drips. Across all the options, the goal is to calm the weather to the point that you hear birds chirping. For each chirp, one receives a "bird" point in the app: the more birds, the calmer the mind.

The soundscape is designed to help individuals control brainwave patterns. Unlike traditional forms of neurofeedback, which use EEG monitors and feedback to help individuals channel specific types of brainwaves (e.g., gamma or alpha waves), Muse "use[s] a unique combination of the various brainwaves to provide valuable insight into the different mind states."[94] Brainwaves are traditionally classified by frequency and fall into five categories that have been associated with particular brain functions. For example, gamma waves that have a frequency between 35 and 100 Hz are equated with high-functioning cognitive tasks and learning. Rather than tracking each of these frequency ranges, Muse breaks brain activity into "calm," "neutral," and "active," providing little information about frequency or the logic behind these categories. This suggests that Muse is less invested in offering individuals an archive of specific brain wave data, and more invested in giving them a sense of their brain patterns throughout the session. While the Muse headband is capable of tracking each of the five frequencies, this data is only available through the Muse Direct app, which requires a paid subscription.[95]

The use of real-time audio feedback suggests that individuals can affect these soundscapes by adjusting their attention or focus through mental efforts or breathing exercises. While the voice-over introduction encourages individuals to treat the soundscape as a reminder to return to the breath or the present state of mind, the experience of these soundscapes poses a challenge to the more traditional meditation principles advertised by the app. Benson and Kippler, along with other meditation and mindfulness guides, tend to stress awareness and passivity: "you should not worry about how well you are performing the technique, because this may prevent the Relaxation Response from occurring."[96] Muse's soundscape, by contrast, seems to foreground technique by constantly drawing attention to the rise and fall of rainfall or wind. For example, as I sit down for a session with Muse, Deepak Chopra's voice-over prompts me to sit comfortably, close my eyes, and focus on the sensation of my breath. However, as the rainforest soundscape takes over, the rush of pouring rain pulls my attention. I've been instructed to use the rising intensity of weather to shift awareness back to the breath, but as I do, I find myself thinking harder, trying to relax the pull in my shoulders and the tension in my neck. While I will my shoulders to release, the rain continues to pour down and my attention returns to the sound. A big inhale through my nose causes a swell of water, but as I exhale it begins to quiet. I hold my breath at the end of the exhale and the rain is reduced to a trickle. I listen closely for a chirp, but the harder I concentrate, the louder the rain swells. My shoulders sag and I try another technique, shifting awareness to my hands in my lap or the shallow bursts of air passing through my nose. Each of these attempts results in the same frustrating dance with quiet: the harder I try to hear the birds, the less frequently they come.

Despite the aim to relax and reduce stress, I found that these sessions often increased my anxiety.[97] The constant struggle to achieve "calm" despite my best efforts led to a degree of skepticism about the device: I found myself questioning whether it was indeed recording my brain patterns. For a few weeks, I experimented with the device, testing it out in different situations and at various times of day, doing my best to note my mood and energy levels. I discovered that on the days when I felt most alert and ready to work, I received the fewest bird points at the end of my session, whereas days when I felt sluggish, tired, and unfocused resulted in my highest scores to date. While my perception of "alert" and "unfocused" may be specific to my experience, this suggests that Muse's categories of "calm" versus "active" perhaps actually reflect brain patterns associated with sleep versus critical thinking. This isn't to say the device is wrong, but instead it points to how these algorithmic processes and data-collection systems can often contradict bodily experience. Indeed, the days when I was most "calm" were often those when I was most frustrated with myself, unable to focus or complete the tasks I'd set out to achieve during the day.[98]

My frustration often emerged from the cause-effect structure of biofeedback, combined with the emphasis on goals, points, and improvement. Muse advertises itself as a tool to "improve mental and physical wellbeing," specifically by creating structures of measurement and feedback that encourage habit formation and productivity. Drawing on scientific studies (including *The Relaxation Response*), Muse claims long-term meditation practice can improve "concentration and problem-solving," and the website advertises several scientific studies using the device, all foregrounding its cognitive benefits, including improved attention and reaction times to complex tasks.[99] Participants in these studies often reported a reduction in stress and an increased ability to trigger relaxation. Like Benson and Kippler's work, these two benefits are always linked: stress reduction and cognitive function. In other words, stress reduction and relaxation are continually linked to "mental performance," or cognitive processes related to productivity.[100] Muse borrows from this logic to suggest that meditation can train one to become more efficient, attentive, and alert.

While research continually stresses the health benefits of meditation, the actual practice is often discussed as an incredibly challenging task that requires a constant pull of the mind away from the state of the body. Over time, individuals learn how to acknowledge these shifts in attention and bring awareness back to the present state of the body and breath.[101] But with Muse, that shifting of attention can become focalized on the sonic intensity of the weather patterns to gain points and rewards. Rather than my mind drifting to the tasks I needed to complete later in the day, I found myself concentrating on the rain patterns, doing my best to find ways to trigger quiet. This was only reinforced through my sense that the device did offer direct access to my brain: I cannot help feeling that if I breathe at this rate and attend to the weight of my hands in my lap, perhaps I'll hear a bird chirp. To be sure, this is my own subjective experience of the device, and Muse's market success suggests that others have an entirely different relationship with it. But the structures of the Muse app and headband can potentially encourage or exacerbate the impulse to allow attention to drift away from the body, particularly when one becomes fixated on the point-based system or specifically aims to "improve" their practice over time (Fig. 17).

Indeed, the point-based system becomes the primary way of reflecting on past meditation experiences. The profile section features a bar graph documenting the individual's meditation history, which can be switched to show the ratio of calm to active brain activity or Muse points to minutes spent in the session. Selecting an individual meditation reveals a graph showing fluctuations in brain waves as they oscillate between calm and active, providing a point breakdown, awards, and below, any notes on the session. The points statistics reflect the number of minutes spent meditating; "recoveries," the movement from active to neutral brain activity, which "represent[s] effort spent noticing your distractions"; and total "birds" that chirp "when you're calm for a long time." Immediately following a meditation session, the interface provides an overview of the session and offers the user a degree of satisfaction through the graph that shows how the fluctuation of brainwaves and rewards them with points. "Calm" appears more concrete when quantified and visualized through a color-coded graph. Moreover, if you didn't earn many bird points, the reveal of the recovery points may ease your worries (which was often the case for my low-scoring sessions). Ideally, individuals improve these statistics over time, through the support of weekly "goals" and "challenges." Each week the app sets a goal for the time spent meditating, while challenges help reinforce habitual practices. For example, the "Level 4 Challenge"

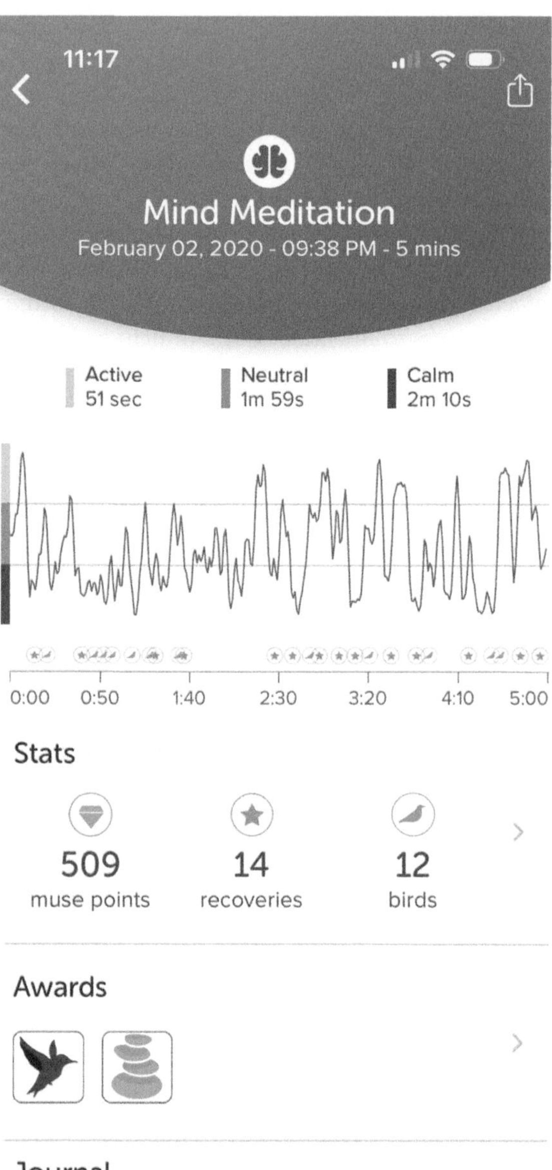

Fig. 17. The result screens for Muse meditation sessions. The left shows a session when I struggled hard to accumulate points, resulting in a low score. The right shows sessions where I read a novel, resulting in a significantly higher score. (Interaxon, "Muse: Meditation and Sleep," vers. 23.5, accessed February 2020.)

asks the individual to meditate on two days in a row at "around the same time of day." Push notifications can be tailored to support these practices, either by setting a reminder for a specific time of day, or providing a nudge when data hasn't been recorded for some time. The goal and challenge structure helps regulate meditation practice and create an archive of data that are comparable and can be tracked over time. Through this structure, meditation is meant to become habitual and satisfying ("tangible") via the accumulation of points and improved data statistics.

Like the point-based systems of Breathesync and Spire, Muse's emphasis on improvement situates meditation in the logic of wellness. While Benson and Kippler's relaxation response similarly invoked the framework of preventative healthcare, it relied on an individual's phenomenological perception of well-being. The benefits were not located in test results, data, or visualization; it was felt in daily experiences compared over time. Individuals may have tracked their daily moods and energy levels, but these qualitative methods did not come with the support of what is perceived as hard scientific data. Instead, they were forced to rely on their own embodied experience to gauge the effects of breathing and meditation. By mediating mindfulness, breathing and meditation technologies appear to train individuals not to listen to their bodies, but to learn from their data: it is not my sense perception that tells me I'm well, but a number or graphic. Indeed, as I discussed in the previous chapter, fitness wearables have been criticized for radically undermining human experience by encouraging people to meet universalized numerical goals rather than attending to the restrictions and affordances of their bodies. Thus, one might argue that meditation and breathing technologies similarly participate in the return to rationalization, reinforcing the division between mind and body.

Drawing on scientific studies on neurofeedback, Muse compares its methods to "physical therapy for the mind." (Indeed, you may compare my systematic attempts to trigger a calm state of mind akin to learning proper form.) I am admittedly new to meditation and do not necessarily ascribe to its principles, but the relationship between quiet and a "calm" state of mind suggested by the Muse's soundscape triggered frustration, often aimed at my own body. The constant struggle to focus on breathing, without *thinking* about breathing (which I found only increased rainfall) made me feel as though I had little control over my mind. Or as my attention shifted to my body, I would grow increasingly frustrated by my inability to relax certain facial muscles or tension in my neck and shoulders, and I would have moments when my body felt like an obstinate obstacle to overcome.

While one might argue that these experiences demonstrate a distancing between body and mind by framing them as objects that can be controlled through conditioning and data collection, these technologies do manage to produce encounters that complicate such a reading. Following Benson, Kippler, and Freldman's attention to the psychosomatic effects of meditation, feelings and experiences that fall outside of the biomedical framework promoted by the device need to be considered. Though I often felt a sense that my body was out of my control, or a constant struggle to take hold of my thoughts, the physical presence of the headband and sonic biofeedback did create a novel form of attention to my body.

As I moved through a meditation session, I often became hyperaware of the pressure of the headband against my forehead and of the micromovements in my facial muscles that may affect the reading. While I know the three sensors across the front of the band are measuring electronic brain waves, the weight and texture of the metal device made it feel as though any twitch, crease, or pinched facial expression could alter the soundscape. In reality, these movements could only cause the sensors to become dislodged from my skin and disrupt the session, but their physical presence combined with the audio feedback often created the sense of a correlation between facial movements and sonic intensity. And though those movements may not influence the reading, they were often indirect indicators of stress or anxiety. The harder I concentrated on my breath, the more I could feel the skin of my forehead contract, my eye muscles squeeze tighter, and my jaw clench. It then would become a test of relaxing the small muscles in my face, which would often trigger a new rush of rain or wind. In other words, attempts to calm the soundscape resulted in increased attention to subtle shifts in my body.

This attention to the body perhaps did not trigger the relaxation response or encourage the traditional meditation practice that emphasizes present, mindful reflection. At the same time, the headband did not alienate me from my body, abstract my experience of meditation into pure data, or subsume my understanding of my health into the preventative framework of wellness. My experience with Muse, rather, demonstrates the complexity of these biofeedback and quantitative methods concerning the experience of the body. Whether this experience exemplifies the unification of mind and body is open to question, but it also does not necessarily reinforce the pure abstraction of the body seen in biomedical models of preventative health and wellness.

From Well-Being to Feeling Health

To understand the experience I describe above, I end by turning to philosophical discussions of health and embodiment. My experience with Muse certainly does not produce the calming, stress-reduction benefits commonly attached to meditation and breathing exercises. But at the same time, the device and quantified feedback system did create novel attunements to the microshifts in my muscles and the sense of the relationship between device and body. As I attempted to meditate with Muse, I did become increasingly aware of my body's movements, boundaries, and borders. Turning to phenomenological descriptions of my experience using Apple Watch's Mindfulness app, I begin to question whether such moments can be understood as the *feeling* of health. While breathing and meditation apps reinforce quantified frameworks from biomedicine and wellness discourse, descriptions reveal how bodily reflexivity can actually be encouraged *through* technological mediation and datafication.[102] I suggest that these moments can perhaps be understood as moments of feeling the health of the body in the present, an account of health not as an existential goal or biostatistical metric, but perhaps as a direct experience of the body itself.

I have used Fitbit's Alta and Apple Watch for more than seven years to track my daily activities. As I discussed in the previous chapter, though I approach these devices as objects of study, over time they have become enfolded into my ordinary experience of the world and have become critical structural devices that, in part, shape my daily movements and behaviors. I primarily use them to monitor exercise goals and validate activity efforts, but the feedback and notification features have also become ambient vibrations that populate my daily routine.

As with a text message or activity reminder, the Apple Watch provides a gentle pulse against the wrist to prompt a breathing exercise. Individuals can customize the duration, frequency, and notification protocol for the breathing exercises to accommodate their schedules, or use the app to mark the beginning or end of a day. Once an hour, I feel a gentle pulse on my wrist. Unlike some of the other technologies discussed in this chapter, Apple Watch does not use quantification techniques to monitor the number of inhalations and exhalations or to suggest a target heart rate: it's merely the challenge of coordinating technology and action.[103] As I tilt my watch toward my gaze, the Mindfulness app icon appears and reminds me to "take a minute to breathe." Selecting the duration of my breathing exercise—anywhere from one to five minutes—I hit "start" to begin the session. A black screen appears with a small, blue dot at the center, and instructions emerge at the bottom of the screen: "Be still and bring your attention to your breath. Now inhale . . ." The blue circle radiates outward, transforming into six overlapping spheres that resemble a flower. As the graphic fills the screen, the watch pulses against my wrist in a series of short, rapid vibrations. "Exhale" appears, the vibrations pause, and the flower shrinks back into the center of the screen. This pattern repeats seven times for one minute, and I try to sync my breath to the pulses and graphics. My gaze focuses on the expanding circles and I concentrate on linking my breath to the haptic feedback of the watch. In these moments my attention shifts from the exterior world to the relationship between image, vibration, and breath. The session ends with congratulations—"well done"—and summarizes my efforts with a reading of my pulse and the number of minutes I spent breathing.

As someone who practices yoga and frequently swims for exercise, I have learned to closely monitor my breathing. However, these fitness-related activities focus on the coordination of movement and breath. I find that my attention to my breath in these situations often serves as an endurance tactic: focused, even breathing can help me hold a balance pose longer or complete a set of laps. But the Mindfulness app's exercises offer a markedly different type of encounter, which I find much more challenging than any fitness-induced practice because it forces me to concentrate on my body and mental state. Whereas breath helped *distract* my mind from my body during exercise—to think of inhalations and exhalations instead of the burning sensation in my muscles and lungs—breathing with my Apple Watch forces me to attend to the sensation of the device vibrating against my wrist and to my feeble attempts to "quiet" my mind. It is hard to say whether my experience is akin to "mindfulness" in the terms discussed in meditation practices or *The Relaxation Response*, but I can attest to the way these practices shift my attention to the present encounter between body and technology. Especially over prolonged use of the app, these breathing practices offered a brief shift in physical and mental attention that felt radically distinct from my everyday habits. If anything, they could be compared to the feeling of "zoning out," or a radical inattention to the world around me. But these moments are filled not with daydreams or distracting thoughts, but with a kind of hypnotic experience of visual and haptic stimulation.

Put another way, breathing with my Apple Watch created moments of attunement to my body's relationship to technology. In his reading of fitness wearables, James Gilmore argues that the quantitative systems of self-tracking can prompt individuals to "re-experience" the "everyday escapes," or the "taken-for-grantedness of everyday movement."[104] The combination of visual and haptic feedback combined with efforts to breathe in coordination with the device created moments of reexperiencing my breath and body's present state. My attention was drawn to the quality of the vibrations, the feeling of air pulled in through my nostrils, and the difference in temperatures between the watch and my skin. In those moments, I found myself *noticing* the small-scale movements, efforts, and qualities of my body in space and time. I felt the weight of my arm as it holds up the watch face to my gaze, the dull pulse of the device against my wrist, and the expansion of my chest as I inhaled and exhaled.

Such experiences can perhaps be compared to what Iris Marion Young describes as an "aesthetic" relationship to the body in her phenomenology of pregnancy. She recounts how the expansion of the body's borders caused her to examine and attend to her body's shifting shape and sensations as she moved through space. This form of attunement is akin to a "splitting" of the self where the body appears as both a part of the self and an object of aesthetic reflection. However, for Young, this split of the self is not a form of self-alienation, but instead a "pleasure" of noticing that "does not divert me from my business."[105] While my experience of bodily attunement with my Apple Watch was not the product of any physical changes in my body, I find Young's use of the term "aesthetic" to be a useful source of comparison. Breathing with Apple Watch led to moments when I would take stock or notice the points of contact, I felt in my body the material weight, and textures of my body, as though it were an object. Like Young, I did not find that this splitting the self resulted in judging my body or in self-alienation, but instead in a momentary taking-in of the body in the world.

I want to suggest that such moments of bodily reflexivity can be compared to a phenomenology of health itself. Often defined as a state of equilibrium, health is understood as the absence of disruption, which makes it incredibly difficult to describe and discern it as a phenomenological state. Gadamer describes health as an "enigma, that 'does not present itself to us,' which only reveals itself in its absence, during illness."[106] But both Gadamer and Svenaeus insist, in somewhat idealistic terms, that despite the hidden nature of health, one can still "feel healthy." Contrary to homeostatic models of health, Gadamer describes it as "a general feeling of well-being. It shows itself above all where such a feeling of well-being means we are open to new things, ready to embark on new enterprises, and forgetful of ourselves, scarcely noticing the remains and strains which are put upon us."[107] In an attempt to clarify and provide greater specificity, Svenaeus characterizes health as a "background attunement, a rhythmic, balancing mood that supports our understanding in a homelike way without caring for our attention."[108] Drawing on Martin Heidegger's theory of being as a "homelike being-in-the-world," Svenaeus argues that health can be understood as the "the way a human being finds its place in the world as a meaning pattern—a being-*in*-the-world. Health is thus not a question of a passive state but rather an active process—*a balancing*."[109] Radically distinct from the preventative definition of health in wellness, Svenaeus considers health to be a position toward the world—"not a state that one feels *in* oneself," or something one possesses, but comportment to the world that can incite action. Breathing with Apple Watch disrupted my daily routine, and forced a momentary reorganization of perception to focus on the present state of my body encountering technology. This pause could be compared to Svenaeus' "active process" of balancing health, one that encourages a shift from unconscious habit to attending to the body's relationship to the world around us.

When breathing with Apple Watch, I felt moments when my body's coordination with the world and technology came to the front of my consciousness, a feeling of "balancing" the physical sensations of my body as it breathes with the technologies and conditions that surround me. Ironically, by way of technology and quantification, one can perhaps achieve this embodied state. While I hesitate to map my singular experience of the Mindfulness app onto a phenomenology of health, Svenaeus and Gadamer offer a way to understand the moments when digital health technologies produce experiences of attunement toward the body and world. Like Muse, the Mindfulness app creates a momentary departure from my relationship with the surrounding environment and my relationship with my body. By disrupting the normative patterns of mental and physical attention that structure my day in favor of attending to an otherwise unnoticed autonomic function, the Apple Watch asks me to *consider* my body. The aesthetics are essential to this process, providing qualitative and quantitative visual and haptic feedback to make the breathing exercises feel "tangible." While my experience of bodily reflexivity is tied to technology—not simply myself as being-in-the-world—the state I describe resembles "a rhythm" of active engagement with my body. For me, this experience is not necessarily comparable to the "benefits" of meditation: I do not feel "calmer" or even a more positive disposition to the world, but it does create a structure of disruption that draws attention to my breath and body at rest. The aesthetics and quantified structures of the app do not replace my lived experience but instead provide a structure that prompts reflection on the feeling of my body being-in-the-world—a feeling of perhaps health itself.

While breathing and meditation technologies' interfaces and design features undoubtedly promote preventative health and wellness models, description shows moments that resist or fall out of the biomedical frameworks they promote. In her Foucaultian study of practices of self-normalization, Cressida Heyes argues that resistance to disciplinary structures requires both experiences of bodily reflexivity and normalization. Attending to the feeling of normalization alongside what she calls "somatic" practices that "permit an openness to becoming without micromanaging our identities" creates a context in which individuals can actively reflect on and understand the embodied impact of disciplinary structures.[110] Descriptions of breathing and meditation technologies reveal experiences of normalization through datafication, but also moments that escape and exceed the structures of the device. In the next chapter, I continue to develop the concept of "feeling health" to question whether digital health technologies may be capable of generating encounters where the normalized body and reflexive body are sensed and experienced alongside one another. Description helps generate an account of digital health that acknowledges how the biomedical structures of health are felt alongside moments of hyper-attunement and bodily awareness, perhaps creating the conditions for critique, consciousness, and resistance to the quantified norms they promote.

CHAPTER 5

Bodies in Action

Measuring Movement and Intensity

I tap the "Fitness" icon on my phone screen's bottom left side. As the app opens, the small graphic on the right showing three concentric rings begins to fill in with color. The red, green, and blue shading indicates my progress toward my daily goals, which is shown in statistical form to the left. With a quick upward swipe of my thumb across the surface of the screen, the app scrolls down to reveal a section titled "Trends." Two columns list various fitness data, ranging from "Cardio Fitness" to "Stand Minutes" and "Running Pace." Each category includes a small up or down arrow on the right and a statistic below. Most of my arrows point down, indicating that my averages have fallen over time. I click the "Show more" button at the top of the list and a new screen appears, breaking down my behaviors into two categories: "Keep it going" and "Worth a look." I skim over the "Worth a look" section, taking in the abstract numbers: "873 cal/day," "114 min/day," and "9 min/hr." My eyes pause on the "873," tracking downward to the small gray text below that suggests a higher calorie burn goal: "If you can stay on track it should take about 8 weeks to flip your arrow up, Mikki." Taking in this information and looking at the list of worsening stats, I feel my shoulders tense as I project into the future, imagining the actions, types of exercise, and energy it would take for me "stay on track."

In 2019, with the iOS 13 update, Apple added a "Trends" section to the Fitness app to allow users to analyze long-term activity patterns.[1] The app tracks statistics for the last ninety days of activity and provides tips on how to improve statistics over time (Fig. 18). "Trends" is designed to encourage individuals to reflect on their health vitals and activity archives and make subsequent changes to "improve" their future health and well-being. In line with the ideology of preventative health, Apple's upgrade reinforces the idea that historical data should be used to imagine and promote a "healthier" version of the self. Within this framework, the present state of the body is displaced in favor of the quantified efforts of the past and the projected numbers for a future, healthy numerical goal. The "Trends" section of the app thus falls in line with many of the technologies described throughout this book that emphasize the use of data and improvement over how an individual feels or experiences their body. But what happens to the body when quantification is meant to prompt reflection on *present* actions or activities? How does real-time data feedback affect one's sense of being a body, or having a body? How does this experience shape an individual's perception of being a healthy body moving through the world?

Critiques of quantification and self-tracking have long emphasized how these devices objectify the body by translating the embodied present into an archive of numbers to be analyzed later.[2] The data archives come to stand in as substitutions for the self, numbers and statistics used in pursuit of health. Of course, this reflective structure for understanding health is not unique to digital health technologies. Philosophers and sociologists of medicine have demonstrated how all individual assessments of health (and identity in general) require a temporary objectification of the body. Or as Nick Crossley and Drew Leder have argued, bringing the body into consciousness requires a perspectival shift from the "I" of immediate experience to the externalized "me."[3] In other words, an assessment of whether I am healthy requires me to think back on *my* body and behaviors. The shift from the present "I" to the external "me" requires the objectification of my body as I shift my attention to a reflective view of my bodily past.[4] Assuming this exterior perspective (and the exterior perspective of others) is essential to understanding our identity,[5] and by extension our health. The danger thus lies not necessarily in the act of objectification itself, but in relying on exterior interpretations of the body—"me"—*and* disassociating this perspective from my bodily sensations.[6] In the case of wearable fitness trackers like Apple Watch and Fitbit, the problem emerges when an individual locates the "me" exclusively in the data sets and statistics—the "Trends" data, for example—rather than in their embodied experiences.

The split between the "I" and "me" in understanding health and the body contributes to the problem of defining health as a present state rather than a condition only recognized when reflecting on its absence. As I dis-

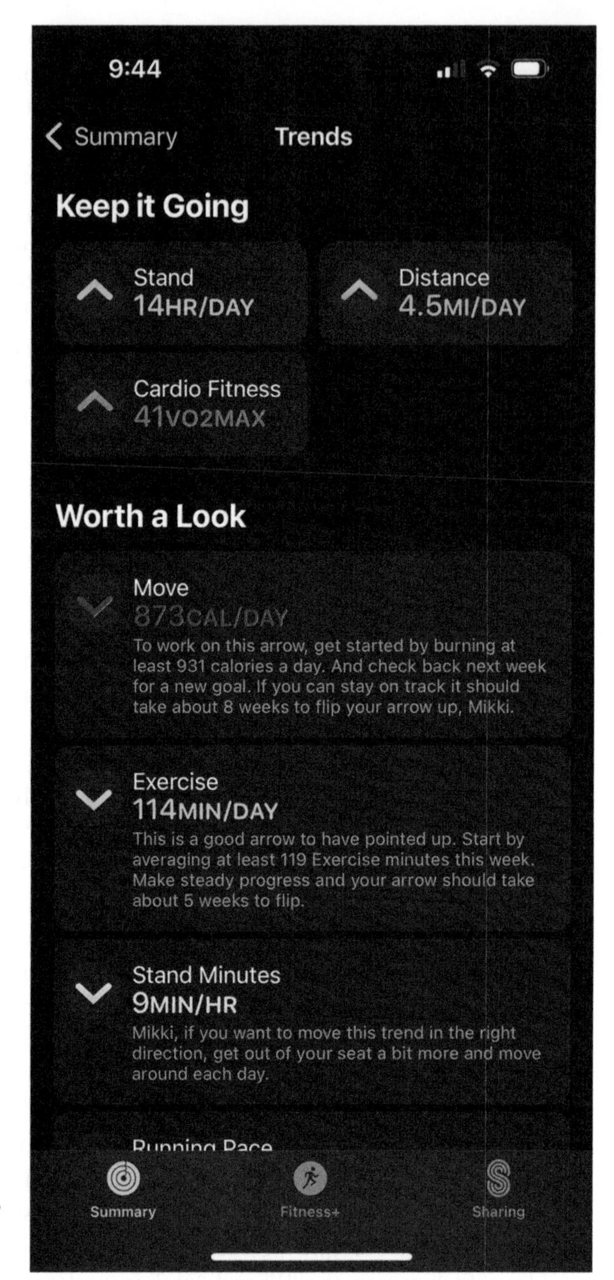

Fig. 18. The "Trends" section of the Apple "Activity" app that summarizes historical data and offers tips to improve. (Apple, "Activity," vers. 13.5.1, accessed January 2023.)

cussed in the previous chapter, health is most often understood as a neutral or unnoticed state, defined negatively as the absence of disease. Leder's influential early work in the phenomenology of medicine has shown that the body ostensibly remains absent in health, going as far as to claim that "in the case of health, the body is alien by virtue of its disappearance, as attention is primarily directed toward the world."[7] In illness or injury, the body "dys-appears," coming into consciousness through pain and discomfort.[8] When this pain is read through medical and scientific frameworks, the ill body is then often interpreted as alien and beyond the individual's control.[9] Drawing on Jean-Paul Sartre, Leder extends his theory to include the "social dys-appearance" of the body to describe how the objectifying look of "the Other" can similarly encourage awareness of the body.[10] For example, he describes the clinical encounter with the physical exam as an example of "social dys-appearance by technical means." Due to unequal power dynamics, the exterior view of the physician brings the body into awareness and encourages the individual to scrutinize themself as an object.[11] This structure could be extended to many digital health technologies, where datafication could cause the body to dys-appear as the revelation of numbers brings the body into consciousness, but is then interpreted through the objectifying lens of statistical analysis and quantification. For example, the "move" statistic reveals that I've failed to increase the number of calories I burn per day. This average could cause me to step back and examine my body and behaviors over the last few weeks and use the Apple Watch's quantified, improvement-based system to interpret my body as "bad" or "lacking."

As I describe, this structure, where the body appears and triggers reflection, is what leaves the body vulnerable to interpretation by universalist statics and metrics. However, self-reflection is neither stable nor static, but rather an ongoing process wherein the body continually emerges as an object with every attempt to evaluate the body—"me."[12] As I demonstrated in chapter 3, wearable fitness trackers often create uneven experiences and encounters with a body that resists generalized critiques of alienation and objectification. Leder's reading of the absent and dys-appearing body helps illustrate how structures of self-reflection open up space alienation and objectification, but also permit revaluation and resistance to the corporate emphasis on productivity and improvement. In other words, the appearance of the body is *always* a potential site of alienation and/or sensuous self-reflection. In the case of smartwatches and other wearable fitness trackers, the appearance of the data archive often generates the appearance of the body, but the historically determined statistical and goal-based structures of the app may encourage self-alienation.

However, I want to consider the status of the body when it appears *during* exercise or activity with digital health technologies. This chapter examines technologies that provide real-time visual, haptic, and auditory feedback and their impact on an individual's immediate sense of their body. I focus on the Moov wearable fitness trainer, Sensoria smart sock, UPRIGHT GO posture wearable, and Orangetheory Fitness heart rate monitor, which are designed to help individuals make in-the-moment adjustments to their form, exercise intensity, and bodily comportment. These devices claim to reveal inaccessible physiological processes, including physical exertion and precise muscular movements, to help individuals improve their form, efficiency, and overall "health." I begin by describing my experience with Orangetheory Fitness and high-intensity interval training (HIIT) to illustrate how quantification and self-tracking through wearable devices are used to navigate the experiential and philosophical problem of measuring "intensity" and "exertion." Placing descriptions of the visual feedback provided through Orangetheory's connected heart rate monitors alongside the philosophy and history of the Rate of Perceived Exertion (RPE) scale used in kinesthesiology and fitness research to measure intensity, I demonstrate how the technological structures of the fitness class privilege numbers over bodily sensation. While Orangetheory's feedback system may lead individuals to self-alienate, the RPE scale's emphasis on small changes in bodily sensation suggests that quantification doesn't universally produce such interpretations of the body. I use this idea to explore how quantification may be used to encourage embodied reflexivity by turning to running and posture wearables, which are designed to track subtle movements and bodily adjustments. Through phenomenological descriptions of Moov, Sensoria smart socks, and UPRIGHT GO, I analyze how haptic and auditory feedback structures can attune individuals to their bodies. I argue that this technologically mediated attention to bodily movements can reveal the "feeling of health" I began to describe in the previous chapter. Building on positive phenomenological definitions of health, I suggest that attending to the phenomenology of digital health can reveal how technologies allow individuals to perhaps access the experience of health as a sense of "homelike being-in-the-world," or the embodied sensation of the body being "in tune" with the world.

This mode of attunement to the relationship between the body and the surrounding world has been described through phenomenologies of athletes' experiences. Activities such as dance, running, and scuba diving all require careful attention to bodily sensations and the world. Through a focus on breathing, heartbeat, or movements, the body may appear and require subsequent adjustments or merely affirm its physical efforts.[13] Much of this research has remained focused on experienced and elite athletes who have the bodily knowledge and skill to create micro-adjustments to muscles, precise movements, and breathing patterns. But for those without years of training and coaching, careful attention to form may prove challenging. It's unlikely that a novice runner has the bodily knowledge or proprioception to control and adjust the angle of their arm or the swing of their leg to cut through wind resistance or release tension in their back. Similarly, to a new participant without experience in gauging intensity during exercise, HIIT's focus on working at specific exertion levels aligned with heart rate zones can prove challenging or opaque. Digital health technologies use quantification to overcome these barriers of expertise and experience through visual, auditory, and haptic feedback. Phenomenological descriptions of running and posture wearables show how these technologies may be capable of attuning individuals to their bodily sensations and their embodied movements through the world.

This isn't to say that any of the technologies described in this chapter increase athletic or physical ability. But phenomenological description can show how they may create encounters with the sensation of the lived body as it moves through the world. As I discussed in the previous chapter, quantification and feedback may be used to draw attention to bodily sensation and can thus help us understand moments of heath as a present state of "balancing." I build on this discussion of health by considering technologies that foreground the relationship between the body *and* the world. Through audio feedback, running wearables draw an individual's attention to incredibly specific movements and patterns, such as landing pressure or the cadence of their steps as their body navigates changing environments throughout a run. Efforts to adjust their behaviors based on feedback require careful attention not only to their body but to their environment: the texture of the terrain, the temperature, and the humidity of the air as they modify their pace. This mode of attention resembles a phenomenological understanding of health that includes the sensorial relationship between bodies and environments, a feeling of "homelike being-in-the-world." While this sense of the body and world continually recedes, Frederik Svenaeus argues that health may be accessible through a focused "attention upon the way you are *in* the world as taking place in meaningful context."[14] This definition aims to move away from homeostatic definitions of health to describe the "characteristics" of health as an experience and to develop a richer vocabulary to describe the dynamic sensations of this ephemeral attunement to the balancing of the body in the world. This chapter participates in this project, building a descriptive vocabulary for how technology may open up encounters with the sensation of health as a present, lived encounter between the body and environment.

"Make Your Body the Sexiest Outfit You'll Ever Own"

—Words of encouragement found on the walls of Orangetheory Fitness studios

Since 2014, high-intensity interval training (HIIT) has been ranked as one of the most popular fitness trends by the American College of Sports Medicine.[15] Following the publication of numerous scientific studies on weight loss and health benefits, HIIT has exploded through apps, online guides and books, and fitness classes. Unlike other fitness crazes such as Pilates, yoga, or cycling, HIIT is not confined to a particular sport or type of exercise. Rather, HIIT is a method of working out geared toward pushing your heart rate into intensity-specific zones. These workouts typically oscillate between short periods of high-intensity work and recovery, aimed to repeatedly spike the heart rate and bring it back down throughout the training. HIIT workouts have been celebrated for their efficiency, with studies showing that ten to twenty minutes of interval training can produce all of the health benefits of a more traditional endurance workout, such as biking or running.[16] While interval training has been practiced by athletes for nearly 100 years, scientific studies of oxygen absorption and muscle fatigue have helped regulate the exercise method, setting clear heart rate zones and ratios between work and rest.[17] The latest research suggests that intervals should push heart rate to at least 80% of max capacity, or "near maximum capacity," to receive the full benefits of the exercise.

While scientific studies emphasize the importance of specific heart rate zones, exercise guides and books have translated these interval ranges into descriptions of "intensity." "Maximum effort" and "80% effort" are gauged through descriptive vocabulary or analogies designed to train the individual to indirectly perceive the heart rate percentage. For example, authors may use tests—an individual should not be able to sustain a conversation while working—or hypothetical scenarios: "Your legs and lungs should be burning, and if someone offered to pay you $100,000 to go for 10 more seconds, you wouldn't do it."[18] Most instructions are based on the Rate of Perceived Exertion (RPE) scale, or a 1–10 rating scale developed to gauge an individual's perception of bodily fatigue during exercise. Developed by Swedish researcher Gunnar Borg in the 1960s, RPE is used across scientific and sociological studies of fitness and movement and has become the standard for measuring exercise experiences in adult populations.[19] Borg's 1–10 scale aims to measure the range of physical, biological, and psychological stimuli that affect an individual's sense of bodily fatigue and endurance. The subjective rating scale runs from 1, indicating no work or exertion, to 10, maximum exertion. Updated versions of the Borg scale couple the rating system with markers of duration—"feels like you can maintain for hours"—and various bodily cues, such as "short of breath" and "unable to talk."[20] Though the connection between Borg's numerical scale and heart rate has never been firmly established, the rating system is meant to roughly correspond to heart rate capacity.[21] For example, if one is working at an "8," their heart rate should be approximately 80% of their maximum heart rate.

While the RPE scale ostensibly allows individuals to indirectly access their heart rate percentage through reflection on bodily sensations, reading and rating those sensations requires practice and the acquisition of bodily knowledge. Though it may be easy to perceive the difference between "light" and "moderate" intensity, or a 3 and 6 on the RPE scale, it becomes much more challenging to determine the threshold between a 7 and 8, or the necessary boundary to cross to maximize an HIIT interval. The RPE scale provides a quantitative means for measuring intensity, but it ultimately relies on the subjective interpretation of exertion by individuals. Only through repeated training combined with active reflection on bodily sensation does one begin to learn to discern the boundaries between numerical structures of the scale. And though over time an individual may begin to be able to quantify their intensity levels, these measurements and assessments of intensity are by no means universal or even consistent.

One solution to the problem of assessing intensity levels during exercise has been the integration of wearable monitors that allow individuals immediate access to precise readings of their heart rate. Studies on intensity and heart rate monitoring have shown that individuals struggle to gauge heart rate based on perceived intensity, often over- or undershooting their target goals. For example, in a study conducted in 2009, participants remarked on how the integration of heart rate monitors into their exercise routines revealed that they were often working too hard, associating difficulty with a target heart rate zone. Indeed, several participants described how relying on the sensorial perception of "high intensity" led them to overexert themselves:

> I didn't think unless I was sweating, or unless I was working really, really hard at working out, then I wouldn't reach my goals. But then I realized, what am I doing? And, with the heart rate monitor, it was just like, okay you're killing yourself here. You're not supposed to be in the 200s.
>
> Before I had a heart rate monitor, I would train just as hard as I could. My heart would be working so fast that I would have to stop because I felt like I was about the pass out. So now with the heart rate monitor, I'm just like, okay, I have to stay within this interval.[22]

Both of these accounts demonstrate how sensorial cues such as sweat, pacing, and muscle fatigue do not necessarily correspond to perceived exertion and heart rate interval. The integration of the wearable devices compensated for the lack of bodily understanding, allowing participants to shift their intensity levels accordingly and reach target heart rate goals. While the 2009 study examined a relatively small population, the responses illustrate the popular conception that by offering real-time readings of vitals, connected heart rate monitors can help individuals "control" their exertion levels and target specific intensity intervals. Indeed, most smartwatches and wearable fitness trackers with screens have integrated in-the-moment heart rate features into the exercise programs and tracking features to support training such as HIIT.[23]

Orangetheory Fitness, a popular boutique exercise studio, has made heart rate monitoring during interval training the core of their exercise program. The company opened its first studio in 2010 and has since expanded to over 1,100 studios across forty-nine states and twenty countries, and it is now valued at over $1 billion.[24] The company claims to have more than a million members, with a target market of middle- and upper-middle-class individuals; pricing packages range from $59 a month to upward of $159 depending on the number of sessions and studio location.[25] The exercise studio distinguishes itself through its connected fitness program, which has individuals wear heart rate monitors in the form of wristbands and chest straps. Visual feedback on screens located across the studio provides visual feedback on their intensity and heart rate zones. Orangetheory's "science-backed, technology-tracked" system is meant to ensure that individuals reach their target zones to "maximize" the benefits of HIIT.[26] During the hour-long class, individuals move between treadmills, rowing machines, and weight exercises, striving to push their heart rates into the "orange zone," or 84% to 91% of maximum heart rate. Rather than relying on a ten-point scale, Orangetheory breaks down intensity into five color-coded heart rate zones and instructs members to aim to work primarily in the green, orange, and red zones throughout the class. For every minute spent in the orange and red zones, members earn a "splat point," with the goal of accumulating at least twelve by the end of the class to trigger the "excess post-oxygen consumption," more commonly known as "afterburn," which supposedly causes your body to continue burning calories for the next thirty-six hours.[27]

The numerical, color-coded system, coupled with heart rate monitoring, claims to solve the problem of ambiguity in HIIT and RPE scale assessment. Offering a heart rate percentage on-screen supposedly lets individuals "know" whether they are working at a 7 or 8, or in the green versus the orange zone. Promotional materials and articles on Orangetheory stress how this system helps eliminate the "guesswork" of exercise to get "the ultimate health benefits." By tracking "every calorie, every splat point gained, every heart beat counted, every second in every color zone," individuals can supposedly better understand and control their progress. In other words, the data are essential to the claimed health benefits of the program: "Can we predict the physiological benefits [of exercise]? You can't if you don't have the data."[28]

Though my Apple Watch can provide similar real-time readings of heart rate, accessing this information is challenging because it requires me to lift my wrist and glance at the tiny numbers on the screen. For example, if I'm completing a set of jumping jacks and would like to check my heart rate, it would require me to lower my hand to my face, attempt to stabilize its position as I continue the movement, squint at the interface, and try to discern the zone in the list of real-time statistics counted on the screen. By contrast, Orangetheory's studio of screens supposedly allows me to see fluctuations in my heart rate as I push through a 300-meter row or complete a three-minute run. To cue individuals to work within specific heart rate zones, the class uses three pace levels, which roughly correspond to color-coded zones: "base pace" to target the green zone, "push" for the orange, and "all-out" for red.[29] Like HIIT intensity prompts, these pacing zones remain relatively ambiguous and hard to decipher. However, coupled with the heart rate system, I can hypothetically begin to learn my unique speed for each pacing prompt. For example, using the visual feedback data on the screen during a run, I might set a "push pace" at 7.0 on the treadmill, only to find that my screen remains green. With a tap, I may increase my speed and watch to see whether the screen turns orange. This immediate feedback can be useful for making adjustments in the middle of short intervals: as I push my feet back during a row, I can look up and see if I need to use a bit more force on the next pull, or I might settle into a steady pace only to discover that my heart rate has dropped back down to the green zone, prompting me to push harder and drive my heart rate up.

Navigating an Orangetheory class requires constant adjustment to bodily movements, machines, and intensity, and the heart rate monitors become an essential way to ground changes in movement and pacing.[30] As a newcomer to HIIT, I lack the reflexive awareness of my body to be able to assess or measure my physical exertion. For example, as I struggle to lift my feet against the backward pull of the treadmill belt, my shoulders hunched and arms swinging in time with my short rapid steps, I can hardly catch my breath. How could I possibly take a moment to consider where my physical and mental state falls along a ten-point scale, or use that number to assess whether I'm reaching my target heart rate? In those moments, all I can think about is surviving the interval: can I manage the next deep breath, or keep my body upright as I wipe the sweat from my forehead? While all of these physical sensations could be used to rate my level of intensity, they do not necessarily map onto a discernable, quantifiable breakdown of my heart rate zones, particularly when I'm caught up in the action of running. However, in an Orangetheory class, I can look up at my screen and watch my number increase as my heart beats faster, feeling the satisfaction of seeing the screen transform from orange to red, indicating that I've reached my "9."

While this may indeed ensure that I reach specific target heart rate zones in pursuit of the "ultimate health benefits" of HIIT, the numerical and color-coded visualizations provided by the screens are often at odds with my embodied experience of exercise during the class. Embodiment in exercise, particularly in group fitness classes, is often shaped by the intersection of social, physical, and emotional conditions that involve both inward reflections on the self and exterior pressures from coaches and fellow participants.[31] In other words, the perception of exercise intensity cannot be reduced to a single vital sign, but instead incorporates a range of physical, environmental, and social factors. The visual feedback on the screens may provide clear targets for pace and "exertion," but it can hardly account for the range of physical sensations I experience as I push through a sprint, or the exterior social pressures I may feel from my neighbor in the class. Though I may be working "hard" according to my heart rate percentage, this vital is only one of several markers of stress and exertion during exercise. Moreover, Orangetheory's classes are so rapidly paced and there is so much emphasis on gaining points and visual feedback that I often find myself forgetting form, straining against the pull of the treadmill as I tap up a level in pursuit of seeing that visual on-screen shift from orange to red. The brief interval periods combined with the emphasis on screens often undermine any reflection on proper running or rowing form, increasing the risk of strain or injury. While coaches periodically offer reminders about form or provide personal corrections during an interval, there is more often a focus on simply surviving: what will it take to reach the orange zone, and can I keep it up until the coach calls time?

Orangetheory concedes that the heart rate displays are often a source of distraction from the difficulty of the HIIT workout: "it keeps you informed but also maybe a little bit distracted."[32] I undoubtedly rely on these screens to keep my attention as I push through a workout. Much like music during exercise, the numbers on the screen can help me move past my body's natural inclination to slow down or stop. But the display consequently also often provides a distraction from the bodily adjustments and sensations that would help me gain the phenomenological awareness of my body that comes with prolonged athletic training and reflection on my physical exertion using the RPE scale. After focusing on the screen and numbers for a long period, I often noticed that I was slouching with my back curved and shoulders tense during a long row, or landing at an odd angle on my foot during a treadmill sprint. Even as I became more familiar with the class structure and pacing, the satisfaction of the quantified feedback was often at odds with small reflexive moments. For example, I found myself over-striding during "all-out" runs on the treadmill, well aware that I was throwing my foot forward with too much force, straining my knee, or landing too hard on my heel. Rather than using these embodied sensations to make adjustments to avoid injury, or to dwell in the rhythm and form of the movements, I found it hard to ignore the visual feedback on the screen and the desire to accumulate points.

Exercise programs and wearable fitness technologies often focus on competition with the self. Increasing distance or duration or reducing pace is framed as a battle to improve one's strength, speed, endurance, or ability. At Orangetheory, the relationship between competition and self-improvement is inextricably linked to data. Founder Ellen Latham argues that quantification is essential to improving health, and promotes the program's emphasis on datafication through slogans such as "guessing does not lead to greatness," or "what you cannot measure, you cannot improve."[33] Latham is referencing that many quantified fitness programs and wearable devices are invested in improving statistics over time as a marker of health and well-being. The focus on personalized heart monitors and a corresponding app where individuals can examine their progress (similar to the "Trends" feature in the Apple Fitness app) suggests that the focus on data analysis can be tailored to specific needs and goals. Indeed, the coaches and creators of Orangetheory stress that "fitness is not a one size fits all," claiming that their program is highly adaptable to levels of experience and health.[34] However, the structure of the class and the focus on heart rate zones do indeed constitute a "size," suggesting that the pursuit of quantifiable exertion levels can be prioritized over individual bodily sensations and the exercise form that keeps the body injury-free.

Because the company stresses data over the body, Orangetheory and other technological systems designed to work toward standardized heart rate zones tend to erase daily shifts in the subjective experience of exertion. My heart rate monitor cannot account for my tight hamstring muscle, the soreness from yesterday's run, or the tiredness I may feel from a restless night of sleep.[35] Rather, it holds me accountable for established numerical zones and an overall point-based goal. I can undoubtedly ignore the class parameters and adjust my exertion levels and focus on maintaining form, but the structures of the class make it incredibly challenging to ignore the numbers. Moreover, the ubiquity of screens surrounding me as I exercise makes the numbers almost impossible to ignore. It is easy to fall back on the quantified sources of distraction and visual feedback to help you push past the fatigue or ignore the twinge in your leg. In other words, Orangetheory's use of visual feedback and monitoring can encourage individuals to prioritize data over their embodied experience of exercise.

Orangetheory's connected heart rate program thus undermines the RPE measurement system, which is traditionally defined as the "*subjective* intensity of effort, strain, and/or fatigue that is felt during exercise."[36] As such, RPE can never technically provide the "objective" measurements or "scientific value" that Latham and Orangetheory promise. The data collected from the RPE scale will always retain a degree of subjectivity.

However, because of the emphasis on subjectivity, RPE is an example of a measurement system that favors individual experience over universalized statistics and numerical standards. While "intensity" is meant to be an indirect measure of physiological processes—such as heart rate—*measurement* of that intensity is located in the subjective interpretation of the embodied experience.

The emphasis on bodily attunement can be found in guides to HIIT workouts that attempt to describe the feeling of "maximum intensity" without relying on heart rate zones. Authors often point to the feeling of breath, sweat, or heat as an indicator of intensity: "You should be extremely breathless, your muscles should be burning, and you know mentally you can't push any harder."[37] A "9" or "10" or "maximum energy" thus becomes understood by carefully reading bodily sensations. Rating intensity is a process of careful and sustained attention to the body, an incredibly keen awareness of the small changes or shifts in temperature, breathing patterns, or muscle strain in a very short period of time. Gauging a HIIT interval using the RPE scale or the RPE method requires me to know the difference between a heavy labored breath and short bursts of air that burn the back of my throat—an indicator that I'm probably working too hard. I have to be able to find a careful balance between the fight against the weight of my legs or the burn of my muscles and the force of my foot during a sprint. While I may not actively think about each and every one of these elements throughout the interval, I am nonetheless forced to confront the range of bodily reactions and sensations in pursuit of a "9" or "10." Moreover, my sense of what a 9 or 10 feels like varies from day to day, affected by a range of behavioral and social conditions that influence my perception of exertion. With a focus on subjective reflection, the RPE scale can account for these shifting conditions.

Quantification is often cited as a source of self-alienation, as individuals attempt to fit their bodies and behaviors into numerical systems. However, RPE offers a counterexample of how a numerical system of self-evaluation can indeed draw attention to bodily sensations. In this respect, RPE resembles many of the epistemological and methodological concerns of the pain scale in medicine. As with "intensity," the pain scale aims to provide a quantified interpretation of a subjective body experience that cannot necessarily be reduced to a single, measurable physiological process: intensity cannot be reduced to heart rate, and likewise, pain cannot be reduced to a single vital sign or metric data point. Physicians, researchers, and philosophers have all grappled with how to communicate the deeply subjective experience of pain, particularly for diagnostic purposes.[38] Since the 1990s, the ten-point pain scale has become a standard measurement taken by most nurses and physicians along with traditional vitals, such as heart rate and blood pressure.[39] As with the RPE scale, patients are asked to reflect on their experience and rate their level of pain using a handful of linguistic cues. Evaluating pain requires careful attention to shifts in the quality and strength of sensations, and often asks individuals to localize the pain and track its frequency, rhythms, and changes. In other words, quantifying pain, much like quantifying intensity, encourages reflection on the lived experience of the body.

RPE and the pain scale may offer examples of how the act of self-quantification can allow individuals to become hyper-attuned to their bodies. However, the pain scale in the context of medicine creates a fundamentally different relationship between self and body. For Leder, pain is the most concrete example of how the body appears to our consciousness but often results in a negative interpretation of the body.[40] Rating pain does draw focused attention to the body, but when that number and the body are interpreted through the framework of biomedicine and the lens of illness, quantifying pain can lead to self-alienation.[41] For example, rating the pain one experiences in the abdomen may cause the body to appear, but interpreted as an illness it can cause an individual to see their body as the "enemy," an object at odds with the self. The RPE scale and reflections on intensity, by contrast, demonstrate a moment when the body appears not as an obstruction or "alien presence," but rather as a collection of bodily affects and sensations.[42] This encounter is facilitated by quantification, not suppressed by it, and indeed suggests that measurement systems can be essential catalysts for reminding us that I don't merely "have" a body, I "am" a body.[43]

Feedback on Form

Comparing Orangetheory and the RPE scale to one another, it is easy to assume that technology (not quantification) is responsible for self-alienation. The integration of wearable heart rate monitors and visual feedback effectively undermines the reflexive possibilities of HIIT and the RPE scale. Or, to put it another way, the exteriorization of heart rate through the wearable device and screens encourages a form of objectification that can lead to bodily alienation. In this sense, Orangetheory's use of wearables reinforces critiques of fitness that claim exercise frames the body as an aesthetic object through an emphasis on improvements to outward appearances and the exterior of the body.[44]

This ideology of fitness is reinforced in the marketing materials for just about any digital health technology that employs the language of exercise or "training." For example, the UPRIGHT GO posture wearable emphasizes the relationship between awareness, improvement, and appearance. Their website advertises that proper posture can make you appear taller, more confident, and slimmer: "upright posture pulls [your stomach] in, giving you the appearance of being inches taller and up to 10 pounds lighter! Who wouldn't want an instant tummy tuck?"[45] Drawing on the language of fitness, UPRIGHT GO describes how posture training and its benefits can affect one's outward appearance and by extension how one is perceived by others. The emphasis on looks and confidence in the marketing materials illustrates how training rhetoric often reinforces the objectification and optimization of the body through a focus on "health" results. In his analysis of the Lumo posture wearable, Brad Millington claims the device operates through "Silicon Valley Syndrome," where neoliberal values such as choice and optimization promote a highly individualized portrait of the "health benefits" of good posture.[46] But this focus on the "payoff" of exercise across all of these technologies overlooks the reflexive possibilities of these experiences.[47] By focusing exclusively on marketing campaigns and the proclaimed benefits and motivations for using technology, Millington argues that the sensations and experiences that are essential to understanding the body during exercises and interactions with these devices are supposedly lost.[48]

In this section, I turn toward the experience of posture and running wearables to examine how forms of technological quantification and feedback may indeed be used to encourage a hyper-attuned relationship to bodily sensations. Drawing on phenomenologies of sport, which have shown how exercise can encourage embodied reflexivity, I demonstrate how in-the-moment haptic and audio feedback can potentially attune individuals to their bodies and the sense of their bodies moving through the world. Like the RPE scale, these devices are used to draw attention to subtle shifts and adjustments in the body in pursuit of a better form and overall "health." Descriptions of these devices illustrate how quantification and technology do not necessarily determine self-alienation, but instead create a range of configurations of the body, self, and world that can bring sensation and embodiment to the fore.

The UPRIGHT GO posture wearable marketing campaign foregrounds the aesthetic benefits of good posture, but places equal emphasis on health and wellness.[49] The company links posture to spinal alignment, breathing, and stress relief:

> [G]ood posture isn't just about appearance and bodily health; it also contributes to overall wellbeing. When you walk with your spine straight and your shoulders back yet relaxed, you frequently look and feel more confident and poised. This has been shown to be linked with less stress, a more positive outlook, more energy, and more productivity at work and outside of the office.[50]

These "benefits" are the product of increased posture awareness that "helps balance your body alignment."[51] Through haptic feedback, the device aims to draw attention to the position of the body and trains individuals to stand and sit upright. Thus, for UPRIGHT GO, "health and wellness" are aligned with sensing the state of the body and the capacity to make small adjustments to the back and shoulders.

Like monitoring intensity and exertion zones, modifying posture requires a keen awareness of the back and shoulder muscles—a sense of how contracting certain parts can release tension or create support for the upper body. UPRIGHT GO uses a gyroscope to read body position and haptic feedback to supposedly help individuals learn to control their muscles. The small device is affixed to an individual's back, just between the shoulder blades, and monitors the angle of the body. When an individual moves outside of a small vertical range of motion, it vibrates to encourage them to adjust their back and shoulders accordingly. The pulsing vibrations emitted from the device bring awareness to the angle of the body and the back and shoulder muscles. The monitoring system begins with the "calibration" of the wearable, which is required with every use. After I affix the wearable to my back and open the app, I'm prompted to "set posture" with the click of a button, which triggers a series of short vibrations to signal that the device is adjusting its tracking features to the current upright position of my body.[52] The pulsing vibrations radiate between my shoulder blades, cueing me to lift my chest, relax my shoulders, and find a comfortable, straight position. Through trial and error, I've discovered that without properly settling into a comfortable upright position, the device will encourage me to sit and stand in positions that cause stress and tension in my shoulders and collarbone. For example, if I begin in a rigid posture, with my lower back caved slightly inward and my shoulders taut, I will have to endure a training session that continually encourages me to push my body back into this stiff and uncomfortable position. This initial phase establishes the baseline for "good" posture on which the remaining time spent wearing the device will be measured. Over time, I've had to learn how to set this initial position, to immediately settle my body into the back of my chair, and to angle my neck and shoulders so I can maintain the position for several hours as I read and write.

The calibration feature distinguishes UPRIGHT GO from other health and fitness wearables because it does not hold the body to universal quantified standards, but instead uses the individual's body as a baseline.[53] However, this is not to say that UPRIGHT GO can accommodate every body, nor is it endlessly customizable.[54] The narrow window for movement often makes it a nuisance to wear while moving or performing tasks. If I get up to grab a glass of water or prepare my lunch while wearing the device, I'm frequently met by irritating vibrations that pull my attention from my task to the technology. UPRIGHT GO cannot make adjustments for basic tasks that may require you to bend down or lean slightly: it reads every major displacement as a violation of "good posture."

Consequently, many times I've found myself frustrated with the device, tensing my shoulders as it vibrates when I lean forward to look closely at the screen or anxiously shift in my chair after sitting in front of my computer for several hours. If I am fatigued, antsy, or anxious, adhering to the structures of the device can feel too restrictive and exacerbate my stress rather than relieve it. However, this feeling is often related to the way it distracts me from the tasks at hand. UPRIGHT GO is marketed as a device to improve productivity by helping "you breathe deeper and more easily, increasing the flow of oxygen to your brain, and enabling you to stay sharp and focused."[55] But phenomenological description of my experiences with UPRIGHT GO shows how that focus is often on the body, or in some cases on the device itself. Hypothetically, over time, holding the body and carefully moving with the device will become unconscious as individuals learn how to sit or stand upright. But in the actual process of developing this muscle memory, the body itself often emerges as a repeated center of focus.

A sense of bodily "awareness" through UPRIGHT GO ultimately lies less in the sense that I have good posture—the resulting action—and more in the groups of muscles that require contraction or relaxation. Learning and maintaining the baseline position requires specific attention to highly specific and deliberate movements. The pulsing vibrations are a reminder to carefully lift my spine and lower back muscles while I relax my shoulder blades and arms: a vertical pulling motion followed by a gentle settling and sagging of my limbs. With each action, my attention scans my back from neck to tailbone, making minor adjustments in preparation for the session.

Some scholars of sport have argued that this kind of sustained attention or awareness can actually undermine one's ability to complete an action.[56] In other words, bodily awareness does not necessarily lead to improvement, or by extension better physical health. With UPRIGHT GO, thinking this hard about my posture may cause me to move my body awkwardly as the act of finding "good" posture comes to be broken down into discrete parts that have to fit together. Particularly in the context of sport or exercise, concentrating too hard on the body or form can interfere with the development of skilled movements, following the clichéd advice, "don't think, just do." At the same time, acquiring any new physical skill often requires sustained attention to the body and action. For example, learning to swim requires paying careful attention to the angle of my body to float, or the shape of my hand as it displaces water and propels me forward. But this does not mean I am consciously breaking down each action and willing my body to act accordingly.[57] To clarify the role of bodily awareness and reflection in sport, sociologists and cognitive scientists have distinguished between cognitive awareness and sensory and kinesthetic forms of awareness.[58] While cognitive awareness tends to focus on *what* one is doing, sensory awareness is focused on the feeling or sensations of the action: while concentrating on the feeling of my buoyant body in the water, I am still thinking about how to balance my weight and position my limbs to stay afloat. This form of sensory awareness does not necessarily provide the same cognitive disruption to completing an action or learning a new skill.

Though UPRIGHT GO claims to train individuals to develop their posture skills by "[discovering] what good posture *feels* like,"[59] the sensory feedback is limited to and depends on the initial calibration stage. As such, the body is held to a (recent) historical, quantified standard. While that standard can be reset for each session, the feedback does necessarily not help develop a sensory awareness of small shifts in the body as it sits or stands over time. In her exploration of movement, philosopher Erin Manning reminds us that posture is "not a position, not something to aim or to attain"[60]; it is a process of continuous micromovements (much like trying to stand still) requiring constant adjustments to maintain a settled, upright position. While the device is precisely designed to acknowledge the work of maintaining "good" posture, UPRIGHT GO cannot account for the way my back muscles tire or sag or the rising tension in my neck that grows as I write and sit at my desk for a prolonged period of time. Instead, I'm encouraged to continually make adjustments to fit that initial ideal.

By contrast, running wearables do not use such rigid feedback structures. These devices, such as the Moov fitness trainer and the Sensoria smart sock, use quantification and audio feedback to offer information on the present state of the body in movement, tracking imperceptible actions and physiological processes such as cadence, foot landing, and range of motion, with the goal of improving form and efficiency and avoiding injury. While other wearables such as Fitbit and Apple Watch provide information on such factors as cadence and pace, this information remains largely inaccessible during the run, or is only provided in the data overview available after completing the exercise.[61] Running wearables are focused on using quantification to prompt individuals to pay attention to specific parts of running form and to make subtle adjustments to the body while in motion.

The audio feedback is designed to reduce the impact of running on the body by encouraging individuals to focus on form, a particularly challenging task for novice runners. Proper form includes the entire body, from the angle and swing of the arms to the tilt of the torso and the pressure of the foot as it lands. For new runners, it can feel like all of one's effort and attention are focused on simply continuing to move: to make it one more block, to go for just five more minutes. Indeed, most apps and programs for new runners often focus exclusively on increasing time or distance, not on the necessary techniques to run safely and efficiently.[62] While they may provide cues for how to pace these runs, there's often little to no emphasis on elements of form, such as arm swing or foot landing. Classes and guides to proper running form often demonstrate ideal body movements, provide tips on how to make adjustments during a run, or allow individuals to practice their form in front of experts who offer suggestions. For example, the running class I attended broke proper form down into its component parts and individuals practiced each element, followed by a final attempt to assemble all of the parts. The final attempt was recorded, and the instructors offered feedback on how to improve. Though this class gave me essential information on where my foot should land and the angle to tilt my body, it's ultimately very challenging to incorporate this information into my runs. Much like the battle against the treadmill in Orangetheory, as an inexperienced runner I'm primarily focused on finishing, and this drive is worsened when I'm tired or struggling, which leads me to ignore the precise sensations and movements associated with proper running form.

Moov and Sensoria monitor the patterns of motion associated with running form and use audio feedback to cue individuals to specific parts of the body, training them to "feel" proper technique and reminding them that running often involves continued reflexive attention to bodily sensations. Inexperienced runners are often overwhelmed by fatigue, which can draw attention away from more acute sensations such as the pressure and placement of the foot. Likewise, for more experienced runners, settling into a pattern of motion can cause the mind to drift away from the body, as unconscious habit takes over.[63] By contrast, phenomenologies of elite and professional runners have shown that they continually reflect on their bodies and the surrounding environment and make adjustments accordingly. Falling into the rhythm of running is unconscious, but still requires "a coordination of body parts as the demands of terrain are negotiated via precise bodily adjustments necessary for the chosen footfall and cadence."[64] The body functions as an essential source of feedback throughout the run, from the quality and sound of the breath to the pull and strain of ligaments and muscles—"[t]hese sensations provide the individual with information about the choices she/he is making about position, balance and pace."[65]

Much like Orangetheory's heart rate monitors, running wearables aim to provide a shortcut to bodily awareness through quantification and audio feedback. The metrics and cues delivered throughout the run are designed to encourage individuals to notice the sensations that typically remain in the background, and to provide instructions on how to make adjustments accordingly. For example, the Moov wearable is a silicone band that tracks precise movements and provides coaching for various exercises, including running, HIIT, and swimming. Strapped to my ankle, it provides real-time feedback on my current cadence and foot landing during a run. Every few minutes, the monotone, computerized voice overtakes the music streaming through my headphones: "your cadence is 183 steps, your foot landing is high. Try to land on the ball of your foot."[66] My attention shifts to the angle of my foot's trajectory. I rotate my knee slightly with the next step, shortening my stride as I aim to land on the front of my foot. "Try to take short, soft steps," rings the voice. I respond by trying to land and swiftly recoil my foot, to reduce the pressure.[67] As I move through these actions, I try to gauge what these sensations feel like—where the ground seems to contact my foot, the swing of my legs and arms—all cues that I can use to settle into the remainder of the run.

These cues are not transparent ways to automatically fix my running form. Rather, they present moments when I'm prompted to attend to subtle sensations and use them to adjust my body and movements. When I hear "160 steps per minute, increase your cadence to 180," I don't automatically adjust the frequency of my steps. Instead, the audio cue draws my attention to the rhythm and sound of my feet as they hit the ground, the feeling of the quick up-and-down of my stride.[68] Only over time have I learned how to use this audio cue to modulate my steps, and even now, this process is by no means automatic or easy. The repeated feedback continually prompts me to attend to the sensations of running and has helped me learn to feel the difference between short, quick steps and a longer stride. Cues to decrease foot landing shift my attention to my knees and ankles, where I begin to sense the effects of my forceful impact. Attempting to decrease this pressure requires careful attention to my legs as they pull upward. My mind shifts to the sensation of my quadriceps and hip joints, which strain as I try to tilt my torso slightly forward and angle to push my foot backward with each step to reduce impact.

Running wearables are most often marketed as tools to reduce or prevent injury and improve efficiency, and consequently they place a great deal of emphasis on foot landing. I often don't feel the impact of running on my body until after the fact, because it's incredibly difficult to sense how the pace or pressure of my foot during a run will cause discomfort or pain later on. The audio feedback on the position and pressure of my foot hitting the ground aims to prevent the future strain on the muscles and joints that often comes with poor form. The Sensoria smart sock is wired with sensors on the base of the foot that monitor the position and pressure of each step and provide audio cues when I'm "heel striking," or landing on the heel of my foot.[69] Unfortunately, as someone with small feet, the sensors of the device often fail to match up with my foot. As I move through a run, the sock slips forward or backward, misaligning the sensors with the bottom of my foot, and thus causes the device to misread my movements. This results in the endless repetition of audio feedback, despite my conscious adjustments to foot landing. Even as I step forward, landing on the ball of my foot, the voice will state, "You are heel striking."[70] In the case of Sensoria, matching my movements to the sensor readings would probably result in injury and improper form.

Like Orangetheory and UPRIGHT GO, the external pressure of the Sensoria sock encourages me to conform to the standards of the device, which can be incredibly frustrating when I know this feedback is based on incorrect readings of my form. However, unlike those moments in class where numbers prove more powerful than my bodily sensations, my awareness of the device's limitations and the feeling of the misplaced sensors on the bottom of my foot can actually help me avoid mindlessly conforming my body to the structures of the device. Instead, I use the audio cue to simply reflect on the position of my foot as it hits the ground. The message causes my focus to shift to the feeling of my shoe as it makes contact with the ground and the way my foot contracts with each step. I try to sense how the base of my shoe bends and becomes flush with the ground and peels back up with each step, aiming to make initial contact with the front section of my foot.

Hypothetically, over time, running no longer requires this kind of hyper-focused attention to precise movements, and the Sensoria cues can simply become reminders for when I find myself fatigued and settling into sloppy form. That is, the feeling of my foot making contact with the ground will become "incorporated" into my embodied knowledge, fading into the background as it becomes habitual, rather than a consciously willed action.[71] Or, in the words of Leder, once the feeling of my foot landing becomes a habit, my body comes to be taken for granted, and my sense of the action transforms from "I can" to "I do."[72] But phenomenological studies of running offer accounts that push back on this overarching description of habit to demonstrate how parts of the body still emerge throughout a run. Elite runners are continually sensing elements of their body and surrounding environment and using this information to make microadjustments. The importance of these sensorial feedback structures is most acutely felt in injury, which often reveals the extent to which individuals rely on their bodily feedback while running. Relearning or "re-incorporating" a skill requires renewed attention to sensations that individuals take for granted, bringing the body and its patterns of movement back to the foreground.[73] Phenomenological description of running wearables demonstrates how this sense of the body can similarly be encouraged via quantification and audio feedback. Reflecting on how these devices draw attention to patterns of movement and track the form of the body illustrates how these devices may help bring embodied sensations to the foreground. While the pain or struggle of a running injury can encourage the body to dys-appear, as the individual faces the limitations of their body movements, running wearables highlight small-scale sensations and adjustments that allow the body to emerge not as an obstruction, but as a site of information.

Health as "Homelike Being-in-the-World"

Like Orangetheory's screens, fitness technologies often function as a source of distraction for individuals as they push through a hard workout. A push notification from a wearable can help draw attention away from the remaining miles in a run or from the increasing heaviness of one's muscles as one climbs a hill. Indeed, the repetitive audio feedback from Sensoria and Moov helped break up any sustained focus on my fatigue that might otherwise tempt me to slow down or stop. However, rather than drawing my attention to externalized data as a source of distraction, diversion is located in the careful adjustments to my body, such as the angle of my arms as they swing at my sides and the repetitive feel for the contact of my foot with the ground. In other words, rather than distracting me from my body's fatigue or strain, the audio feedback helps me adjust my focus to the sense of my body as it moves through the world.

Such an account of distraction during a run acknowledges the way attention and experience shift throughout the activity. However, discourses on running and running form often emphasize a sustained, continuous rhythm. Running form is essential precisely because the body is meant to fall into a steady pattern of movement for the duration of the run, and as a result, running often appears to simply be a repetitive, unconscious motion.[74] While running involves a standardized, cyclical action, that does not mean that movements or the body remain uniform or constant in the rhythmic action of running. The body can emerge through fatigue, pain, or other sensorial cues and require small shifts. But, importantly, these adjustments to form are not confined to the body, but instead are most often related to the surrounding environment. Runners may need to attend to a shift in foot pressure during a descent, to the length of stride for an uphill climb, or even to small-scale changes to the underlying terrain and trajectory of the route. Phenomenologies of sport have argued that athletes have a "heightened awareness of the body as it moves"; every action is "highly specific and [a] much practiced one, combining pressure between the sporting body, terrain and equipment."[75] In other words, elite training involves developing an active, reflexive relationship with the body as it interacts with the surrounding environment. While this form of embodiment has primarily been discussed in studies of athletes, phenomenological descriptions of running wearables demonstrate how these devices can likewise encourage a highly attuned relationship to the body as it moves through space and adjusts to shifts in the world around it.

Running, walking, and standing all require unconscious adjustments to the surrounding environment. While the mind may consciously focus on the total action—the complete act of taking a step forward—this action is composed of countless micro-adjustments and actions related to the specific qualities of the ground or surrounding space that one has incorporated into one's embodied knowledge through past experiences: "for most of us, taking a step is not an issue. We know the ground is there," we trust our capacity to gauge space.[76] But this doesn't mean the action is entirely automatic or unconscious: "movement always begins with a certain degree of open improvisation mixed with a certain degree of habit."[77] That is, moving through an environment is always relational, a combination of automatic actions and an active negotiation of the surrounding environment.

This hybrid of habit and improvisation is revealed in sociological studies of distance running, which stress the highly spatial nature of the action. John Hockey, for example, describes how running involves a "combination of corporeal and cognitive [work that] interacts with a particular physical environment to create a particular form of 'emplacement,'" or the sensuous reaction of the body to place.[78] Hockey's subsequent phenomenological studies have described how the sport continually requires corporeal awareness of terrain and a keen sense of how one's body relates to the texture and density of the ground.[79] While runners may not have to think about every step or movement, they must remain focused on the sensations of their feet within the shoes, the pressure of their step, and slight changes to the conditions underfoot.

The feedback on cadence, foot-landing position, and pressure provided by running wearables draws attention to the point of contact between the body and terrain. As I shift focus to the repetitive feeling of my steps as I aim to increase my cadence, this causes me to consider the quality of the ground beneath my feet, to feel for an even texture, and to look ahead slightly to see if my adjusted rhythm will work for the upcoming section of the route. Or when the Sensoria device reminds me that I'm "heel striking," I aim my leg beneath my body and feel for the pressure of the sidewalk on the front of my foot. In these moments, I reflect not only on the sensations in my feet and legs but also on the properties of the underlying ground. I can feel the different stress points on my ankles as I move from the concrete of the sidewalk to the dirt shoulder, or sense the pull in my calves and the angle of my body as I push up an incline. In drawing attention to these elements, running wearables attune me to the surrounding environment and remind me that running is a fundamentally reflexive, embodied experience.[80] In their phenomenological study of running, Hockey and Jacquelyn Allen-Collinson draw on geographer Paul Rodaway to describe the haptics of running not merely as touch, but as a "combination of tactile and locomotive properties [that] provide information about the character of objects, surface, and whole environments as well as our own bodies."[81] In other words, a runner's "touch" provides sensorial information not only about the body but the world around them.

Though a running wearable may attune me to the reflexive experience of running, I don't yet know how to use this "touch" to precisely adjust the force of my foot as I move between hard and soft surfaces, nor do I have a sense of how an off-kilter stone may affect the angle of my foot as it makes contact with the ground. I may unconsciously adapt to upcoming changes in my path as I tilt my body slightly in anticipation of an upcoming bend in the trail, or slow my pace as I see a hill rise ahead, but I have not yet gained the phenomenological awareness of the more subtle shifts between my body and environment. Moreover, regardless of whether I settle into the proper form or consider the sensuous relationship between my foot and the ground, my attention always returns to the stronger feeling of physical fatigue, or an object that catches my eye, or the music streaming through my headphones. But the audible interruptions of a running wearable do provide a small reminder to sense the relationship between my feet, patterns of movement, and the underlying terrain. Quantification and feedback, in these instances, continually pull my attention back to the sensation of my body as it moves through the world.

This is not to say that Moov or Sensoria have made me a faster or stronger runner. While the marketing of these devices stresses improved speed and "maximized" performance, they have not helped me reduce my mile time or increase the distance of my runs.[82] But by drawing increased attention to the precise movements of running, they have helped me avoid the small injuries and pain that I often experienced when running without the aid of a device. However, the real "benefit," I would argue, lies in the moments when I feel a sense of cooperation between my body and the world underfoot. Over time, the short, technology-supported interludes of focused attention have helped me recognize a "soft step," the feeling of my foot as it quickly makes contact with the ground, lightly springs up, and pushes backward to propel me forward. The feeling of "good form" has largely emerged from the almost buoyant sensation of displacement of my feet as they lift off and gently "pat" the ground to create a subtle, audible beat that underlines the music streaming through my headphones. This "buoyancy" is accompanied by a striking sense of ease and control over my body as it moves through space, a feeling of coordination with my surrounding environment.

This description of buoyancy or "balance" helps build on the definition of health introduced in the previous chapter. There, I described how the Apple Watch Mindfulness app disrupts my day-to-day activities and directs my attention to the present state of my body: it reminds me to consider myself as a body in the world. The audio feedback and quantification features of running wearables provide an extension of this encounter to notice not only my body but also the embodied feeling of moving through the world. In his phenomenological redefinition of health, Frederik Svenaeus emphasizes the importance of considering the environment. For phenomenologists, individuals are not separate from the world, but instead are fundamentally shaped and affected by the surrounding environment, and this extends to the experience of illness and health.[83] By drawing on Heideggerian phenomenology, he describes health as a state of balance between the individual and world through the metaphor of riding a bicycle: "In the same way as you do not think of your homelike being-in-the-world when you are healthy, you do not think of your physical balance when you are riding a bicycle."[84] While biking, one does not consciously think about how to keep upright—the ongoing process of balancing remains in the background. Nonetheless, it creates the conditions and feel of the capacity to propel oneself forward through the world. As with health, it is only when one falls off the bike that one realizes the careful balancing of the body, machine, and world.

The bicycle metaphor resembles traditional definitions of health that juxtapose health and illness. However, Svenaeus revises this dichotomy, which tends to focus on health as something "lost," by describing health as a "homelike being-in-the-world." In contrast to the sense of being "at home" in health, the "unhomelike" experience of illness involves the loss of a transparent, healthy attunement to the world, or creates the feeling of being "out of tune" with the body and the world.[85] Just as falling off a bicycle reveals the limitations of the body's movement through the world, so too does illness.[86] Though health and illness remain opposed in this configuration, Svenaeus turns to "homelike being-in-the-world" to stress that states of health and illness exist along a spectrum: "health and illness . . . must be seen as graded phenomena, since both homelikeness and unhomelikeness are always present to some degree in our being-in-the-world."[87] Thus, to become ill is to gradually lose a grasp of an unconscious being-in-the-world. This helps move health away from negative definitions that understand health as something one possesses, or illness as a radically distinct embodied state.[88] It breaks down the boundary between the sick and the healthy offered by homeostasis models that have historically supported a moralized, exclusionary understanding of health, to instead focus on how the experience of health and illness is continuously present and intertwined within an embodied experience of the world.[89]

While Svenaeus often relies on illness as a contrast to define health, his phenomenological exploration is still useful for developing a vocabulary to describe the experience of health itself. Svenaeus suggests that despite its background nature, health can be accessed through "focused attention on the way you are *in* the world."[90] The "homelike" state of health is a "non-apparent attunement," or a sense of placedness and "possibility."[91] The use of the term "homelike" helps incorporate the environmental component of health through its emphasis on the world, but it also suggests the sense of contentment or ease that creates the opportunity for action in health. While this emphasis on attunement and "ability" risks suggesting that health should be associated with a sense of able-bodiedness, Svenaeus argues that a phenomenological approach is not concerned with exterior standards of ability, but rather with the individual's homelike perception of being-in-the-world.[92] Differently abled bodies still experience homelikeness; they have "reached a transcendence that undoubtedly is different from that of most other people (consider the way the blind use their sense of touch, for instance), but that still enables them to perform their activities in a way that makes sense to them in their life."[93] To be "at-home" in health thus describes an individual's subjective sense of being "in-tune," a feeling of openness and possibility that enables meaningful participation in everyday actions: it describes a sense of the capacity to act, do, and be in the world.[94]

Phenomenologies of running wearables help clarify this philosophical discussion and offer a possible site to experience this "homelike" feeling of health as it pertains to exercise. The experience of "good form" that I describe is related to feeling the capacity to control and propel my body through space, or what I might call a "homelike" feeling that comes from the "ability to act."[95] This is not a reflective understanding of my fitness skill, but the experience of my present ease of movement, a sense that I can carry out the rhythm of the action in the immediate future.[96] The feeling of "buoyancy" is related to the sense that I can move myself forward in this moment of action, and comes from the synchronicity between my body and the surrounding environment as sensation, action, and the ground momentarily feel in balance. In these moments, I am attuned to my capacity to move through the world. This feeling is not the same thing as "feeling fit" or experiencing running as "effortless," nor is it the same as "enjoying exercise." Svenaeus clarifies that the attunement of health does not simply describe a "good or bad feeling,"[97] but rather a sense of being and moving through the world. Though attunement in health is attached to "ability," it has less to do with skill and more with a subjective facility for action.[98] In moments when Moov directs my attention to my moving body as it coordinates with space, I feel satisfaction in the rhythmic balance and the momentum to continue to propel myself forward. This action is still quite challenging, both mentally and physically, but I momentarily grasp at a feeling that I *can* keep moving.

Of course, this experience is ephemeral, mere minutes, if not seconds of my run. While the audio feedback can cue this experience, it is not necessarily required, nor does it guarantee this form of attunement. For example, sometimes as I transition from the concrete running trail to the sandy shoulder, the give of the softer surface and the satisfying crunch of my feet against the ground can similarly draw my attention to my body and environment.[99] Or perhaps a more common example is that when Moov directs my attention to the sensations in my lower legs, I become aware of my lack of coordination or clumsiness, the strange twinge in the top of my foot or the awkward angle of my stride. In these moments, I feel myself at odds with my body, grasping to correct and control my course of action, and failing. However, this is not the same as the alienating experience of pain. I don't feel an uncanny rift between myself and my body, but instead, simply feel less "at home" in my body and strive to make adjustments that will return me to that sense of balance.

In these moments, when the device draws my attention to the present state of my body in motion, I am reminded of not only the fact of my body—that I am a body and have a body—but also that I am a body moving through the world. In other words, these are moments when a sense of being-in-the-world comes to the foreground, when the transparent attunement of health becomes perhaps sensible. This mode of attention is made possible by way of quantification and technology, revealed through the practice of description. Of course, my account of running wearables is unique to my own experience of the devices, but the sensations and forms of embodiment I describe help provide an account of how description can articulate the sensations of health that typically remain remote in our everyday movements through the world.

Referring to health as "homelike" describes a constant push and pull, a "rhythmic balancing," of existence.[100] This understanding of health is neither stable nor clearly defined, but instead always receding, with varying degrees of attunement to the world. A focus on being, bodies, and environment reveals how health and illness are often felt in one's capacity and will to action. Phenomenological descriptions of running wearables show how quantification and feedback can potentially point an individual to this capacity. By encouraging hyper-focused attention to bodily sensation and movement, they create a context in which this "homelike" health can be felt and described. Rather than providing universal models or statistical standards of health in line with biomedical definitions, accounts of the experiences of these technologies help characterize an active understanding of health that does not rely on the opposition to illness. As a result, a phenomenology of running wearables—and digital health, more generally—builds a vocabulary to trace how injury and illness subtly shift or alter the sense of being-in-the-world, the feeling of being at home in a body in the world. Like Svenaeus, I do not suggest that these descriptions of health are meant to replace existing biomedical approaches to health and illness, but attending to these technologically mediated encounters can help us understand health as a lived, active experience of moving through the world.[101] Indeed, only through accounts of experience can researchers and scholars truly understand how digital health technologies shift, shape, and reveal an embodied perception of health.

Of course, this book is only the beginning. The analytical tools and philosophical frameworks I discuss throughout this book are meant to serve as a starting point for scholars to further examine the rapidly expanding array of devices and platforms used to monitor and interpret the "healthy" and "well" body. The descriptive techniques I offer can be used by any scholar or creative interested in exploring the impact of technology on the body. Because of the focus on tracing the relationship between particular design features and the sensorial experience, the methods are particularly useful for those working at the intersection of design and critical analysis, such as scholars in critical design studies and human-computer interaction design. Description is a useful tool at any stage of the process, whether emerging interfaces are being investigated or existing technologies are being explored. At the same time, I hope I have also laid the foundation for more systematic explorations of the experience of digital health. Social scientists may find the descriptive tools in this book to be a resource for exploring larger populations and experiences within specific communities. Phenomenological description has historically been used to show the lived experiences of those who exist outside of the norm, and the methods I've offered can be employed by social scientists to collect information on how the design features I trace may affect a range of different bodies. The descriptions in this book are limited to my embodied experience and a small sample of students, but the practice can be used widely to examine the multiplicity of sensorial encounters and forms of embodiment afforded by digital health technologies. It is essential that this work be extended through sociological work to truly grasp how individuals use and interpret these increasingly influential and ubiquitous technologies.

My hope is that this book will serve as a launching point for critical attention to embodied experiences of design, technology, and health. I offer a set of tools, but truly grasping the impact of digital health and the possibility of creating technologies that avoid or resist the normalizing structures of quantification and biostatistical analysis will require continued efforts on the part of scholars, creators, and the individuals who use these platforms and devices. Description functions as a first step toward such goals, as an analytical tool that can be used to reveal and reflect on how individuals experience, interact with, and perceive their bodies through the aesthetic and biomedical frameworks of digital health.

Notes

Introduction

1. World Health Organization. "Agenda item 12.4. Digital health resolution." Seventy-First World Health Assembly, Geneva, 26 May 2018, accessed January 2023.

2. "aesthetic, n. and adj," OED Online. Oxford University Press, accessed 10 January 2022, https://www-oed-com.electra.lmu.edu/view/Entry/3237

3. "Move More; Sit Less," Centers for Disease Control, June 2, 2022, https://www.cdc.gov/physicalactivity/basics/adults/index.html

4. Several major national health insurance companies offer reduced rates and rewards for sharing fitness-tracking data. Sigrid Forberg, "Can a Fitness Tracker Save You Money on Your Health Insurance?" *Yahoo Finance*, 22 January 2021, https://finance.yahoo.com/news/heres-could-free-fitbit-insurance-151900485.html

5. "Buy Apple Watch SE," Apple, n.d., https://www.apple.com/shop/buy-watch/apple-watch-se

6. Olivia Banner, *Communicative Biocapitalism* (University of Michigan Press, 2017); Deborah Lupton, "The Digitally Engaged Patient: Self-Monitoring and Self-Care in the Digital Health Era," *Social Theory & Health* 11, no. 3 (2013): 256–70; Arthur D. Soto-Vásquez, "Moving with Fitbit: Body Narratives, Fit Subjectivities, and Racialized Discipline," *Communication Studies* 72, no. 6 (2021): 1112–28; Christopher Till, "Commercialising Bodies: The New Corporate Health Ethic of Philanthrocapitalism," *Quantified Lives and Vital Data: Exploring Health and Technology Through Personal Medical Devices*, edited by Rebecca Lynch and Conor Farrington (Palgrave MacMillan, 2018), 229–49; Jennifer R. Whitson, "Foucault's Fitbit: Governance and Gamification," *The Gameful World*, edited by Steffen P. Walz and Sebastian Deterding (MIT Press, 2014), 339–58.

7. Nick J. Fox makes a similar argument in his analysis of personal health technologies. Nick J. Fox, "Personal Health Technologies, Micropolitics, and Resistance: A New Materialist Analysis," *Health* 21, no. 2 (2017): 143.

8. My approach follows Minna Ruckenstein and Natasha Dow Schüll claim that scholars need to explore the tensions and contradictions of datafication and technology. Minna Ruckenstein and Natacha Dow Schüll, "The Datafication of Health," *Annual Review of Anthropology* 46 (2017): 270.

9. Kirsten Ostherr, "Digital Medical Humanities and Design Thinking," *Teaching Health Humanities* (2019): 245–60.

10. While "aesthetic analysis" has been foundational to the medical and health humanities, the use of aesthetics largely refers to narrative analysis, borrowed from literary traditions. Although many collections do include chapters on the study of media and popular culture, they primarily focus on the analysis of character and story. Paul Crawford and colleagues have brought an expanded definition of aesthetics to the health humanities, acknowledging the connection between text and spectatorial experience, but this method is reserved for the study of the performing arts without considering the extension to media and mediated experiences. Paul Crawford, Brian Brown, Charlie Baker, Victoria Tischler, and Brian Abrams, *Health Humanities* (Palgrave McMillan, 2015), 60–81; Paul Crawford, Brian Brown, and Andrea Charise, *Routledge Companion to Health Humanities* (Routledge, 2020); Anne Hudson Jones, "Literature and Medicine: Traditions and Innovations," *The Body and the Text*, edited by Bruce Clarke and Wendell Aycok (Texas Tech University Press, 1990), 11–24; Therese Jones, Delese Wear, and Lester D. Friedman, *Health Humanities Reader* (Rutgers University Press, 2014).

11. Svenaeus, Fredrik. *The Hermeneutics of Medicine and the Phenomenology of Health: Steps Towards a Philosophy of Medical Practice*, International Library of Bioethics, 97 (Springer, 2022), 112.

12. Vaike Fors, "Sensory Experiences of Digital Photo-Sharing 'Mundane Frictions' and Emerging Learning Strategies," *Aesthetics and Culture* 7 (2015): 9.

13. Banner, *Communicative Biocapitalism*; Lupton, "The Digitally Engaged Patient"; Brad Millington, "Quantifying the Invisible: Notes Toward a Future of Posture," *Critical Public Health* 26, no. 4 (2016): 405–17; Julie Passanante Elman, "Find Your Fit: Wearable Technology and the Cultural Politics of Disability," *New Media and Society* 20, no. 10 (2018): 3760–77; Alessandra Mularoni, "Feminist Science Interventions in Self Tracking Technology," *Catalyst* 7, no. 1 (2021): 1–21; Rachel Sanders, "Self-Tracking in the Digital Era: Biopower, Patriarchy, and New Biometric Body Projects," *Body and Society* 23, no. 1 (2017): 36–63; Chris Till, "Exercise as Labour: The Quantified Self and the Transformation of Exercise into Labour," *societies* 5 (2014): 446–62.

14. Elman, "Find Your Fit," 3761.

15. Scholars have made this argument through a number of approaches, from the focus on the relationship between fitness and weight, to the analysis of the "lifestyle" promoted by digital health technologies. Jennifer Smith Maguire has also argued that the fitness industry more generally promotes a white, middle-class lifestyle. Banner, *Communicative Biocapitalism*, 77–102; Katelyn Esmonde and Shannon Jette, "Assembling the 'Fitbit Subject': A Foucauldian-Sociomaterialist Examination of Social Class, Gender and Self-Surveillance on Fitbit Community Message Boards," *Health* 24, no. 3 (2020): 299–314; Mularoni, "Feminist Science Interventions in Self Tracking Technology"; Soto-Vásquez, "Moving with Fitbit," 1123; Jennifer Smith Maguire, *Fit for Consumption* (Routledge, 2008).

16. Elman, "'Find Your Fit'": Sanders, "Self-Tracking in the Digital Era," 10–11.

17. My method resembles Fotopoulou and O'Riordan's work, which combines interface analysis with auto-ethnography. However, their work is largely focused on the rhetoric of the interface design—what "messages" or ideas about fitness are promoted—and the auto-ethnographies are more reflective rather than working in the tradition of phenomenology. Aristea Fotopoulou, and Kate O'Riordan, "Training to Self-Care: Fitness Tracking, Biopedagogy and the Healthy Consumer," *Health Sociology Review* 26, no. 1 (2017): 54–68.

18. This idea of description as a method of quotation and analysis in film studies has been theorized perhaps most famously in Raymond Bellour's "The Unattainable Text." Bellour, "The Unattainable Text," *Screen* 16, no. 3 (1975): 19–28.

19. Julian Hanich and Christian Ferencz-Flatz, "What Is Film Phenomenology?" *Studia Phaenomenologica* 16 (2016): 11–61.

20. Phenomenology in film and media studies can loosely be defined as "an attempt that describes *invariant structures* of the film viewer's *lived experience* when watching moving images in a cinema or elsewhere. Here the emphasis can either lie on the *film*-as-intentional-object or the *viewer*-as-experiencing-subject." Hanich and Ferencz-Flatz, "What Is Film Phenomenology?" 13.

21. The earliest critiques of medically determined definitions of health specifically focused on disability. Ivan Illich, most famously, focused on how biomedical definitions of health exclude or frame the disabled as "disordered." Ivan Illich, *Limits to Medicine: Medical Nemesis*. (Marion Boyars, 1976).

22. S. Kay Toombs, *The Meaning of Illness: A Phenomenological Account of the Different Perspectives of Physician and Patient*. Vol. 42. Springer Science & Business Media, 2013, xiii.

23. Simone de Beauvoir, *The Second Sex*, edited and translated by H. M. Parshley (Jonathan Cape, 1956).

24. Sara Ahmed extends Fanon's work to classical theories in phenomenology to show how his early works on race drew on similar frameworks and ideas. Sara Ahmed, "A Phenomenology of Whiteness 1," *Fanon, Phenomenology, and Psychology* (Routledge, 2021), 152; Frantz Fanon, *Black Skin, White Masks* (Paladin, 1970), 112.

25. While I do not focus my analysis on specific identity categories, examples of this approach to self-tracking can be found in the 2021 *Catalyst* special issue, "Self-Tracking, Embodied Differences and Intersectionality."

26. Deborah Lupton, "How Does Health Feel? Towards Research on the Affective Atmospheres of Digital Health," *Digital Health* 3 (2017): 2.

27. I use phenomenology, rather than post-phenomenology, affect theory, or other "entanglement theories," because of phenomenology's attachment to the *structures of experience*. While phenomenology denies a causal relationship between an empirical a priori reality and experience, it is invested in tracking the relationship between sense perception and the world's social, cultural, and material conditions. This attention to structure makes it a more useful methodology for scholars and researchers invested in exploring a given technology's design and user experience. While the above theoretical frameworks can help examine the conditions of embodiment and relations between humans and technology, they are often attached to claims of "relationality," "flow," and "networks" that make it challenging

to pinpoint the specific conditions of experience. Havi Carel, *Phenomenology of illness* (Oxford University Press, 2016), 19–24.

28. Here, I invoke Annemarie Mol's claim that experiences of health and illness reveal the multiple ontologies of the body, which coexist simultaneously, often in contradiction to one another. One ontology is not more "correct" than any other; rather it is only by attending to these multiple ontologies that scholars can work to improve the healthcare system. Annemarie Mol. *The Body Multiple: Ontology in Medical Practice* (Duke University Press, 2002).

29. Maurice Merleau-Ponty, *Phenomenology of Perception* (Routledge, 2013), 95.

30. Following Mol, I contend that the descriptive practices may reveal contradictions and the impossibility of a perfect solution, but nonetheless draw attention "to the possibility of alternative configuration." Mol, *The Body Multiple*, 164.

31. Elselijn Kingma, "Health and Disease: Social Constructivism as a Combination of Naturalism and Normativism," *Health Illness and Disease: Philosophical Essays* (Taylor Francis Group, 2018), 40–43.

32. Drew Leder, *The Absent Body* (University of Chicago Press, 1990).

33. Merleau-Ponty, *Phenomenology of Perception*, 147.

34. Iris Marion Young, "Pregnant Embodiment," *On Female Body Experience: "Throwing Like a Girl" and Other Essays* (Oxford University Press, 2005), 57.

35. Patricia Benner, "The Phenomenon of Care," *Handbook of Phenomenology and Medicine*, edited by S. Kay Toombs (2001), 351–69; James Brennan, "Transitions in Health and Illness: Realist and Phenomenological Accounts of Adjustment to Cancer," *Health, Illness and Disease* (Routledge, 2014), 141–54; Antonio Casado da Rocha and Arantza Etxeberria, "Towards Autonomy-Within-Illness: Applying the Triadic Approach to the Principles of Bioethics," *Health, Illness and Disease* (Routledge, 2014), 69–88; Linda Fisher, "The Illness Experience: A Feminist Phenomenological Perspective," *Feminist Phenomenology and Medicine* (2014): 27–46; Elizabeth Lindsey, "Health within Illness: Experiences of Chronically Ill/Disabled People," *Journal of Advanced Nursing* 24, no. 3 (1996): 465–72.

36. Svenaeus, *The Hermeneutics of Medicine*, 101.

37. Phenomenological description has been used to show that the experience of exercise is often highly variable and reflexive, but such description has not been extended to health, wellness, or digital health. Jacquelyn Allen-Collinson and John Hockey, "Feeling the Way: Notes toward a Haptic Phenomenology of Scuba Diving and Running," *International Review for the Sociology of Sport*, 46, no. 3 (2010): 330–45; Jacquelyn Allen-Collinson and Helen Owton, "Take a Deep Breath: Asthma, Sporting Embodiment, the Senses and 'Auditory Work,'" *International Review for the Sociology of Sport* 49, no. 5 (2014): 592–608; John Hockey, "Sensing the Run: The Senses and Distance Running," *Senses and Society* 1, no. 2 (2006): 183–202; James Morley, "Inspiration and Expiration: Yoga Practice Through Merleau-Ponty's Phenomenology of the Body," *Philosophy East and West* 51, no. 1 (2001): 73–82.

38. Akin to Young's account of the "aesthetic" relationship to the body in pregnancy, this form of bodily reflexivity takes the form of a noticing or even curiosity: "I do not feel myself alienated from [my body], as in illness. I merely notice its borders, rumblings with interest, sometimes with pleasure." Young, "Pregnant Embodiment," 52.

39. "Leading Causes of Death," Centers for Disease Control, updated 17 March 2017, accessed 16 July 2020, https://www.cdc.gov/nchs/fastats/leading-causes-of-death.htm

40. Illich, *Limits to Medicine*; Johnathan Metzl, "Why 'Against Health?'" *Against Health* (New York University Press, 2010), 1–12; Nancy Tomes, *Remaking the American Patient: How Madison Avenue and Modern Medicine Turned Patients into Consumers* (University of North Carolina Press, 2015).

41. Examples of this public health messaging can be found on all major public health institution websites. "Physical Activity: Why It Matters," Centers for Disease Control, accessed 11 January 2022, https://www.cdc.gov/physicalactivity/about-physical-activity/why-it-matters.html; Department of Health and Human Services, *Physical Activity Guidelines for Americans*, 2nd ed., 2018, PDF; World Health Organization, "Physical Activity," accessed 11 January 2022, https://www.who.int/news-room/fact-sheets/detail/physical-activity

42. Shelly Mckenzie, *Getting Physical: The Rise of Fitness Culture in America* (University of Kansas Press, 2013); Maguire, *Fit for Consumption.*

43. Carl Cederström and André Spicer, *The Wellness Syndrome* (Polity Press, 2015); David Dranove, *The Economic Evolution of American Health Care* (Princeton University Press, 2000); Carl Elliott, *Better than Well: American Medicine Meets the American Dream* (Norton, 2004); James William Miller, "Wellness: The History and Development of a Concept," *Heft* 1 (2005): 84–102.

44. Examples of histories of quantification applied to holistic and reproductive approaches to health can be found in Herbert Benson and Miriam Z. Klipper, *The Relaxation Response* (Avon, 1976); Louise Lander, *Images of Bleeding: Menstruation as Ideology* (Orlando Press, 1988).

45. Adele E Clarke, Laura Mamo, Jennifer Ruth Fosket, Jennifer R. Fishman, and Janet K. Shim, eds., *Biomedicalization: Technoscience, Health, and Illness in the US* (Duke University Press, 2010), 2.

46. Clarke et al., *Biomedicalization*, 49.

47. Clarke et al., *Biomedicalization*, 52, 55.

48. Clarke et al., *Biomedicalization*, 40.

49. Illich, *Limits to Medicine.*

50. Clarke et al., *Biomedicalization*, 65.

51. Department of Health and Human Services, *Physical Activity Guidelines for Americans*, 2.

52. Clarke et al., *Biomedicalization*, 40.

53. Tomes, *Remaking the American Patient.*

54. Countless historians of medicine have argued that health and medical standards are often established through the study of white male bodies. Thus, critiques have largely been waged against the biomedical model for reinforcing a highly classed, gendered, able-bodied, raced model of health. Examples of how this critique has been extended to digital health can be found in Luna Dolezal and Venla Oikkonen, "Introduction: Self-Tracking, Embodied Differences, and Intersectionality," *Catalyst: Feminism, Theory, Technoscience* 7, no. 1 (2021): 1–15.

55. Johnathan Metzl and Anna Kirland's *Against Health* focuses on the intersection of health, personal responsibility, and morality. Johnathan Metzl and Anna Kirkland, *Against Health* (New York University Press, 2010).

56. Articles that emphasize the relationship between digital health and self-care include Fotopoulou and O'Riordan, "Training to Self-Care"; Brad Millington, "Fit for Prosumption: Interactivity and the Second Fitness Boom," *Media, Culture & Society* 38, no. 8 (2016): 1184–200; Gina Neff and Dawn Nafus, *Self-Tracking* (MIT Press, 2016), 56.

57. Scholars have argued that gamification in digital health reinforces neoliberal ideology. For example, see Paulo Ruffino, "Engagement and the Quantified Self: Uneventful Relationships with Ghostly Companions," *Self-Tracking* (Palgrave Macmillan, Cham, 2018), 11–25; Whitson, "Foucault's Fitbit."

58. Banner, *Communicative Biocapitalism*, 12–14.

59. Banner, *Communicative Biocapitalism*, 12.

60. Digital health companies often promote their products by drawing on medical and scientific expertise. Fitbit and Apple both highlight their partnerships with research labs and academic institutions. Many of these companies also hire academic and medical consultants, whose names are proudly displayed in their "About Us" sections. Examples of these marketing devices can be found on "IOS—Research App," Apple, accessed July 2022; https://www.apple.com/ios/research-app/; "About Us," Fitbit, accessed 11 January 2022, https://www.fitbit.com/global/us/about-us

61. This is particularly apparent in Google's purchase of Fitbit in 2021. By acquiring the company, Google gained access to user health data that can be used to sell products or support Google's own predictive health analytics research. Jon Porter and Nick Statt, "Google Completes Purchase of Fitbit," *The Verge*, 14 January 2021, https://www.theverge.com/2021/1/14/22188428/google-fitbit-acquisition-completed-approved

62. The expansion of the medical gaze was originally theorized through telemedicine. Deborah Lupton has since extended this configuration both to digital health technologies that emerge through medical institutions and to popular technologies. Scholars have taken Lupton's framework and applied it to the discussion of a range of wearable devices and workplace wellness programs. Bithaj Ajana, "Digital Health and the Biopolitics of the Quantified Self." *Digital Health* 3 (2017): 2055207616689509; Deborah Lupton, "The Digitally Engaged Patient"; Millington, "Quantify the Invisible."

63. Ajana, "Digital Health"; Lupton "The Digitally Engaged Patient"; Tamar Sharon, "Healthy Citizenship Beyond Autonomy and Discipline: Tactical Engagements with Genetic Testing," *BioSocieties* 10 (2015): 295–316; Tamar Sharon, "Self-tracking for Health and the Quantified Self: Re-Articulating Autonomy, Solidarity, and Authenticity in an Age of Personalized Healthcare," *Philosophy and Technology* 30 (2017): 93–121; Whitson, "Foucault's Fitbit."

64. For this reason, scholars have applied the concept of the "data double" to the analysis of self-tracking. Minna Ruckenstein, "Visualized and Interacted Life: Personal Analytics and Engagements with Data Doubles," *societies* 4 (2014): 68–84; Whitson, "Foucault's Fitbit."

65. The quantified self webpage includes forums to share work and information about meetups and events. "Homepage," Quantified Self, n.d., accessed 3 January 2022, https://quantifiedself.com/

66. Ajana, "Digital Health"; Farzana Dudhwala, "Redrawing Boundaries around

the Self: The Case of Self-Quantifying Technologies," In *Quantified Lives and Vital Data* (Palgrave Macmillan, 2018): 97–123; Deborah Lupton, *The Quantified Self* (Polity Press, 2016); Ruffino, "Engagement and the Quantified Self"; Ruckenstein, "Visualized and Interacted Life"; Sanders, "Self-Tracking in the Digital Era"; Till, "Exercise as Labour."

67. Suneel Jethani, "Mediating the Body: Technologies, Bodies, and Epistemologies of the Self," *Communication, Politics, and Culture* 47, no. 3 (2015): 34–43; Millington, "Quantify the Invisible"; Jamie Sherman, "Data in the Age of Digital Reproduction: Reading the Quantified Self through Walter Benjamin," *Quantified: Biosensing Technologies in Everyday Life*, edited by Dawn Nafus (MIT Press, 2016): 27–42; Gavin J. D. Smith, "Surveillance, Data and Embodiment: On the Work of Being Watched," *Body and Society* 22, no. 2 (2016): 108–39; Gavin J. D. Smith and Ben Vonthethoff, "Health by Numbers: Exploring the Practice and Experience of Datafied Health," *Health Sociology Review* 26, no. 1 (2017): 6–21.

68. This assumption has, in part, been reinforced by the disproportionate attention to the quantified self movement as the standard for the self-tracking subject and digital health user. Quant selfers remain at the far end of the spectrum and are not the majority of digital health users. Moreover, sociological studies have increasingly shown that quant selfers engage with and understand digital health technologies in incredibly diverse ways. Deborah Lupton, "The Diverse Domains of Quantified Selves: Self-Tracking Modes and Dataveillance," *Economy and Society* 45, no. 1 (2016): 101–22; Neff and Nafus, *Self-Tracking*; Tamar Sharon and Dorien Zanderbergen, "From Data Fetishism to Quantifying Selves: Self-Tracking Practices and the Other Values of Data," *New Media and Society* 19, no. 11 (2017): 1695–709; Smith and Vonthethoff, "Health by Numbers."

69. Abhishek Pratap, Elias Chaibub Neto, Phil Snyder, Carl Stepnowsky, Noémie Elhadad, Daniel Grant, Matthew H. Mohebbi, et al., "Indicators of Retention in Remote Digital Health Studies: A Cross-Study Evaluation of 100,000 Participants," *NPJ Digital Medicine* 3, no. 1 (2020): 1–10.

70. Ramesh Srinivasan, *Whose Global Village?* (NYU Press, 2017), Kindle ebook, chapter 3.

71. Srinivasan, *Whose Global Village?* Kindle ebook conclusion.

Chapter 1

1. "FDA Allows Marketing of First Direct-to-Consumer App for Contraceptive Use to Prevent Pregnancy," FDA, 10 August 2018, https://wayback.archive-it.org/7993/20190207210732/https://www.fda.gov/NewsEvents/Newsroom/PressAnnouncements/ucm616511.html

2. Those who use the device to get pregnant are rewarded with a narrower and presumably more accurate fertility window. Indeed, the app and thermometer are primarily marketed as fertility tools. "Homepage," Natural Cycles, accessed July 2021, https://www.naturalcycles.com/

3. "Typical use" refers to the pregnancy prevention rates under average conditions. This is contrasted with "perfect use," which describes individuals who religiously abstained from sexual activity on "red days." Natural Cycles, "Homepage."

4. Like most novel forms of contraception, Natural Cycles has faced criticism from medical practitioners and individuals alike. Since the FDA's announcement, numerous women have blamed the company for unwanted pregnancies, and doctors have cautioned individuals against the app, claiming that the loosening of FDA certification standards ultimately leaves individuals at risk. Natural Cycles was under investigation for reported unwanted pregnancies at the time of the FDA's announcement, though it should be noted that all forms of contraception (except abstinence) are associated with reports of unwanted pregnancy under typical use. The discussion of FDA standards is related to the administration's 2018 introduction of the De Novo approval process for Class II medical devices, which offers a shortened approval timeline. Examples of this critique can be found in Natasha Lomas, "Natural Cycles App Told to Clarify Pregnancy Risk," *Tech Crunch*, 17 September 2018, https://techcrunch.com/2018/09/17/natural-cycles-contraception-app-told-to-clarify-pregnancy-risks/; Natural Cycles, "Homepage"; Tessa Ruff, "An App Is Not Birth Control: Natural Cycles' Approval Raises Serious Questions," *Women's Health Activist* 44, no. 1 (January-February 2019): 6; Amy Scanlin, "Expanded Use of De Novo Pathway Offers Opportunity for Device Manufacturers," *Med Tech Intelligence*, 23 April 2018, https://www.medtechintelligence.com/feature_article/expanded-use-of-de-novo-pathway-offers-opportunity-for-device-manufacturers/; Kaitlyn Tiffany, "Period Tracking Apps Are Not for Women," *Vox*, 16 November 2018, https://www.vox.com/the-goods/2018/11/13/18079458/menstrual-tracking-surveillance-glow-clue-apple-health

5. "About," Natural Cycles, accessed November 2020, https://www.naturalcycles.com/about/

6. Rachel Louise Healy, "Zuckerberg, Get Out of My Uterus! An Examination of Fertility Apps, Data-Sharing and Remaking the Female Body as a Digitized Reproductive Subject," *Journal of Gender Studies* 30, no. 4 (2021): 406–16; Maria Novotny and Les Hutchinson, "What Our Body Tells: Toward Critical Feminist Action in Fertility and Period Tracking Applications," *Technical Communication Quarterly* 28, issue 4 (2019): 332–60; Gareth Thomas and Deborah Lupton, "Threats and Thrills: Pregnancy Apps, Risk and Consumption," *Health, Risk and Society* 17, no. 7–8 (2016): 499.

7. Examples of this discussion can be found in Emily Martin, *The Woman in the Body: A Cultural Analysis of Reproduction* (Beacon Press, 2001); Iris Marion Young, *On Female Embodied Experience: Throwing Like a Girl and Other Essays* (Oxford University Press, 2005).

8. Precedence Research, "Fertility Market Size to Hit Around US $47.9 Billion by 2030," *Global Newswire*, 10 February 2021, https://www.globenewswire.com/news-release/2021/02/10/2173389/0/en/Fertility-Market-Size-to-Hit-Around-US-47–9-Billion-by-2030.html

9. Gabriella Weigel, "Coverage and Use of Fertility Services in US," *Women's Health Policy*, 15 September 2020, https://www.kff.org/womens-health-policy/issue-brief/coverage-and-use-of-fertility-services-in-the-u-s/#:~:text=Many%20fertility%20treatments%20are%20not,others%20(e.g.%2C%20IVF)

10. Natural Cycles, "About."

11. Natural Cycles, "Homepage."

12. Mikki Kressbach, "Period Hacks: Menstruating in the Big Data Paradigm," *Television and New Media* 22, no. 3 (2021): 241–61.

13. Flo similarly claims self-tracking can help you "take full control of your health." "Flo," Apple App Store, accessed April 2019, https://itunes.apple.com/us/app/flo-period-ovulation-tracker/id1038369065?mt=8

14. Paula J. Adams-Hillard and Marija Valjic Wheeler, "Data from Menstrual Cycle Tracking App Informs Knowledge of Menstrual Cycle in Adolescents and Adults," *Journal of Pediatric and Adolescent Gynecology* 30 (April 2017): 268–74; Daniel A. Epstein, Nicole B. Lee, Jennifer H. Kang, Elena Agapie, Jessica Schroeder, Laura R. Pina, James Fogarty, Julie A. Kientz, and Sean A. Munson, "Examining Menstrual Tracking to Inform the Design of Personal Informatics Tools," *Proceedings of the 2017 CHI Conference on Human Factors in Computing Systems* (2017): 6876–88; Kate Gambier-Ross, David J. McLernon, and Heather M. Morgan, "A Mixed Methods Exploratory Study of Women's Relationships with and Uses of Fertility Tracking Apps," *Digital Health* 4 (January-December 2018): 2055207618785077; Ruff, "An App Is Not Birth Control"; Mary Summer Starling, Zosha Kandel, Liya Haile, and Rebecca G. Simmons, "User Profile and Preferences in Fertility Apps for Preventing Pregnancy: An Exploratory Pilot Study," *MHealth* 4:21 (30 June 2018).

15. Minna Ruckenstein and Natasha Dow Schüll, "The Datafication of Health," *Annual Review of Anthropology* 46 (October 2017): 261–78.

16. Laetitia Della Bianca, "The Cyclic Self: Menstrual Cycle Tracking as Body Politics," *Catalyst: Feminism, Theory, Technoscience* 7, no. 1 (2021): 15.

17. Jane M. Ussher and Janette Perz, "PMS as a Process of Negotiation: Women's Experience and the Management of Menstrual Distress," *Psychology and Health* 28, no. 8 (2013): 910.

18. Flo is primarily marketed toward heterosexual women who aim to get pregnant. "Homepage," Flo, accessed November 2020, https://flo.health/

19. Marina Khidekel, "The Race to Hack Your Period Is On," *Elle*, 25 June 2018, https://www.elle.com/beauty/health-fitness/a21272099/clue-period-app/

20. Victoria Louise Newton, *Everyday Discourses of Menstruation* (Palgrave McMillan, 2015), 145.

21. Marija Vlajić Wheeler, Tabor Vedrana Högqvist, Kayleigh Teel, and Mike LaVigne, "The Science of Your Cycle: Evidence-Based App Design," Clue, 12 October 2015, https://helloclue.com/articles/about-clue/science-your-cycle-evidence-based-app-design

22. "New in Clue: Our Sex Icons Got a Makeover," Clue, 8 January 2018, accessed November 2020, https://helloclue.com/articles/about-clue/new-in-clue-our-sex-tracking-icons-got-makeover

23. For examples of this discussion see Deborah Lupton, "Quantifying Sex: A Critical Analysis of Sexual and Reproductive Self-Tracking Using Apps," *Culture, Health and Sexuality* 17, no. 4 (2014): 1–17; Sophie Laws, *Issues of Blood: The Politics of Menstruation* (Palgrave McMillan, 1990); Newton, *Everyday Discourses*.

24. While most scholars agree that menstrual euphemisms uphold gendered stereotypes and create shame around menstrual discourse, Newton notes that sociological studies have revealed that euphemisms can be used to give the speaker

power. According to Newton, shared vernacular language for menstruation can help make the experience "familiar," or even shift the power dynamics of a conversation. For example, she details how women using menstrual euphemisms in a space where such talk is deemed "impolite" can use coded language to break the social rules and "gain control of the situation." Newton, *Everyday Discourses*, 136, 143.

25. Sigmund Freud famously distinguished between the hostile joke and the obscene joke: hostile jokes exhibit aggression toward a subject or a defensive parody of the topic, while obscene jokes aim to uncover or expose the taboo. Sigmund, Freud, *Sigmund Freud: Jokes and Their Relation to the Unconscious* (Penguin Book, 1976), 139–40.

26. Janice Delaney, Mary Jane Lupton, and Emily Toth, *The Curse: A Cultural History of Menstruation* (University of Chicago Press, 1976), 128; Newton, *Everyday Discourses*, 147.

27. Camilla Mørk Røstvik, "Mother Nature as Brand Strategy: Gender and Creativity in Tampax Advertising 2007–2009," *Enterprise & Society* 21, no. 2 (2020): 413–52.

28. Newton, *Everyday Discourses*, 149.

29. Laws, *Issues of Blood*, 208.

30. Newton, *Everyday Discourses*, 158.

31. Theresa E. Jackson and Rachel Joffe Falmagne, "Women Wearing White: Discourses of Menstruation and the Experience of Menarche," *Feminism and Psychology* 23, no. 3 (2013): 389.

32. In her analysis of Bodyform's "Natural Blood" campaign, Røstvik likewise points to how jokes and references do not necessarily subvert cultural stereotypes surrounding menstruation. She argues that the campaign's recreation of the shower scene in *Carrie* ultimately reinforces the alignment of menstrual suppression with cleanliness and hygiene. Camilla Røstvik, "Crimson Waves: Narratives About Menstruation, Water, and Cleanliness," *Visual Culture and Gender* 13 (2018): 54–63.

33. Epstein et al., "Examining Menstrual Tracking," 6883.

34. Epstein et al., "Examining Menstrual Tracking," 6883.

35. Epstein et al., "Examining Menstrual Tracking," 6884.

36. Jackson and Falmagne, "Women Wearing White"; Ingrid Johnson-Robledo, Jessica Barnack, and Stephanie Wares, "'Kiss Your Period Good-Bye': Menstrual Suppression in the Popular Press," *Sex Roles* 54 (2006): 353–60; Elizabeth Kissling, *Capitalizing on the Curse: The Business of Menstruation* (Lynne Reinner Publishers, 2006); Janet Lee and Jennifer Sasser-Cohen, *Blood Stories: Menarche and the Politics of the Female Body in Contemporary U.S. Society* (New York: Routledge, 1996); Louise Lander, *Images of Bleeding: Menstruation as Ideology* (Orlando Press, 1988); Newton, *Everyday Discourses*; Hanna Sveen, "Lava or Code Red: A Linguistic Study of Menstrual Expressions in English and Swedish," *Women's Reproductive Health* 3, no. 3 (2016): 145–59; Jane M. Ussher, *Managing the Monstrous Feminine: Regulating the Reproductive Body* (Routledge, 2006).

37. Young, *On Female Embodied Experience*, 106.

38. J. C. Chrisler, "2007 Presidential Address: Fear of Losing Control: Power, Perfectionism, and the Psychology of Women," *Psychology of Women Quarterly* 32

(2008): 1–12; Ussher, *Managing the Monstrous Feminine*; Young, *On Female Embodied Experience*.

39. Ussher, *Managing the Monstrous Feminine*, 6.

40. Lara Freidenfelds, *The Modern Period* (Johns Hopkins University Press, 2009), 137.

41. Freidenfelds, *The Modern Period*, 137.

42. For Kotex, wrapping the boxes created basic distribution challenges, as the wrapped box became associated with menstrual products and thus undermined any attempt at concealment: "I think we're enslaving women with this thing. We've created a monster that we can't get rid of. . . . [Y]ou have to keep changing the package every three months because pretty soon this has a symbolic status. Anything wrapped in a plain bag has to be sanitary napkins. It can't be anything else. You're in the trap of an eternity of package change if you're going to try to hide what's in there." Quoted in Freidenfelds, *The Modern Period*, 140.

43. "Spot On Period Tracker," Planned Parenthood, accessed February 2023, https://www.plannedparenthood.org/get-care/spot-on-period-tracker

44. Gareth Thomas and Deborah Lupton make a similar argument about pregnancy-monitoring apps. Their sociological study argues that the pregnant body is figured as a site of risk and entertainment, in which "users of the apps are encouraged to view pregnancy as an embodied mode of close monitoring and surveillance, display and performance." Thomas and Lupton, "Thrills and Threats," 495.

45. Epstein et al., "Examining Menstrual Tracking," 6880.

46. Ovulation is sometimes marked by a contraction or pain in the lower abdomen accompanied by an "egg white" discharge, but this is not necessarily always the case. Amanda Laird, *Heavy Flow* (Dundurn, 2019), 55.

47. Lauren C Houghton and Noémie Elhadad, "Practice Note: 'If Only All Women Menstruated Exactly Two Weeks Ago': Interdisciplinary Challenges and Experiences of Capturing Hormonal Variation Across the Menstrual Cycle," *Palgrave Handbook of Critical Menstruation Studies* (2020): 726.

48. Clue and other menstrual tracking apps have the option to remove the fertile window section of the cycle visualization. For example, by designating that an individual is using pharmaceutical contraceptives, the app removes the possibility of fertilization or ovulation.

49. "Fertile Window," Clue, vers. 5.13., 2019, accessed November 2020.

50. Apple App Store, "Clue."

51. Laird, *Heavy Flow*, 57.

52. Laird, *Heavy Flow*, 57; "What to Know about Clue's Analysis Features," Clue, 31 March 2019, https://helloclue.com/articles/about-clue/introducing-enhanced-analysis-understand-what-your-period-is-telling-you

53. Clue, "What to Know."

54. "Your Menstrual Cycle and Your Health," Department of Health and Human Services, 16 March 2018, https://www.womenshealth.gov/menstrual-cycle/your-menstrual-cycle-and-your-health

55. Jerilynn C Prior, "The Menstrual Cycle: Its Biology in the Context of Silent Ovulatory Disturbances," *Routledge International Handbook of Women's Sexual and Reproductive Health* (Routledge, 2019), 40.

56. Houghton and Elhadad, "If Only All Women," 729.

57. Department of Health and Human Services, "Your Menstrual Cycle and Your Health."

58. Sarah E. Fox, Amanda Menking, Jordann Eschler, and Uba Backonja, "Multiples over Models: Interrogating the Past and Collectively Reimagining the Future of Menstrual Sensemaking," *ACM: Transactions on Human-Computer Interaction* 27, no. 4, article 22 (September 2020): 1–24; Sarah E. Fox and Daniel A. Epstein, "Monitoring Menses: Design-Based Investigations of Menstrual Tracking Applications," *The Palgrave Handbook on Critical Menstruation Studies* (Palgrave MacMillan, 2020), 733–50.

59. Katie Ann Hasson, "Not a 'Real' Period? Social and Material Constructions of Menstruation," *Palgrave Handbook on Critical Menstruation Studies* (2020), 763–86; Martin, *The Woman in the Body*, 46.

60. Thomas and Lupton, "Thrill and Threats," 499.

61. Celia Roberts and Catherine Waldby, "Incipient Infertility: Tracking Eggs and Ovulation across the Life Course," *Catalyst: Feminism, Theory, Technoscience* 7, no. 1: 5.

62. As Roberts and Waldby note, this promise is always "dwindling," and thus requires further investment and intervention. Roberts and Waldby, "Incipient Infertility," 17.

63. Fox et al., "Multiples over Modules," 8.

64. Laird, *Heavy Flow*, 43.

65. Chris Bobel, *New Blood: Third-Wave Feminism and the Politics of Menstruation* (Rutgers University Press, 2010), 84.

66. Prior, "The Menstrual Cycle," 40.

67. Prior, "The Menstrual Cycle," 40.

68. Epstein et al., "Examining Menstrual Tracking," 6885.

69. Della Bianca, "The Cyclic Self," 13.

70. Ussher and Perz, "PMS as a Process," 916.

71. Clue does include an optional "notes" section for the log, however, this module is organized through a tag system, where the individual must design specific tags to be logged each day. The default tags suggest this section is primarily designed for monitoring fertility. Biowink, "Clue."

72. Flo Health, Inc., "Flo," vers. 4.31, 2019, accessed November 2019.

73. Clue, "Homepage."

74. Epstein et al., "Examining Menstrual Tracking," 6884.

75. Epstein et al., "Examining Menstrual Tracking," 6884.

76. Epstein et al., "Examining Menstrual Tracking," 6879.

77. Joan Chrisler and Paula Caplan go as far as to suggest that PMS can function as a mode of "self-handicapping," by "setting up insurmountable (or nearly so) obstacles to success so the inevitable failure can later be attributed to the obstacles rather than to one's own lack of effort or ability." Making PMS known to others can function as a "catch-all excuse." Joan C. Chrisler and Paula Caplan, "The Strange Case of Dr. Jekyll and Ms. Hyde: How PMS Became a Cultural Phenomenon and a Psychiatric Disorder," *Annual Review of Sex Research* 13, no. 1 (2002): 289.

78. Epstein et al., "Examining Menstrual Tracking," 6882.

79. Kathryn Strother Ratcliff, *Women and Health: Power, Technology, Inequality, and Conflict in a Gendered World* (Pearson 2002), 158.

80. Joan C. Chrisler and Jenifer A. Gorman, "The Menstrual Cycle: Attitudes and Behavioral Contaminants," *Routledge International Handbook of Women's Sexual and Reproductive Health*, edited by Jane M. Ussher (Rutledge, 2020), 58; B. Sommer, "How Does Menstruation Affect Cognitive Competence and Psychophysiological Response?" *Women & Health* 8, no. 2/3 (1983): 53–90.

81. Robert T. Frank, "The Hormonal Cause of Premenstrual Tension," *Arch Neuropsychology* 26, no. 5 (1931): 1053–57.

82. Chrisler and Caplan, "The Strange Case," 283.

83. Chrisler and Caplan, "The Strange Case," 283.

84. Several scholars have noted how surges in PMS research have coincided with women entering the workforce. Maria Gurevich, "Rethinking the Label: Who Benefits from the PMS Construct?," *Women and Health*, 23, no. 2 (1995): 78–79.

85. Chrisler and Caplan, "The Strange Case," 283.

86. In the 1980s and '90s, PMS as a condition was further legalized with the establishment of premenstrual dysphoric disorder. The American Psychiatric Society added this condition to the *Diagnostic and Statistical Manual of Psychiatric Disorders–4* (*DSM-4*), further fomenting the biomedical model for premenstrual distress. Kissling, *Capitalizing on the Curse*, 50.

87. Lander, *Images of Bleeding*, 79.

88. Kissling, *Capitalizing on the Curse*, 41–42.

89. Kissling, *Capitalizing on the Curse*, 41–42.

90. Chrisler and Caplan, "The Strange Case," 289.

91. This can also be seen in studies of menopause and hormone replacement therapy, which "promised to keep women biologically sound so they could participate more fully in changing society." Rather than questioning the social standards of femininity, HRT offered a pharmaceutical "solution" to the disruption of feminine norms in menopause. Judith Houck, *Hot and Bothered: Women, Medicine and Menopause in America* (Harvard University Press, 2006), 169.

92. Ida Tin, "5 Unexpected Benefits of Period Tracking," Clue, 22 January 2019, https://helloclue.com/articles/cycle-a-z/5-reasons-you-should-pay-attention-to-your-period

93. Della Bianca, "The Cyclic Self," 13.

94. Della Bianca, "The Cyclic Self," 13.

95. Ussher, *Managing the Monstrous Feminine*, 52.

96. Lee and Sasser-Cohen, *Blood Stories*, 14; Martin, *The Woman in the Body*, 20.

97. Chrisler and Caplan, "The Strange Case," 281.

98. Lander 1988, *Images of Bleeding*, 101.

99. "MyFlo Period Tracker," Flo Living, 2023, accessed February 2023, https://myflotracker.com/

100. My Flo Living, "MyFlo Period Tracker."

101. Elizabeth Kissling, "Bleeding Out Loud: Communicating About Menstruation," *Feminism and Psychology* 6, no. 4 (1996): 481–504; Kissling, *Capitalizing on the Curse*; Young, *On Female Embodiment*, 101.

102. Martin, *The Woman in the Body*, 21.

103. Kissling, *Capitalizing on the Curse*, 55.
104. Kissling, *Capitalizing on the Curse*, 55.
105. Chrisler and Caplan, "The Strange Case," 278; Gurevich, "Rethinking the Label," 72; Kissling, *Capitalizing on the Curse*, 39.
106. Chrisler and Caplan, "The Strange Case," 278.
107. Chrisler and Caplan, "The Strange Case," 301.
108. Gurevich, "Rethinking the Label."
109. Chrisler and Caplan, "The Strange Case," 284.
110. Ussher and Perz, "PMS as a Process," 910.
111. Swann and Ussher, "A Discourse Analytic Approach"; Houck, *Hot and Bothered*, 162; Ussher and Perz, "PMS as a Process"; Jane M. Ussher and Janette Perz, "Resisting the Mantle of the Monstrous Feminine: Women's Construction and Experience of Menstrual Embodiment," *Palgrave Handbook on Critical Menstruation Studies*, 213–32.
112. Ussher and Perz, "PMS Is a Process, 911"; Samantha Ryan, J. Ussher, and J. Perz, "Women's Experiences of the Premenstrual Body: Negotiating Body Shame, Self-Objectification, and Menstrual Shame, *Women's Reproductive Health* 7, no. 2 (2020): 107–26.
113. Ussher and Perz, "PMS Is a Process," 914, 920.
114. Ela Przybylo and Breanne Fahs advocate for "menstrual crankiness," which acknowledges the challenges of the menstrual experience as a way to push at sexist and transphobic discourses around bodies and embodiment—"arguing that menstrual crankiness is vital to thinking about the material pains and pleasures of menstrual bleeding." Ela Przybylo and Breanne Fahs, "Empowered Bleeders and Cranky Menstruators: Menstrual Positivity and the 'Liberated' Era of New Menstrual Product Advertisements," *Palgrave Handbook on Critical Menstruation Studies*, 376.
115. Ussher and Perz, "Resisting the Mantle," 226.
116. Ussher and Perz, "PMS Is a Process," 919.
117. Della Bianca, "The Cyclic Self," 10.
118. Della Bianca, "The Cyclic Self," 15.
119. Discussion of diagnosis and validation can be found in studies on PMS, menopause, and PMDD. See Katie Ann Hasson, "From Bodies to Lives, Complainers to Consumers: Measuring Menstrual Excess," *Social Science & Medicine* 75, no. 10 (2012): 1729–36; Houck, *Hot and Bothered*; Ussher and Perz, "PMS Is a Process"; Ussher and Perz, "Resisting the Mantle."
120. Fox and Epstein, "Monitoring Menses."
121. Fox and Epstein, "Monitoring Menses," 745.
122. Fox and Epstein, "Monitoring Menses," 746; Fox et al., "From Multiples to Modules."
123. Ussher and Perz, "PMS Is a Process," 915.
124. Women of color, in particular, remain overlooked in menstrual health research. For example, there is still no medical explanation for why Black women often experience heavier flows or are less likely to be diagnosed with endometriosis despite showing symptoms. Staff BWHI, "I've Got What? Figuring Out Endometriosis," Black Women's Health Collective, 25 July 2017, https://bwhi.org/2017/07/25/ive-got-figuring-endometriosis/

125. Sam Schechner and Mark Secada, "You Give Apps Sensitive Personal Information. Then They Tell Facebook," *Wall Street Journal*, 22 February 2019, https://www.wsj.com/articles/you-give-apps-sensitive-personal-information-then-they-tell-facebook-11550851636

126. Epstein et al., "Examining Menstrual Tracking."

127. The Supreme Court decision to overturn Roe vs. Wade revealed how the privacy features of menstrual tracking apps can place people at risk for legal action. While apps currently reassure users that their data cannot be shared with outside parties, most privacy policies include a clause that allows data to be shared with a warrant. Since the apps are not protected by HIPPA, the data collected remains in a gray zone that is at risk in states without protection. Kashmir Hill, "Deleting Your Period Tracker Won't Protect You," *New York Times*, 2 July 2022.

128. "Do Menstrual Cycles Sync? Unlikely, finds Clue Data," Clue, 8 March 2017, https://helloclue.com/articles/cycle-a-z/do-menstrual-cycles-sync-unlikely-finds-clue-data; FIGO, "Period Syncing Myth Debunked," *FIGO: International Federation of Gynecology and Obstetrics*, 13 April 2017, https://www.figo.org/news/period-syncing-myth-debunked-0015541

129. "Clue Period Tracker," Apple App Store, accessed April 2019, https://itunes.apple.com/us/app/clue-period-tracker-ovulation/id657189652?mt=8

130. While I note the economic incentive for app developers, this argument operates in line with debates on the "ethics of coding," which emphasize the ethical responsibilities of creators. I follow Colman and colleagues' claim that developers should adjust their code according to "fluctuations in social coding," and argue that menstrual tracking app developers should be held responsible for how these technologies encourage harmful relationships with menstruation and should adjust their products accordingly. Felicity Colman, Vera Bühlmann, Aislinn O'Donnell, and Iris van der Tuin, *Ethics of Coding: A Report on the Algorithmic Condition*, 2018, H2020-EU.2.1.1-Industrial Leadership. https://cordis.europa.eu/project/rcn/207025_en.html, 45.

Chapter 2

1. "How Does Our Technology Work?" Lioness, accessed April 2021, https://lioness.io/pages/how-it-works

2. Andrea Barrica, *SexTech Revolution* (Lioncrest Publishing, 2019), epub, chapter 1.

3. "Episode 681: Escape from the Lab Transcript," *This American Life*, accessed March 2021, https://www.thisamericanlife.org/681/transcript

4. Li Cornfeld, "Videotape and Vibrators: An Industry History of Techno-Sexuality," *Feminist Media Histories* 6, no. 4 (2020): 95.

5. Cornfeld, "Vibrators and Videotapes," 101.

6. Cornfeld describes how this legitimization has manifested itself materially, by quite literally distancing the companies from the stigmatized adult entertainment industry, which is now sequestered in a separate, enclosed space at the annual conference. Cornfeld, "Vibrators and Videotapes," 111–12.

7. *This American Life*, "Episode 681: Escape from the Lab Transcript."

8. Cornfeld, "Vibrators and Videotapes," 113.

9. Hallie Lieberman and Eric Schatzberg, "A Failure of Academic Quality Control: *The Technology of the Orgasm*," *Journal of Positive Sexuality* 4, no. 2 (August 2018): 30.

10. Lieberman and Schatzberg, "The Failure of Academic Quality Control," 26; Rachel P. Maines, *The Technology of the Orgasm: Hysteria, the Vibrator, and Women's Sexual Satisfaction* (Johns Hopkins University Press, 1999), 108.

11. Lynn Comella, *Vibrator Nation* (Duke University Press, 2017), 92.

12. While this discourse aims to reunite mind and body, participates in sex-positive movements, and like midcentury sexology aims to destigmatize sexual pleasure, it simultaneously presents a model of health (and pleasure) dependent on continuous bodily maintenance. Thea Cacchioni, "Heterosexuality and the 'Labour of Love': A Contribution to Recent Debates on Female Sexual Dysfunction," *Sexualities* 10, no. 3 (2007): 299–320; Kristina Gupta, "'Screw Health': Representations of Sex as Health-Promoting Activity in Medical and Popular Literature," *Journal of the Medical Humanities* 32 (2011): 127–40; Kristina Gupta and Thea Cacchioni, "Sexual Improvement as If Your Health Depends upon It: An Analysis of Contemporary Sex Manuals," *Feminism and Psychology* 23, no. 4 (2013): 442–58.

13. Stuart Brody, "The Relative Benefits of Different Sexual Activities," *International Society for Sexual Medicine* 7, no. 4, pt. 1 (2010): 1336–361; Breanne Fahs and Elena Frank, "Notes from the Back Room: Gender, Power and (In)visibility in Women's Experiences of Masturbation," *Journal of Sex Research* 51, no. 3 (2014): 241–52; François Kraus, "The Practice of Masturbation for Women: The End of a Taboo?" *Sexologies* 26 (2017): e35–41; Harriet Hogarth and Roger Ingham, "Masturbation Among Young Women and Associations with Sexual Health: An Exploratory Study," *Journal of Sex Research* 46, no. 6 (2009): 558–67.

14. Gupta, "Screw Health," 128.

15. Thomas Lacquer, *Making Sex: Body and Gender from the Greeks to Freud* (Harvard University Press, 1992), 4.

16. Sigmund Freud, "Three Essays on the Theory of Sexuality," *The Freud Reader* (Norton, 1989), 279.

17. Wilhelm Reich, *The Function of the Orgasm* (York: Farrar, Straus and Giroux, 1973), 91.

18. Reich, *The Function of the Orgasm*, 371.

19. Reich, *The Function of the Orgasm*, 378.

20. Reich, *The Function of the Orgasm*, 379.

21. Janet Irvine, *Disorders of Desire* (Temple University Press, 1990), 43–44.

22. Early descriptions of the orgasm often focus on the language of "release" or finality, in line with the presumption that ejaculation functions as the end of the sexual experience. Freud, for example, defined the culmination of sexual pleasure as "the discharge of sexual products." Freud, "Three Essays," 279.

23. Alfred C. Kinsey, Wardell B. Pomeroy, Clyde E. Martin, and Paul H. Gebhard, *The Sexuality of the Human Male* (Harper & Row, 1972), 158.

24. Alfred C. Kinsey, Wardell B. Pomeroy, Clyde E. Martin, and Paul H. Gebhard, *The Sexuality of the Human Female* (Pocket Books, 1953), 102.

25. Irvine, *Disorders of Desire*, 46–47.

26. Irvine, *Disorders of Desire*, 51.

27. Hannah Frith, *Orgasmic Bodies: The Orgasm in Contemporary Western Culture* (Springer, 2015), 10–12.

28. Irvine, *Disorders of Desire*, 49.

29. Kinsey et al., *Human Male*, 209.

30. Frith, *Orgasmic Bodies*, 12.

31. American Psychiatric Association, *Diagnostic and Statistical Manual of Mental Disorders*, 5th ed. (2013), 302.73 (F52.31).

32. In an attempt to acknowledge the experiential and subjective dimensions of "female orgasmic disorder," *DSM-5* added "distress or interpersonal difficulty." However, as Frith and others have pointed out, it's not clear whether "distress" is produced by the orgasmic absence or a host of other cultural factors, including social and cultural expectations around orgasmic presence. Frith, *Orgasmic Bodies*, 36–37.

33. American Psychiatric Association, 302.73 (F52.31).

34. Kinsey et al., *Human Male*, 110.

35. Irvine, *Disorders of Desire*, 49–50.

36. Irvine, *Disorders of Desire*, 51.

37. John R. Wheatley and David A. Putz, "The Evolutionary Science of the Female Orgasm," *The Evolution of Sexuality*, edited by T. K. Shackelford and R. D. Hansen (Springer International Publishing, 2015): 128–32.

38. Wheatley and Putz, "The Evolutionary Science," 141.

39. Kinsey et al., *Human Male*, 202.

40. Kinsey et al., *Human Male*, 5.

41. Kinsey et al., *Human Male*, 5.

42. Irvine, *Disorders of Desire*, 37.

43. Janet Irvine, "From Difference to Sameness: Gender Ideology in Sexual Science," *Journal of Sex Research* 27, no. 1 (1990): 16.

44. Elizabeth A. Mahar, Laurie B. Mintz, and Brianna M. Akhar, "Orgasm Equality: Scientific Findings and Societal Implications," *Current Sexual Health Reports*, 24 (2020): 25.

45. An example of this can be found in "About Us," Dame, accessed April 2021, https://www.dameproducts.com/pages/about-us; Katriona Harvey-Jenner, "The Orgasm Gap Is REAL—Women Are Losing Out," *Cosmopolitan Magazine UK*, 25 March 2015, https://www.cosmopolitan.com/uk/love-sex/sex/news/a34410/female-orgasm-survey/; Laurie B. Mintz, "The Orgasm Gap: Simple Truth and Sexual Solutions," *Psychology Today*, 4 October 2014; Vox Creative, "Women Are Having Fewer Orgasms. But Why?" *Vox*, 7 December 2020, https://www.vox.com/ad/21564023/women-pleasure-pornography-bellesa-streaming

46. Katherine Rowland, *The Pleasure Gap: American Women and the Unfinished Sexual Revolution* (Seal Press, 2020), epub, chapter 2.

47. Frith, *Orgasmic Bodies*, 13.

48. Irvine, *Disorders of Desire*, 40.

49. "About Us," Lora DiCarlo, accessed April 2021, https://www.loradicarlo.com/about-us

50. "What Is the Pleasure Gap?" Dame, 4 April 2019, https://swell.damewellness.co/what-is-the-pleasure-gap/

51. In their discussion of postfeminism and health, Riley and colleagues also highlight how the rhetoric of equality effaces difference and the structural conditions that lead to inequality in the first place. Sarah Riley, Adrienne Evans, and Martine Robson, *Postfeminism and Health* (Routledge, 2019), 84.

52. “Homepage,” Lora DiCarlo, accessed April 2021, https://www.loradicarlo.com/

53. Through the analysis of self-help and marriage manuals scholars have noted the shift from an emphasis on reproduction toward sexual pleasure and reciprocity in the mid-twentieth century. Jessamyn Neuhaus, “The Importance of Being Orgasmic: Sexuality, Gender, and Marital Sex Manuals in the United States, 1920–1963,” *Journal of the History of Sexuality* 9, no. 4 (2010): 447–73; Frith, *Orgasmic Bodies*, 25.

54. Frith notes that the “right” to pleasure was symbolized by an orgasm for many second-wave feminist movements. Frith, *Orgasmic Bodies*, 25.

55. Anne Koedt, “Myth of the Vaginal Orgasm,” *Notes from the First Year* (New York Radical Feminists, 1968).

56. Jane Gerhard, “Revisiting ‘The Myth of the Vaginal Orgasm’: The Female Orgasm in American Sexual Thought and Second-Wave Feminism,” *Feminist Studies* 26, no. 2 (2000): 450.

57. Gerhard, “Revisiting the Myth.”

58. Koedt, “Myth of the Vaginal Orgasm.”

59. Kinsey et al., *Human Female*, 492; William Masters and Virginia Johnson, *Human Sexual Response* (Little Brown, 1966), 66.

60. William Masters and Virginia Johnson, *Heterosexuality* (Harper Collins, 1994), 42.

61. Gerhard, “Revisiting the Myth,” 465–66.

62. Koedt, “The Myth of the Vaginal Orgasm,” 41.

63. Koedt, “The Myth of the Vaginal Orgasm,” 38.

64. Comella, *Vibrator Nation*, 26.

65. Comella, *Vibrator Nation*, 36–37.

66. Comella, *Vibrator Nation*, 36.

67. Comella, *Vibrator Nation*, 35.

68. Comella, *Vibrator Nation*, 26.

69. Comella, *Vibrator Nation*, 99.

70. Comella, *Vibrator Nation*, 96.

71. Comella, *Vibrator Nation*, 95.

72. Frith, *Orgasmic Bodies*, 27; Riley et al., *Postfeminism and Health*, 77.

73. Barrica, *SexTech Revolution*, chapter 1.

74. Frith, *Orgasmic Bodies*, 23.

75. Barrica, *SexTech Revolution*, chapter 1, introduction.

76. Cindy Gallop, “What Is Sextech and Why Is Everyone Ignoring It?” Hottopics.ht, 30 March 2020, accessed April 2021, https://www.hottopics.ht/14192/what-is-sextech-and-why-is-everyone-ignoring-it/

77. Barrica, *SexTech Revolution*, chapter 1; Hallie Lieberman, *Buzz: A Stimulating History of the Sex Toy* (Simon and Schuster, 2017), 292.

78. This is exemplified by the earlier discussion of Cornfeld's work on the DiCarlo CES scandal. Cornfeld, "Videotapes and Vibrators."

79. "Homepage," Lioness, accessed April 2021, http://Lioness.io

80. Dame, "About Us."

81. Jeffery Bardzell and Shaowen Bardzell, "'Pleasure Is Your Birthright': Digitally Enabled Designer Sex Toys as a Case of Third-Wave HCI," *Conference: Proceedings of the International Conference on Human Factors in Computing Systems*, CHI 2011, Vancouver, BC, Canada, May 7–12, 2011, 4.

82. "iroha+," Iroha, accessed April 2021, https://iroha-tenga.com/en/plus/; "iroha stick," Iroha, accessed April 2021, https://iroha-tenga.com/en/stick/

83. "Concept," Iroha, accessed April 2021, https://iroha-tenga.com/en/concept/

84. Bardzell and Bardzell, "'Pleasure Is Your Birthright,'" 2.

85. Dame and Iroha foreground the language of self-care, while Maude likewise emphasizes the benefits of stress relief.

86. "FAQs: Do You Offer Discrete Shipping?" Maude, accessed April 2021, https://getmaude.com/pages/faq#products

87. Fahs and Frank, "Notes from the Back Room," 241.

88. Comella, *Vibrator Nation*, 1.

89. The creator of Lioness, Liz Klinger, describes how her company offers women a "classier" alternative to traditional sex shops: "I've had women tell me they don't want to go to a sex shop and have a 20-something recommend a toy. These are mature women taking control of their sexuality—we want to give them an experience that's as cool and classy as they are." Shannon Perry, "The Lioness Vibrator: Learn to Love Your Body," *Genev*, 25 March 2021, https://gennev.com/education/lioness-vibrator-sex-toy

90. Companies like Maude, Dame, and Lora DiCarlo all attempt to address queer populations and remain relatively gender-neutral. However, they do primarily target individuals with a vulva.

91. Diane Negra and Yvonne Tasker, *Interrogating Postfeminism* (Duke University Press, 2007), 2.

92. While Comella argues that feminism can be expressed through commodity choices and entrepreneurial endeavors, Riley and colleagues argue that "understanding sexuality through consumerism masks the vested interest in selling sex in ways that make money. Women's most intimate desires are thus structured through capitalism." I likewise agree that selling and purchasing feminist products or promoting sex-positive and more diverse companies does not address the way neoliberal capitalism has structured contemporary sexuality and health. Comella, *Vibrator Nation*, 13; Riley et al., *Postfeminism and Health*, 96.

93. Frith similarly defines the postfeminist woman as "constantly seeking to develop their sexual knowledge, understanding and experience, and investing in their sexual skills to achieve the ultimate orgasm." Frith, *Orgasmic Bodies*, 28.

94. Frith, *Orgasmic Bodies*, 27.

95. Rossalind Gill, "Mediated Intimacy and Postfeminism: A Discourse Analytic Examination of Sex and Relationships Advice in a Women's Magazine," *Discourse & Communication* 3, no. 4 (2009): 345–69.

96. Riley et al., *Postfeminism and Health*, 79.

97. Liz Klinger, "How Does Lioness Help Me Have Better Sex/Orgasms?" Lioness, accessed May 2021, https://help.lioness.io/en/articles/3873563-how-does-lioness-help-me-have-better-sex-orgasms

98. Lioness, "Homepage."

99. Gill, "Mediated Intimacy," 365; Frith, *Orgasmic Bodies*, 28.

100. Frith, *Orgasmic Bodies*, 29.

101. Kinsey et al., *Human Male*, 202; Kinsey et al., *Human Female*, 591–93.

102. Irvine, *Disorders of Desire*, 56.

103. Masters and Johnson, *Human Sexual Response*, 285.

104. Masters and Johnson, *Human Sexual Response*, 127.

105. Masters and Johnson, *Human Sexual Inadequacy*, 9.

106. Masters and Johnson, *Human Sexual Response*, 4.

107. Irvine, *Disorders of Desire*, 91.

108. Irvine, *Disorders of Desire*, 91.

109. Toni Ayers, Maggi Rubenstein, and Carolyn Haynes Smith, *Masturbation Techniques for Women* (Multimedia Resource Center, 1972), 6.

110. "Homepage," Bodysex, Betty Dodson and Carlin Ross, n.d., accessed May 2021. https://dodsonandross.com/

111. Comella, *Vibrator Nation*, 22.

112. Quoted in Comella, *Vibrator Nation*, 27.

113. Frith makes a similar claim, arguing that in contemporary sex self-help, "the body is depicted as having both 'natural' orgasmic capabilities . . . and as a machine which can be made to work more effectively and efficiently." Frith, *Orgasmic Bodies*, 90; Cacchioni, "Labour of Love," 306.

114. Frith, *Orgasmic Bodies*, 87.

115. While the homepage links to appointments with a "wellness coach," the scheduling portal describes the meeting as a "product coaching consultation." This suggests that the "coaching" sessions are directly attached to buying and using their products. Lora Di Carlo, "Homepage."

116. Lioness, "Homepage."

117. "Workshops," Dame, accessed April 2021, https://damewellness.co/pages/workshops?utm_source=swell&utm_medium=blog&utm_campaign=nav

118. Lioness, "Homepage."

119. "Lioness: Sexual Health Tracker," Apple App Store, accessed May 2021, https://apps.apple.com/us/app/lioness-sexual-health-tracker/id1177248589

120. "Guide to Good Vibes with Lioness," Lioness, 28 July 20218, https://blog.lioness.io/guide-to-good-vibes-with-the-lioness-vibrator-8d73962829e9?gi=256c4d6a4cf4

121. Lioness, "Lioness Health and Sex Tracker," vers. 2.0.07, accessed June 2021.

122. Irvine, *Disorders of Desire*, 68, 78–79.

123. Masters and Johnson, *Human Sexual Response*, 6.

124. Masters and Johnson, *Human Sexual Response*, 6.

125. Masters and Johnson, *Human Sexual Response*, 132.

126. Frith, *Orgasmic Bodies*, 128.

127. Lioness "Homepage."

128. Lioness "Homepage."
129. Lioness, "Homepage."
130. Lioness, "How Does Our Technology Work?"
131. Frith, *Orgasmic Bodies*, 22.
132. Fahs and Frank, "Notes from the Back Room," 246.
133. Frith, *Orgasmic Bodies*, 128.
134. Frith, *Orgasmic Bodies*, 129.
135. A range of studies on the correlation between orgasms and other bodily processes have been examined. Orgasms have been shown to decrease stress and pain, and to improve self-esteem, depression, and indicators of cancer and heart disease. Some examples include Carl Charnetski and Francis X. Brennan, *Feeling Good Is Good for You: How Pleasure Can Boost Your Immune System and Lengthen Your Life* (Rodale Books, 2001); D. J. Weeks, "Sex for the Mature Adult: Health, Self-Esteem, and Countering Agist Stereotypes," *Sexual and Relationship Therapy* 17 (2002): 231–40; Harry Feldman, Catherine B. Johannes, Andre B. Araujo, Beth A. Mohr, Christopher Longcope, and John B. McKinlay, "Low Dehydroepiandrosterone Sulfate and Heart Disease in Middle-Aged Men: Cross-Sectional Results from the Massachusetts Male Aging Study," *Annals of Epidemiology* 8 (1998): 217–28; Randolph W. Evans and R. Couch, "Orgasm and Migraine," *Headache* 41 (2001): 512–14; Beverly Whipple and Brian R. Komisaruk, "Brain (PET) Responses to Vaginal-Cervical Self-Stimulation in Women with Complete Spinal Cord Injury: Preliminary Findings," *Journal of Sex and Marital Therapy* 28 (2002): 79–86.
136. Barry R. Komisaruk, Carlos Beyer-Flores, and Beverly Whipple, *The Science of Orgasm* (Johns Hopkins University Press, 2006), 47.
137. This can potentially also reinforce the medicalization of sexuality by encouraging individuals to compare themselves to datafied norms.
138. Alex Cranz, "Hands on with the Vibrator that Wants to Be the Smartest Sex Toy in the World," *Gizmodo*, 16 August 2017, https://gizmodo.com/hands-on-with-the-vibrator-that-wants-to-be-the-smartes-1797868452; Liz Klinger, "How People Have Explored with Lioness," Lioness, 10 March 2019, https://lioness.io/blogs/sex-guides/how-people-have-explored-with-lioness-smart-vibrator
139. Klinger, "How People Have Explored."
140. Rowland, *The Pleasure Gap*, 133.
141. Fahs and Frank, "Notes from the Back Room," 248.
142. It should be noted that many studies of women's experiences of masturbation survey primarily cis white women. Hogarth and Ingham note that the frequency of masturbation is relatively lower among Black women, but further research needs to be done to understand the reasons for this difference. Hogarth and Ingham, "Masturbation among Young Women," 559.
143. Lioness partners with research labs and institutions that run studies on a range of topics, from pelvic floor health to device verification. Individuals can share their anonymized data with a selected study. However, it's unclear whether these data are used to revise the data or platform. In other words, these studies primarily treat the device as a scientific tool, rather than reflecting on how assumptions about orgasmic presence or how the device operates may inform the results. "Research," Lioness, accessed May 2021, https://lioness.io/pages/user-faq-lioness-research-platform

144. Karen Holly, "Pelvic Rehab Health—My One Year Lioness Vibrator Experiment—Why Vibrators Matter," updated 2019, n.d. publication, accessed May 2021, https://www.karenkholly.com/blog/pelvic-rehab-health-my-one-year-lioness-vibrator-experiment-why-vibrators-matter

145. Leder argues that solo pleasures are still largely aimed toward projecting an image for others. I disagree. Many sociological studies of masturbation have shown that women often engage in masturbation for a variety of reasons, ranging from relaxation to performative reasons closer to Leder's reading. Likewise, studies of "tantric orgasm" draw on Reich and Taoist practices to promote an energy-based theory of the orgasm. These accounts have tried to expand definitions of the orgasm to include intrapersonal and intrasubjective factors that contribute to the experience of an orgasm. Drew Leder, *The Absent Body* (University of Chicago Press, 1990); Mike Lousada and Elena Angel, "Tantric Orgasm: Beyond Masters and Johnson" *Sexual and Relationship Therapy* 6, no. 24 (2011): 389–402.

146. Drew Leder, *The Absent Body*, 75.

147. Simone de Beauvoir, *The Second Sex* (Jonathan Cape, 1956), 388.

148. Indeed, de Beauvoir's discussion of sexual pleasure is premised from her claim that the "goal" of sexual pleasure is "uncertain from the start, and more psychological than physiological in nature." de Beauvoir, *The Second Sex*, 387.

Chapter 3

1. The manifesto no longer appears on the Fitbit "About Us" section of the webpage, but remained a central feature until the end of 2018. I have not been able to find a reason for the change. "Why Fitbit," Fitbit, accessed May 2017, http://www.fitbit.com/whyfitbit

2. Adrienne E. Hardman and David J. Stensel, *Physical Activity and Health: Evidence Explained* (Routledge, 2009), 13; Jeremy Howell and Alan Ingham, "From Social Problem to Personal Issue: The Language of Lifestyle," *Cultural Studies* 15, no. 2 (2010): 342.

3. Jürgen Martschukat "The Age of Fitness: The Power of Ability in Recent American History," *Rethinking History* 23, no. 2 (2019): 160.

4. Examples of this discussion can be found in David Armstrong and Elizabeth Metzger Armstrong, "Fitness: The Ultimate Cure," *The Great American Medicine Show: Being an Illustrated History of Hucksters, Healers, Health Evangelists, and Heroes from Plymouth Rock to the Present* (Prentice Hall, 1991), 257–67; Harvey Green, *Fit for America: Health, Fitness, Sport, and American Society* (Pantheon, 1986); Bruce Haley, *The Healthy Body and Victorian Culture* (Harvard University Press, 1978); R. J. Shepard, *A History of Health and Fitness: Implications for Policy Today* (Spring International Publishing, 2018); Jennifer Smith Maguire, *Fit for Consumption: Sociology and the Business of Fitness* (Routledge, 2008); James C. Whorton, *Crusaders for Fitness: The History of American Health Reformers* (Princeton University Press, 1982).

5. Green, *Fit for America*, 23–24; Whorton, *Crusaders for Fitness*, 5, 271.

6. Vassilis Charitsis, "Survival of the (Data) Fit: Self-Surveillance, Corporate Wellness and the Platformization of Healthcare," *Surveillance and Society* 17, nos. 1/2 (2019): 140.

7. Examples of these arguments can be found in Mary Louise Adams, "Step-Counting in the 'Health Society': Phenomenological Reflections on Step-Counting in the Era of Fitbit," *Social Theory of Health* 17 (2018): 109–24; Charitsis, "Survival of the (Data) Fit"; Kate Crawford, Jesse Lingel, and Tero Karppi, "Our Metrics, Ourselves: A Hundred Years of Self-Tracking from the Weight Scale to the Wrist Wearable Device," *European Journal of Cultural Studies* 18, nos. 4–5 (2015): 479–96; Deborah Lupton, *The Quantified Self: A Sociology of Self-Tracking* (John Wiley and Sons, 2016); Chris Till, "Exercise as Labour: Quantified Self and the Transformation of Exercise into Labour," *societies* 4, no. 3 (2014): 446–62; Jennifer R. Whitson, "Foucault's Fitbit: Governance and Gamification," *The Gameful World*, edited by Steffen P. Walz and Sebastian Deterding (MIT Press, 2014), 339–58.

8. Susannah Fox and Maeve Duggan, "Tracking for Health," Pew Research Center Internet & American Life Project, 2013, http://www.pewinternet.org/2013/01/28/main-report-8; Abbey Lunny, Nicole R. Cunningham, and Matthew S. Easton, "Wearable Fitness Technology: A Structural Investigation into Acceptance and Perceived Outcomes," *Computers in Human Behavior* 65 (2011): 114–20; Lotfi Chaari, *Digital Health Approach for Predictive, Preventive, Personalised and Predictive Medicine* (Springer, 2019); "White Paper on Connected Health: The Case for Medicine 2.0," Withings Health Institute, n.d.

9. The most famous assessment of American health comes from a report compiled by the US Department of Health and Human Services once a decade called, "Healthy People." Since 1980, these reports have served as summative, authoritative assessments of the current state of American health. The report repeatedly identifies "lifestyle diseases" as a key point of concern. "History of Healthy People," Department of Health and Human Services, updated 2 December 2020, accessed July 2021, https://health.gov/our-work/healthy-people/about-healthy-people/history-healthy-people

10. Shelly McKenzie, *Getting Physical: The Rise of Fitness Culture in America* (University Press of Kansas, 2013), 2.

11. Bithaj Ajana, "Digital Health and the Biopolitics of the Quantified Self," *Digital Health* 3 (2017): 2055207616689509; Farzana Dudwala "Redrawing Boundaries Around the Self," *Quantified Lives and Vital Data: Exploring Health and Technology Through Personal Medical Devices*, edited by Rebecca Lynch and Conor Farrington (Palgrave MacMillan, 2018), 97–123; Deborah Lupton, *The Quantified Self*; Paulo Ruffino, "Engagement and the Quantified Self: Uneventful Relationships and Ghostly Companions," *Self-Tracking: Empirical and Philosophical Investigations*, edited by Btihja Ajana (Palgrave MacMillan, 2018), 11–25; Minna Ruckenstein, "Visualized and Interacted Life: Personal Analytics and Engagements with Data Doubles," *societies* 4 (2014): 68–84; Chris Till, "Exercise as Labour: The Quantified Self and the Transformation of Exercise into Labour," *societies* 5 (2014): 446–62.

12. My research was conducted at three universities, each with unique IRB standards. At two of the universities, the project was considered "exempt," and the third granted IRB approval to complete the study (LMU IRB 2020 SU 17 R). In all classes, students were given informed consent, including information on how their material would be used, stored, and reproduced. It was made clear that they had no obligation to agree to share their work, and it would have no impact on their grade

in the class. I have received written, informed consent from all the participating students cited here to share their work anonymously.

13. Kenneth M. Cooper, *The New Aerobics* (Bantam, 1970), 26.

14. Hardman and Stensel, *Physical Activity and Health*, 3.

15. Maguire, *Fit for Consumption*, 26.

16. Green, *Fit for America*, 10.

17. Michael S. Goldstein, *The Health Movement: Promoting Fitness in America* (Twayne Publishers, 1992), 78.

18. Quoted in Maguire, *Fit for Consumption*, 30.

19. Goldstein, *The Health Movement*, 80; Smith Maguire, *Fit for Consumption*, 31.

20. Quoted in Whorton, *The Kingdom of Health*, 287.

21. Whorton, *The Kingdom of Health*, 282–85.

22. Martschukat, "The Age of Fitness," 160.

23. Examples of these discourses have been discussed by Martschukat, "The Age of Fitness," 164; Whorton, *The Kingdom of Health*, 299–301.

24. McKenzie, *Getting Physical*, 136.

25. McKenzie, *Getting Physical*, 5.

26. McKenzie, *Getting Physical*, 3, 83.

27. McKenzie, *Getting Physical*, 136.

28. McKenzie, *Getting Physical*, 139.

29. McKenzie, *Getting Physical*, 139.

30. McKenzie, *Getting Physical*, 99–101, 104.

31. McKenzie, *Getting Physical*, 102.

32. McKenzie, *Getting Physical*, 102.

33. McKenzie, *Getting Physical*, 106.

34. Bowerman's use of military experience shows how despite the move toward medical and scientific frameworks for fitness, fitness training remained tied to practices associated with masculinity and nationalism.

35. William J. Bowerman and W. E. Harris, *Jogging* (Charter Books, 1967), 65–151.

36. McKenzie, *Getting Physical*, 118–19.

37. Eileen Kennedy and Pirkko Markula, *Women and Exercise: The Body, Health and Consumerism* (Routledge, 2012). Maguire, *Fit for Consumption*, 40; Phillip White, Kevin Young, and James Gillet, "Bodywork as a Moral Imperative: Some Critical Notes on Health and Fitness," *Leisure and Society* 15, no. 2 (2015): 162.

38. Bowerman and Harris, *Jogging*, 9.

39. Smith Maguire, *Fit for Consumption*, 40.

40. Kenneth H. Cooper, *Aerobics* (Bantam Books, 1968), 165.

41. Cooper, *Aerobics*, 53–55.

42. Cooper adds this note about pedometers in the second edition of *The New Aerobics*, published in 1970. Cooper, *The New Aerobics*, 30.

43. Cooper, *The New Aerobics*, 16.

44. Cooper, *Aerobics*, 30.

45. In the preface to the new edition, *The New Aerobics*, Cooper states, "My most earnest hope is that the wisdom gained from testing and training tens of thousands

of men and women can be imparted to people everywhere who are still seeking healthier, more productive and more effective lives." Cooper, *The New Aerobics*, 9.

46. Cooper, *The New Aerobics*, 16.

47. Cooper, *The New Aerobics*, 16–17; Cooper, *Aerobics*, 21.

48. McKenzie, *Getting Physical* 1; Smith Maguire, *Fit for Consumption*, 49.

49. Smith Maguire, *Fit for Consumption*, 10.

50. Quoted in Smith Maguire, *Fit for Consumption*, 45.

51. The expansion of workplace wellness programs is also attributed to the establishment of the Occupational Health and Safety Administration (OSHA) in 1970.

52. Martschukat, "The Age of Fitness," 159.

53. Till, "Exercise as Labour"; Brad Millington, "Fit for Prosumption: Interactivity and the Second Fitness Boom," *Media Culture & Society* 38, no. 2 (2016): 1184–1200.

54. Millington, "Fit for Presumption," 85.

55. Maguire, *Fit for Consumption*, 111.

56. Charitsis, "Survival of the (Data) Fit"; James N. Gilmore, "Everywear: The Quantified Self and Wearable Fitness Technology," *New Media & Society* 18, no. 11 (2016): 2524–39; Lupton, *The Quantified Self*; Till, "Exercise as Labour"; Whitson, "Foucault's Fitbit."

57. Charitsis, "Survival of the Data Fit," 140; Gilmore, "Everywear," 2530–31; Deborah Lupton, *Digital Health: Critical and Cross-Disciplinary Perspectives* (Routledge, 2017), 47, 103; Deborah Lupton, "Beyond Techno Utopia: Critical Approaches to Digital Health Technologies," *societies* (2014): 707; Whitson, "Foucault's Fitbit," 342.

58. Several scholars have discussed fitness-tracking technologies through the ideology of gamification, arguing that the competition and award structure of these apps condition neoliberal subjects. An example of this argument can be found in Whitson, "Foucault's Fitbit."

59. "Activity," Apple, vers. 14.6 (2021), accessed June 2021.

60. There are countless interviews and news articles on doctors' and researchers' criticisms of fitness-tracking technologies. Some recent examples include Dalvin Brown, "Doctors Say Most Metrics Provided by Your Apple Watch and Fitbit Are Not Useful to Them," *USA Today*, 14 August 2019, https://www.usatoday.com/story/tech/2019/08/14/how-doctors-really-feel-data-your-apple-watch-fitbit/1900968001/; Daily Telegraph, "Fitbit Devices Could Be Harmful to Heart Patients, Researchers Warn," *Daily Telegraph*, 17 August 2020; Randi Hutter Epstein, "Can a Smartwatch Save Your Life?" *New York Times*, 28 May 2021, https://www.nytimes.com/2021/05/20/well/live/smartwatch-heart-rate-monitor.html; Zina Moukheiber, "I Asked 20,000 Doctors About Fitbit and Apple's HealthKit and Here's the Answer," 24 November 2014, https://www.forbes.com/sites/zinamoukheiber/2014/11/24/i-asked-20000-doctors-about-fitbit-and-apples-healthkit-and-heres-the-answer/?sh=4bd4501251a7

61. Rob Kitchin, "Big Data, New Epistemologies and Paradigm Shifts," *Big Data & Society* 1 (2014): 4–5.

62. Over the last decade, a handful of meta-analyses have explored studies testing the accuracy of commercial fitness trackers. Results often highlight the lack of a standardized way to assess accuracy, which in turn affects the ability to compare studies. Most highlight the strengths and weaknesses of the device, claiming that certain metrics are more accurate than others. Examples of these meta-analyses include Kelly R. Evanson, Michelle M. Goto, and Robert D. Furberg, "Systematic Review of the Validity and Reliability of Consumer-Wearable Activity Trackers," *International Journal of Behavioral Nutrition and Physical Activity* 12, no. 159 (2015): 1–22; Lynne M. Feehan et al., "Accuracy of Fitbit Devices: Systematic Review and Narrative Syntheses of Quantitative Data," *JMIR mHealth and uHealth* 6, no. 8 e10527, 9 August 2018, *doi:10.2196/10527*; Jessica Gorzelitz, Chloe Farber, Robert Gangnon, and Lisa Cadmus-Bertram, "Accuracy of Wearable Trackers for Measuring Moderate- to Vigorous-Intensity Physical Activity: A Systematic Review and Meta-Analysis," *Journal of Measurement of Physical Behavior* 3 (2020): 346–57.

63. danah boyd and Kate Crawford, "Critical Questions for Big Data," *Information, Communication & Society* 15, no. 5 (2012): 663.

64. Halpern's use of the term "communicative objectivity" draws on Loraine Daston and Peter Galison's historicization of scientific objectivity, which helps demonstrate how standards of objectivity have shifted over time. Lorraine Daston and Peter Galison, *Objectivity* (Princeton University Press, 2007).

65. Orit Halpern, *Beautiful Data: A History of Vision and Reason since 1945* (Duke University Press, 2015), 60.

66. Halpern, *Beautiful Data*, 95.

67. Lisa Gitelman similarly argues that data visualization enhances the rhetorical power of big data: "Not only are data abstract and aggregative, but also data are mobilized graphically. That is, in order to be used as part of an explanation or as a basis for an argument, data typically require graphical representation and often involve a cascade of representations. . . . Data visualization amplifies the rhetorical function of data." Lisa Gitelman, *"Raw Data" Is an Oxymoron* (MIT Press, 2013), 12.

68. Helen Kennedy and Rosemary Lucy Hill, "The Feeling of Numbers: Emotions in Everyday Engagements with Data and Their Visualization," *Sociology* 52, no. 4 (2018): 381.

69. This is in line with Kennedy and colleauges' work on data visualization aesthetics, where they identify four primary conventions that designers use to communicate authority: "(a) two-dimensional viewpoints; (b) clean layouts; (c) geometric shapes and lines; (d) the inclusion of data sources." Helen Kennedy, Rosemary Lucy Hill, Giorgia Aiello, and William Allen, "The Work that Visualization Conventions Do," *Information, Communication, and Society* 19, no. 6 (2016): 716.

70. Edward Tufte, *The Visual Display of Quantitative Information* (Graphics Press, 2001), 13.

71. Edward Tufte, *Visual Explanations: Images and Quantities, Evidence and Narrative* (Graphics Press, 1997), 48.

72. Tufte, *Visual Explanations*, 53.

73. Giorgia Aiello, "Theoretical Advances in Critical Visual Analysis: Perception, Ideology, Mythologies, and Social Semiotics," *Journal of Visual Literacy* 26, no. 2 (2006): 89–102; Nick Cawthon and Andrew Vande Moere, "The Effect of

Aesthetic on the Usability of Data Visualization," *11th International Conference on Information Visualization* (2007); Kennedy et al., "The Work"; Alexander Vande Moere and Helen Purchase, "On the Role of Design in Information Visualization," *Information Visualization* 10, no. 4 (2011): 356–71.

74. Tufte, *Visual Explanations*, 48.

75. Fitbit uses similar visualization strategies but places greater emphasis on numbers. The interface uses the same circular visualization to measure progress, but it includes the calorie count below. "Fitbit App," Fitbit, vers. 3.43.1 (2021), accessed June 2021.

76. Apple does include a "Trends" section that offers information about behaviors over time, however, this requires navigating to the "Fitness" app on the Apple phone. None of these statistical data are accessible via the watch platform. Moreover, there is often a lag when you open the app, delaying the appearance of the information, which can encourage individuals to navigate away before processing. "Trends" allows individuals to monitor whether their daily move goal has been increasing, or their running pace has decreased. A list of statistical averages is coupled with an up or down arrow, and the platform encourages individuals to keep their "arrows up!" "Activity," Apple, iOS 8.1, accessed June 2021.

77. Paolo Ruffino, "Engagement and the Quantified Self: Uneventful Relationships and Ghostly Companions," *Self-Tracking*, edited by B. Ajana (Palgrave McMillan, 2018), 11–25; Gavin J. D. Smith and Ben Vonthethoff, "Health by Numbers? Exploring the Practice and Experience of Datafied Health," *Health Sociology Review* 26, no. 1 (2017): 6–21; Till, "Exercise as Labour"; Jacqueline Wernimont Ruffino, *Numbered Lives: Life and Death in Quantum Media* (MIT Press, 2019), 96.

78. This is in line with many weight- and BMI-based definitions of health, which have been critiqued for reinforcing the connection between appearance and health. Maguire, *Fit for Consumption*, 25.

79. Hyunho Lee and Youngseok Lee, "A Look at Wearable Abandonment," *18th IEEE International Conference on Mobile Data Management (MDM)*, (2017), 392–93; Neff and Nafus, *Self-Tracking*, 24; Valencell, "National Wearables Survey Reveals Accelerating Convergence of Consumer Wearables and Personal Health & Medical Devices," 2018, https://valencell.com/news/national-wearables-survey-shows-convergence-of-wearables-and-health-devices/

80. Patrick Allen, "Five Ways to Cheat Your Way to 10,000 Steps Every Day," *Lifehacker*, 27 October 2016, https://lifehacker.com/five-ways-to-cheat-your-way-to-10-000-fitbit-steps-ever-1788302045; Mike McPhate, "Just How Accurate Are Fitbits? The Jury Is Still Out," *New York Times*, 25 May 2016, https://www.nytimes.com/2016/05/26/technology/personaltech/fitbit-accuracy.html; Erin MacPherson, "How Accurate Are Apple Watch Calories? How to Make them as Accurate as Possible," *iPhone Life*, 17 May 2021, https://www.iphonelife.com/content/how-accurate-are-apple-watch-calories-how-to-ensure-theyre-accurate; Jake Peterson, "Cheat Your Apple Watch Rings," *Gadget Hacks*, 13 December 2018, https://ios.gadgethacks.com/how-to/cheat-your-apple-watch-rings-0191261/; Michael Swah, "Transform Your Fitbit's Accuracy: Step Count, Heart Rate and Sleep," *Wearable*, 21 December 2020, https://www.wareable.com/fitbit/how-to-calibrate-fitbit-3031

81. Kennedy and Hill, "The Feeling of Numbers," 488. Emphasis my own.

82. "In data some things get communicated while others get lost. There is much room for people to maneuver in the imperfect translation." Neff and Nafus, *Self-Tracking*, 25.

83. Dawn Nafus and Jamie Sherman, "Big Data, Big Questions, This One Does Not Go Up to 11: The Quantified Self Movement as an Alternative Big Data Practice," *International Journal of Communication* 8 (2014): 1793.

84. For the full assignment instructions and student's accounts of the reflection see Mikki Kressbach, Ivan Martinez-Medina, and Thomas Streed, "Strategies for Teaching Ephemeral Media: Phenomenological Description," *Journal of Interactive Technology and Pedagogy*, 12 October 2022, https://jitp.commons.gc.cuny.edu/strategies-for-analyzing-ephemeral-media-phenomenological-description/

85. This assignment was accompanied by a lesson on privacy policies that required students to read through the policy of their respective app or device. Students completed a quiz to ensure they understood the way the app used and shared their data. Those who were uncomfortable with the privacy policies could opt out of the activity.

86. Sarah Pink and Vaike Fors, "Being in a Mediated World: Self-Tracking and the Mind-Body Environment," *Cultural Geographies* 24, no. 3 (2017): 379.

87. Student paper, Los Angeles, 2020.

88. Student paper, Chicago, 2017.

89. Gilmore "Everywear," 2533.

90. Lupton, *Digital Health*, 59.

91. Student, exit survey, Los Angeles 2020; student paper, Los Angeles 2020.

92. Both Fitbit and Apple Health have departments that market their devices for clinical studies. "Fitbit Health Solutions" provides resources for researchers to purchase and use Fitbit devices in ongoing studies. Apple Health Kit allows individuals to opt in to current studies on a range of conditions, including heart health and hearing. In addition to research developed in partnership with these companies, many university and lab-based studies incorporate the technology to monitor subjects' vitals. "Apple Announces Three Groundbreaking Health Studies," Apple, 10 September 2019, https://www.apple.com/newsroom/2019/09/apple-announces-three-groundbreaking-health-studies/; "Fitbit Health Solutions," Fitbit, accessed July 2021, https://healthsolutions.fitbit.com/researchers/

93. As of 2021, several leading American insurance companies offered discounts for syncing fitness tracker data. Some major names include Blue Cross Blue Shield, Kaiser Permanente, and John Hancock. Sigrid Forberg, "Can a Fitness Tracker Save You Money on Health Insurance?" *MoneyWise*, 22 January 2021, https://www.yahoo.com/now/heres-could-free-fitbit-insurance-151900485.html?guccounter=1

Chapter 4

1. Fitbit staff, "Here's Why You'll Love Relax, Fitbit's New Guided Breathing Experience," Fitbit Blog, 9 April 2020, https://blog.fitbit.com/heres-why-youll-love-fitbits-new-guided-breathing-experience/

2. For example, see Robert D. Brook, Lawrence J. Appel, Melvyn Rubenfire,

Gbenga Ogedegbe, John D. Bisognano, William J. Elliott, Flavio D. Fuchs, et al., "Beyond Medications and Diet: Alternative Approaches to Lowering Blood Pressure," *American Heart Association* 61, no. 6 (2013):1360–83.

3. "Homepage," Breathesync, accessed February 2018, https://www.breath esync.com/. This logic has been reinforced across wearables, meditation apps, blog posts, and TEDx Talks. Examples include recent TED Talks by Max Strom and Christian de la Huerta. The American Psychiatric Association has published endorsements of breath work, citing research studies on heart rate variability. The American Institute of Stress additionally endorses breathing exercises for better health. Kellie Marksberry, "Take a Deep Breath," *American Institute of Stress*, 10 August 2012, https://www.stress.org/take-a-deep-breath/; TEDx Talks, "The Power of Breath: Christian De La Huerta," 23 April 2013, https:// www.youtube .com/watch?v=VLAziEkvUT8; TEDx Talks, "What Is Your Breath Telling You? Neema Moraveji," 22 December 2014, https://www.youtube.com/watch?v=tRAg7 YfCpGc; TEDx Talks, "Breathe to Heal: Max Strom," 7 December 2015, https:// www.youtube. com/watch?v=4Lb5L-VEm34

4. Robert Crawford, "Healthism and the Medicalization of Everyday Life," *International Journal of Health Services* 10, no. 3 (1980): 365–88; Carl Elliot, *Better Than Well: American Medicine Meets the American Dream* (W. W. Norton Company, 2003); Jonathan M. Metzl and Anna Kirkland, *Against Health* (New York University Press, 2010); Deborah Lupton, "Beyond Techno-Utopia: Critical Approaches to Digital Health Technologies," *societies* 4, no. 711 (2014): 706–11.

5. Frederik Svenaeus, *The Hermeneutics of Medicine and the Phenomenology of Health* (Springer Science + Business Media, 2000), 88.

6. Donald B. Ardell, *High Level Wellness: An Alternative to Doctors, Drugs, and Disease* (Rodale Press,1977), 2; Donald B. Ardell, *The History and Future of Wellness* (Kendall Hunt Publishing Co., 1985), 2–3.

7. The National Wellness Institute, for example, claims that "wellness is the active process through which people become aware of, and make choices toward, a more successful existence." "Six Dimensions of Wellness," National Institute of Wellness, accessed July 2020, https://nationalwellness.org/resources/six-dimensio ns-of-wellness/

8. Quoted in Ardell, *High Level Wellness*, 5.

9. Quoted in James William Miller, "Wellness: The History and Development of a Concept," *Spektrum Freizeit* 1 (2005): 90.

10. Hans Georg Gadamer, *The Enigma of Health: The Art of Healing in a Scientific Age* (Stanford University Press, 1996); Svenaeus, *The Hermeneutics of Medicine*; Fredrik Sveneaus, "Phenomenology of Health and Illness," *Handbook of Phenomenology and Medicine*, edited by S. Kay Toombs (Kluwer Academic Publishers, 2001), 87–108.

11. A version of this argument appears in Mikki Kressbach, "Breath Work: Mediating Health through Breathing Apps and Wearable Technologies," *New Review of Film and Television Studies* 16, no. 2 (2018): 184–206. https://doi.org/10.10 80/17400309.2018.1444459

12. Jonathan Metzl, "Why 'Against Health?'" *Against Health*, edited by Jonathan M. Metzl and Anna Kirkland (New York University Press, 2010), 2.

13. Drew Leder, *The Absent Body* (University of Chicago Press, 1990), 119.

14. For example, see Leder, *The Absent Body*, 1993; Kay S. Toombs, *The Meaning of Illness: A Phenomenological Account of the Different Perspectives of Physician and Patient* (Kluwer Academic Publishers, 1992).

15. The National Wellness Institute, for example, defines wellness as "multidirectional . . . encompassing lifestyle, mental and spiritual wellbeing." Through the "Six Dimensions of Wellness," the institute offers strategies to become "aware of the interconnectedness of each dimension and how they contribute to healthy living." National Wellness Institute, "Six Dimensions of Wellness."

16. Examples of Myers and Sweeney's wheel can be found in Jane E. Meyers and Thomas J. Sweeny, *Counseling for Wellness* (American Counseling Association, 2005); Brett Kyle Gleason, *A Phenomenological Investigation of Wellness and Wellness Promotion in Counselor Education Programs*, Old Dominion University, 2015; Thomas J. Sweeney, C. S. Gill, C. B. Minton, and J. Myers, "Five Factor Wellness Inventory," *Adultspan Journal* 14, no. 2 (2015): 66–76.

17. Designed to examine the economic viability of workplace wellness programs, the RAND study showed a correlation between workplace wellness programs and decreased healthcare costs. Soeren Mattke, Hangsheng Liu, John Caloyeras, Christina Y. Huang, Kristin R. Van Busum, Dmitry Khodyakov, and Victoria Shier, "Workplace Wellness Programs Study," *Rand Health Quarterly* 3, no. 2 (2013).

18. Universities were some of the first institutions to adopt wellness practices and programs. The first wellness program was launched at the University of Wisconsin–Stevens Point in 1977. Miller, "Wellness," 96.

19. Miller, "Wellness," 84.

20. Nancy Tomes and Carl Elliot are among many scholars who have discussed how medical care shifted to framing care through the language of consumption. Carl Elliot, *Better than Well*; Nancy Tomes, *Remaking the American Patient: How Madison Avenue and Modern Medicine Turned Patients into Consumers* (University of North Carolina Press, 2015).

21. In his attempt to write a history of wellness, James William Miller notes the challenge of assembling such a history. Given wellness's affiliation with a broad range of treatments, philosophical approaches, and economic policies, it's often invoked through a range of terms, including "holistic health," "alternative health," and "self-care." Each of these terms has its own history, so to try and define and trace a coherent lineage of an umbrella term like "wellness" feels almost impossible. Miller, "Wellness," 100–101.

22. Cederström and Spicer and Miller all call wellness an "ideology" rather than a movement. Carl Cederström and André Spicer, *The Wellness Syndrome* (Polity Press, 2015); Miller, "Wellness."

23. Miller, "Wellness."

24. Miller, "Wellness," 86.

25. Tomes, *Remaking the American Patient*, 291–92.

26. By 1947, the WHO amended their constitution to define health as a "state of complete physical, mental and social wellbeing and not merely the absence of disease or illness." While the WHO's definition moves toward a more inclusive definition of health, it fails to address the increasing importance of prevention.

"Frequently Asked Questions," World Health Organization, accessed July 16, 2020, https://www.who.int/about/who-we-are/frequently-asked-questions

27. Quoted in Miller, "Wellness," 92.

28. In 1962, thalidomide, a drug prescribed to women to reduce nausea, was found to cause severe fetal deformation. This spurred a great public panic and drug testing and approval reform. For a longer discussion, see Tomes, *Remaking the American Patient*, 254.

29. In 1964, the surgeon general first published the report on the harmful effects of smoking, which radically shifted professional and popular understanding of the habit. "The Surgeon General's Report on Smoking and Tobacco," Centers for Disease Control, accessed July 2020, https://www.cdc.gov/tobacco/data_statistics/sgr/index.html

30. Historical examples of this discussion can be found in the edited collection by Ivan Illich, Irving K. Zola, John McKnight, Jonathan Caplan, and Harley Shaiken, *Disabling Professions* (Marion Boyars, 1977).

31. Stuart Sarbacker, *Tracing the Path of Yoga: The History and Philosophy of Indian Mind-Body Discipline* (SUNY Press, 2021), 200.

32. Sarbacker, *Tracing the Path of Yoga*, 185.

33. For histories of the feminist health movements in this period, see Karen Baird, Dana-Ain Davis, and Kimberly Christensen, *Beyond Reproduction: Women's Health, Activism, and Public Policy* (Fairleigh Dickinson University Press, 2009); Wendy Klein, *Bodies of Knowledge: Sexuality, Reproduction, and Women's Health in the Second Wave* (University of Chicago Press, 2010).

34. For a discussion of Black health activism in this period, see Alondra Nelson, *Body and Soul: The Black Panther Party and the Fight Against Medical Discrimination* (University of Minnesota Press, 2013).

35. Mike Saks, "Medicine and the Counter Culture," *Companion Encyclopedia of Medicine in the Twentieth Century*, edited by Roger Cooter and John Pickstone (Routledge, 2016), 119.

36. Miller, "Wellness," 97.

37. Ardell, *High Level Wellness*, 186.

38. United States Office of the Assistant Secretary for Health, *Healthy People: The Surgeon General's Report on Health Promotion and Disease Prevention* 79, no. 55071, US Department of Health, Education, and Welfare, Public Health Service, Office of the Assistant Secretary for Health and Surgeon General; Washington, DC, 1979, 1.

39. Tomes, *Remaking the American Patient*, 257.

40. Tomes, *Remaking the American Patient*, 252.

41. Tomes, *Remaking the American Patient*, 263.

42. Mauro Turrini, "A Genealogy of 'Healthism': Healthy Subjectivities between Individual Autonomy and Disciplinary Control," *Journal of Medical Humanities & Social Studies of Science and Technology* 7, no. 1 (June 2015): 18.

43. Turrini, "A Genealogy," 17; Crawford, "Healthism," 390.

44. Turrini, "A Genealogy," 21–22.

45. Ardell, *The History and Future*, 9–13.

46. Ardell offers an overview of historical texts that exhibit these values in *The History and Future of Wellness*.

47. Tomes, *Remaking the American Patient*, 286.

48. Cederstrom and Spicer, *The Wellness Syndrome*, 3.

49. David L. McMahan and Erik Braun, “Introduction: From Colonialism to Brainscans: Modern Transformations in Buddhist Traditions,” *Meditation Buddhism and Science*, edited by David L. McMahan and Erik Braun (Oxford: Oxford University Press, 2017), 9.

50. McMahan and Braun, “Introduction,” 10.

51. Erik Braun, “Mindful but Not Religious: Meditation and Enchantment in the Work of Jon Kabat-Zinn,” *Meditation Buddhism and Science*, edited by David L. McMahan and Erik Braun (Oxford University Press, 2017), 174.

52. Benson and Kippler, *The Relaxation Response*, 17.

53. Benson and Kippler, *The Relaxation Response*, 17–18.

54. McMahan and Braun, “Introduction,” 1–2.

55. Benson and Kippler, *The Relaxation Response*, 15.

56. Benson and Kippler, *The Relaxation Response*, 55.

57. Benson and Kippler, *The Relaxation Response*, 58.

58. Benson and Kippler, *The Relaxation Response*, 114.

59. Benson and Kippler, *The Relaxation Response*, 19.

60. Benson and Kippler, *The Relaxation Response*, 17.

61. Benson and Kippler, *The Relaxation Response*, 19.

62. For example, see Sara W. Lazar, George Bush, Randy L. Gollub, Gregory L. Fricchione, Gurucharan Khalsa, and Herbert Benson, “Functional Brain Mapping of the Relaxation Response and Meditation.” *NeuroReport* 11, no. 7 (2000): 1581–85.

63. Manoj K. Bhasin, Jeffery A. Dusek, Bei-Hung Chang, Marie G. Joseph, John W. Denninger, Gregory L. Fricchione, Herbert Benson, and Towia A. Libermann, “Relaxation Response Induces Temporal Transcriptome Changes in Energy Metabolism, Insulin Secretion and Inflammatory Pathways,” *PLoS ONE* 8, no. 5, (2013): e62817.

64. Benson and Kippler, *The Relaxation Response*, 19.

65. “mindfulness, n.” OED Online, accessed June 2020, https://electra.lmu.edu:5402/view/Entry/118742?redirectedFrom=mindfulness

66. Benson and Kippler, *The Relaxation Response*, 119.

67. Benson and Kippler, *The Relaxation Response*, 117–22.

68. Herbert Benson and Richard Friedman, “Harnessing the Power of the Placebo Effect and Renaming It ‘Remembered Wellness,’” *Annual Review of Medicine* 47, no. 1 (1996): 198.

69. Benson and Friedman, “Harnessing the Power,” 195.

70. Benson and Friedman “Harnessing the Power,” 198.

71. Benson and Friedman “Harnessing the Power,” 198.

72. Tainya C. Clarke, Patricia M. Barnes, Lindsey I. Black, Barbara J. Stussman, and Richard L. Nahin, “The Use of Yoga, Meditation, and Chiropractic Services in the United States,” US Department of Health and Human Services, Centers for Disease Control and Prevention, National Center for Health Statistics, November 2018.

73. For example, see “Relax, Take a Deep Breath,” American Psychological

Association, 21 June 2017, https://www.psychiatry.org/news-room/apa-blogs/apa-blog/2017/06/relax-take-a-deep-breath

74. For example, Margaret Chapman-Clarke, *Mindfulness in the Workplace: An Evidence-Based Approach to Improving Wellbeing and Maximizing Performance* (Kogan Page, 2016); Daniel Goleman, *The Meditative Mind: The Varieties of Meditative Experience* (Tarcher/Putnam, 1996); Liza Varvogli and Christina Darviri, "Stress Management Techniques: Evidence-Based Procedures That Reduce Stress and Promote Health," *Health Science Journal* 5, no. 2 (2011): 74–89; Christiane Wolf and J. Greg Serpa, *A Clinician's Guide to Teaching Mindfulness: The Comprehensive Session-by-Session Program for Mental Health Professionals and Health Care Providers* (New Harbinger Publications, 2015).

75. "What Should I Know about Fitbit's Relax Feature?" Fitbit, 18 November 2017, https://help.fitbit.com/articles/en_US/Help_article/2077

76. Spire does not discuss the science behind its flash heart-rate detector on its website or the app page. I would assume it works similarly to the Apple Watch's photoplethysmography. This process uses LED green light coupled with "with light-sensitive photodiodes to detect the amount of blood flowing through your wrist at any given moment." The device registers this movement and translates it into a heart rate. Given that iPhone flash does not use the same LED frequency, I'm skeptical about the accuracy of Breathesync's data. Nonetheless, on testing this app, it provided a remarkably accurate reading of my heart-rate range (inferred through the "WQ" data). "Your Heart Rate. What It Means, and Where on Apple Watch You'll Find It," Apple, 4 December 2017, https://support.apple.com/en-us/HT204666

77. "Breathesync," App Advice, accessed February 2018, https://appadvice.com/app/breathesync/722304193

78. BreatheSync, "Homepage."

79. Benson and Kippler, *The Relaxation Response*, 75.

80. "Homepage," SpireHealth, accessed July 2020, https://spirehealth.com/pages/stone

81. "Science," SpireHealth, accessed February 2018, https://spirehealth.com/pages/science-behind-spire

82. Head researcher Neema Moraveji claims that Spire is designed to combat the fight-or-flight response through mindfulness and breathing. TEDx, "What Is Your Breath?"

83. SpireHealth, "Homepage."

84. SpireHealth, "Science."

85. SpireHealth, "Science."

86. James N. Gilmore, "Everywear: The Quantified Self and Wearable Fitness Technologies," *New Media & Society* 18, no. 11 (2016): 2532.

87. "Core," Hyperice, accessed February 2023, https://www.hellocore.com/

88. Gilmore "Everywear," 2533, emphasis mine.

89. Benson and Friedman, "Harnessing the Power," 198.

90. Muse explicitly aligns EEG measurements with heart rate, which can be used to assess stress: "Muse is a brain fitness tool that measures brain signals much like a heart rate monitor senses your heartbeat." "What It Measures," Muse, accessed May 2020, https://choosemuse.com/what-it-measures/

91. Muse, "What It Measures."

92. Muse notably often uses the word "performance" to describe meditation in contrast to the common emphasis on "practice." This slight rhetorical shift is in line with the device's emphasis on training and improvement.

93. "How It Works," Muse, accessed May 2020, https://choosemuse.com/how-it-works/

94. "What Is Neurofeedback and Biofeedback?" Muse, accessed July 2020, https://choosemuse.com/blog/what-is-neurofeedback-and-biofeedback/?store_id=ca&utm_source=google&utm_medium=cpc&gclid=Cj0KCQiAnL7yBRD3ARIsAJp_oLaCO0TnOoO9BFkbQJemfEwBupmoytKD3H5UuM-folMGSoOBJ6U0iK0aAgGfEALw_wcB

95. The Muse Direct app is not designed for popular audiences. It is primarily a tool used by researchers and scientists. To extract information from the app, one must know how to read EEG wave patterns.

96. Benson and Kippler, *The Relaxation Response*, 74.

97. At first, this led me to doubt the legitimacy of the device. However, after repeated use, I did get the sense that the device was recording brain patterns. To discern this, I tested the device through multiple experiences, including writing, reading, and watching television. From what I can tell, the reading of "calm" was most frequently recorded when I felt tired, whereas "active" was more commonly recorded when I felt most alert (rather than merely stressed). However, the structure of the soundscape and the graphs provided make it seem as though activity may be affiliated with "distraction."

98. While Muse's promotional materials and in-app instructions never use the language of "success" and "failure," it's hard to ignore the correlation between quiet and chirping birds and a calm mind or peaceful meditation practice.

99. Muse, "What Is Biofeedback?"; "Muse Research," Muse, accessed February 2020, https://choosemuse.com/muse-research/

100. "Why Muse?" Muse, accessed February 2020, https://choosemuse.com/why-muse/

101. This structure can be found across popular meditation guides. For example, David Gelles, "How to Meditate," *New York Times*, n.d., https://www.nytimes.com/guides/well/how-to-meditate

102. While I turn to phenomenology to analyze the experience of breathing, it should be noted that breath and breathing have increasingly been explored through the lens of affect theory in English and media studies. Recent works have examined how audiovisual media represent, exploit, and politicize breath and embodiment by drawing on philosophical work closely tied to affect theory, such as Gilles Deleuze and Félix Guattari, and Luce Irigaray. Works on breath and affect theory in media include Liz Greene, "The Labour of Breath." *Music, Sound, and the Moving Image* 10, no. 2 (2016): 109–33; Davina Quinlivan, *The Place of Breath in Cinema* (University of Edinburgh Press, 2012); Jean-Thomas Trembley, "Breath Image and Sound, An Introduction," *New Review of Film and Television* 16, no. 2 (2018): 93–97; Jean-Thomas Tremblay, *Breathing Aesthetics* (Duke University Press, 2022).

103. Fitbit's Relax app is slightly different in that it claims to be able to track an

individual's breathing rate during the exercise. Sparkles appear on the screen when the user meets the correct breathing rate, which is determined through the device's heart rate monitor. Fitbit "What Should I Know?"

104. Gilmore, "Everywear," 2533–34.

105. Iris Marion Young, *On Female Body Experience: "Throwing Like a Girl" and Other Essays* (Oxford University Press, 2005), 52.

106. Gadamer, *The Enigma of Health*, 107.

107. Gadamer, *The Enigma of Health*, 112.

108. Svenaeus, *The Hermeneutics of Medicine*, 96.

109. Sveneaus, *The Hermeneutics of Medicine*, 95.

110. Cressida Heyes, *Self-Transformations: Foucault, Ethics, and Normalized Bodies* (Oxford University Press, 2007), 131.

Chapter 5

1. "Track Your Trends in the Activity App," Apple, 19 October 2019, https://support.apple.com/en-us/HT210343

2. Overviews of this critique can be found in Deborah Lupton, *The Quantified Self* (Polity Press, 2016); Gina Neff and Dawn Nafus, "What Is at Stake? The Personal Gets Political," *Self-Tracking* (MIT Press, 2016), 37–68.

3. Nick Crossley, *Reflexive Embodiment in Contemporary Society* (Open University Press, 2006), 87; Drew Leder, *The Absent Body* (University of Chicago Press, 1990), 50.

4. Moreover any understanding of the present "I" relies on a historical reflection on the self/"me:" "I always reflect on a historical reconstruction of the self; that is, upon 'me'. . . . [H]istory . . . might be a matter of microseconds but there is a gap nonetheless, and it is important because it means that the I, the agent in the present tense, is elusive. It only ever knows itself through the mode of historical reconstruction." Crossley, *Reflexive Embodiment*, 94.

5. Crossley, *Reflexive Embodiment*, 95.

6. Leder, *The Absent Body*, 152–53.

7. Leder, *The Absent Body*, 91.

8. Leder, *The Absent Body*, 91.

9. For Leder, the receding, healthy body has indeed facilitated dualist interpretations of the body and the continued objectification of bodily experiences. Leder, *The Absent Body*, 50.

10. Leder, *The Absent Body*, 96.

11. Leder draws on Foucault here to describe how the clinical gaze encourages bodily dys-appearance. Leder, *The Absent Body*, 98.

12. Crossley, *Reflexive Embodiment*, 95.

13. Jacquelyn Allen-Collinson and John Hockey, "Feeling the Way: Notes toward a Haptic Phenomenology of Scuba Diving and Running," *International Review for the Sociology of Sport*, 46, no. 3 (2010): 330–45; Jacquelyn Allen-Collinson and Helen Otwon, "Take a Deep Breath: Asthma, Sporting Embodiment, the Senses, and 'Auditory Work,'" *International Review for the Sociology of Sport* 49, no. 5 (2014): 592–608; John Hockey, "Sensing the Run: The Senses and Distance Run-

ning," *Senses and Society* 1, no. 2 (2006): 183–202; James Morley, "Inspiration and Expiration: Yoga Practice through Merleau-Ponty's Phenomenology of the Body," *Philosophy East and West* 51, no. 1 (2001): 73–82.

14. Fredrik Svenaeus, *The Hermeneutics of Medicine and the Phenomenology of Health* (Springer Science + Business Media, 2000), 95.

15. Walter R. Thompson, "Now Trending: Worldwide Survey of Fitness Trends for 2014," *ACSM's Health and Fitness Journal* 17, no. 6 (November/December 2013): 10–20.

16. The first scientific study on HIIT was published in 1959. Since then, countless studies have explored the health benefits of HIIT, focused on heart health, weight loss, and athletic training. Overviews of these studies can be found in Andrea Nicolo and Michele Giradi, "The Physiology of Interval Training: A New Target to HIIT," *Journal of Physiology* 594.24 (2016): 7169; Paul Larsen and Martin Bucheit, *Science and Application of High Intensity Interval Training: Solutions to the Programming Puzzle* (Human Kinetics, 2019); H. Reindell and H. Roskamm, Ein Beitrag zu den physiologischen Grundlagen des Intervalltrainings unter besonderer Berücksichtigung des Kreislaufes [A Contribution to the Physiological Basics of Interval Training with Special Regard to Circulation]. *Schweiz Z Sportmed*, 7 (1959): 1–8.

17. Larsen and Bucheit, *Science and Application*, 7.

18. Stephanie Smith, "5 Ways to Know You're Going Hard Enough with HIIT," *Fitbit Blog*, 7 December 2017, https://blog.fitbit.com/5-ways-know-youre-going-hard-enough-hiit/

19. Luke Haile, Michael Gallagher, and Robert J. Johnson, *Perceived Exertion Laboratory Manual* (Springer Verlag, 2016).

20. "RPE Scale," Fit Tutor, accessed May 2020, https://thefittutor.com/rpe-scale/

21. Haile, Gallagher, and Johnson, *Perceived Exertion*, 16.

22. Katarina Segerståhl and Harri Oinnas-Kukkonen, "Designing Personal Exercise Monitoring Employing Multiple Modes of Delivery: Implications from a Qualitative Study on Heart Rate Monitoring," *International Journal of Medical Informatics* 80 (2011): E208.

23. Both Fitbit and Apple Watch, for example, provide heart rate data while tracking exercise. The individual simply needs to lift their wrist and tap the screen to receive a reading.

24. Anthony Dominic, "Orangetheory Fitness Exceeds 1 Billion in 2018 System-wide Revenue," *Club Industry*, 4 February 2019, https://www.clubindustry.com/news/orangetheory-fitness-exceeds-1-billion-2018-system-wide-revenue

25. Orangetheory is a franchise business, so pricing is determined by individual studios. Pricing is not advertised on studio websites, so the recent pricing scale relies on member-reported information. Ryan Jons, "Orangetheory Fitness Costs and Orangetheory Membership Costs," *Gym Price List 2022*, https://gympricelist.com/orangetheory-fitness-prices/

26. "Homepage," Orangetheory Fitness, accessed April 2020, https://www.orangetheory.com/en-us/

27. Orangetheory qualifies their suggested twelve "splat point" goal, suggesting that individuals should make adjustments based on their personal fitness levels:

"Here at Orangetheory, each minute in the red or orange heart rate zones, where the heart is working at its highest levels, equals one splat point. The goal for each workout is at least a dozen such points. But if you feel like you're working as hard as possible and even the 12 seems elusive—or if you easily pile up 30 with breath to spare—the tried-and-true heart rate formula may not be tried-and-true for you." Leslie Barker, "Do You 'Fit' the Heart Rate Equation?" Orangetheory Fitness, n.d., https://www.orangetheoryfitness.com/apps/blog/post/661

28. "Data is the key. The longer we work with someone who has a measurable Burn device, the more specifically we can see the results of what we're trying to accomplish." Leslie Barker, "We Have a Heart: The 'Why' Behind Our Heart Rate Monitors," Orangetheory Fitness, n.d., https://www.orangetheory.com/en-au/articles/the-why-behind-our-heart-rate-monitors/

29. Orangetheory breaks these paces down further depending on athletic ability. They provide pacing for "power walkers," "joggers," and "runners," with "runner" defined as anyone with a mile time under ten minutes.

30. Like other circuit training and exercise classes, Orangetheory requires a base level of knowledge about the mechanics and social dynamics of the class. This is often manifested in embodied knowledge as those familiar with the flow of the class instinctually move through the prompts: "[Moving through the class] isn't a reflexive calculation, however, it is an embodied feel, partial sense of the self and world derived from immersion in practice." Nick Crossley, "The Circuit Trainer's Habitus: Reflexive Body Techniques and the Sociality of the Workout," *Bodies and Society* 10, no. 1 (2004): 49.

31. "Physical exercise is experienced first and foremost within the individual's body, but the physical environment, which is controlled by the service provider, and other customers also influence the total experience. Thus, [the group fitness experience] is the sum of the customer's interpretations through the lived body." Tiina-Kaisa Kuuru and Elina Närvänen, "Embodied Interaction in Customer Experience: A Phenomenological Study of Group Fitness," *Journal of Marketing Management* 35, no. 13–14 (2019): 1242.

32. "What Makes Orangetheory Work: Technology," Orangetheory Fitness, online video clip, uploaded to YouTube 18 October 2018, https://www.youtube.com/watch?v=4n6hZzsXXOs

33. Orangetheory Fitness, "What Makes Orangetheory Work: Technology."

34. Orangetheory Fitness, "What Makes Orangetheory Work: Technology."

35. Though it's possible that these factors indirectly affect heart rate, the technology does not calibrate for these exterior factors, and it would not necessarily be possible to do so.

36. Emphasis mine. Haile et al., *Perceived Exertion*, 11.

37. Jessica Migella, "7 HIIT Mistakes You're Probably Making," *Daily Burn*, 7 August 2017, https://dailyburn.com/life/fitness/hiit-workout-mistakes/. Another example that combines a scenario with bodily cues: "10 equal to running for your life as you are chased by a rabid beast. You should be working almost that hard during a HIIT workout, pushing yourself to a level 8 or 9. Remember that HIIT is hard. Your heart should be pounding, your breathing should be heavy, you should be sweating." Sean Bartram, *High Intensity Interval Training for Women* (DK, 2016), 16.

38. The pain scale in medicine has been discussed in fields including philosophy, science and technology studies, English, and sociology. Some examples include Wim Dekkers, "Pain as a Subjective and Objective Phenomenon," *Handbook of the Philosophy of Medicine* (2017): 169–87; Bill Nobel, David Clarke, Marcia Meldrum, Henk Ten Have, Jane Seymour, Michelle Winslow, and Silvia Paz, "The Measurement of Pain, 1945–2000," *Journal of Pain and Symptom Management* 29, no. 1 (2005): 14–21; Elaine Scarry, *The Body in Pain: The Making and Unmaking of the World* (Oxford University Press, 1987).

39. Nobel et al., "The Measurement of Pain," 18–19.

40. Leder claims pain has an "affective call" or demand to be named that ruptures the "general neutrality [of] well-being." While pain remains one of the most challenging experiences to communicate, the pain scale attempts to render the sensation sharable through a metric scale. That is, the pain scale aims to "name" that pain in a way that renders it communicable to physicians and the public without relying on language. Leder, *The Absent Body*, 73.

41. Leder, *The Absent Body*, 84.

42. Leder, *The Absent Body*, 77.

43. My phrasing plays on Leder's discussions of pain, which argues that in pain, the subject shifts from being a body to having a body-object. Leder, *The Absent Body*, 77.

44. Critiques of fitness often stress how exercise more generally encourages individuals to self-alienate. Through an emphasis on the "slimming," "toning," and "sculpting" effects of fitness, exercise frames the body as an aesthetic object. Consequently, fitness—and by extension, health—can be determined by outward physical appearances encouraging individuals to fashion their bodies in pursuit of the ideal physical manifestation of health. Examples of this argument can be found in Debra Gimlin, *Body-Work: Beauty and Self-Image in American Culture* (University of California Press, 2002); Jennifer Smith Maguire, *Fit for Consumption* (Routledge, 2008).

45. "The Benefits of Upright Posture," UPRIGHT GO, accessed January 2023, https://www.uprightpose.com/en-nz/benefits/?afmc=1k

46. Brad Millington, "Quantify the Invisible: Notes toward a Future of Posture," *Critical Public Health* 26, no. 4 (2016): 412–13.

47. Indeed, in one of the only studies of posture wearables, Brad Millington claims that the marketing materials of the devices figure posture as a way to "optimize" the human. Millington, "'Quantify the Invisible."

48. I follow Nick Crossley's critique of "grand theories" of body reflexivity, which he claims tend to focus exclusively on "manuals and ignore lived experience." Crossley, *Reflexive Embodiment*, 82.

49. The device appears to be largely marketed toward individuals required to sit for long portions of the day for work. As a result, there is great emphasis on the way these health benefits improve productivity. "The Benefits of Upright Posture," accessed April 2020.

50. "Why Does Posture Matter?" Help Center, UPRIGHT GO, accessed April 2020, https://help.uprightpose.com/en/articles/3346617-why-does-posture-matter

51. UPRIGHT GO, "The Benefits of Upright Posture."

52. Upright Technologies. "UPRIGHT GO." vers. 1.8.0, accessed April 2020.

53. The calibration feature makes it easy for individuals to "cheat" or may undermine learning "good" posture if they fail to set their device to an upright position. However, as I discussed in chapter three, individuals are often more interested in what they can learn from the device despite its problems or failures.

54. Millington notes that the emphasis on "personalized" posture supports the neoliberal ideology of individual empowerment and choice. Millington, "Quantify the Invisible," 413.

55. UPRIGHT GO, "Benefits of Upright Posture."

56. Sian Beilock, *Choke: What the Secrets of the Brain Reveal About Getting It Right When You Have To* (Free Press, 2010); Sian L. Beilock and Thomas H. Carr, "From Novice to Expert Performance: Attention, Memory, and the Control of Complex Sensorimotor Skills," *Skill Acquisition in Sport: Research, Theory and Practice*, edited by A. M. Williams, N. J. Hodges, M. A. Scott, and M. L. J. Court (Routledge, 2004), 309–28; Edward Slingerland, *Trying Not to Try: The Art and Science of Spontaneity* (New York: Crown Publishers, 2004).

57. With the example of learning to swim, this action requires the coordination of several elements simultaneously. An individual may be required to monitor the shape of their hands, the angle of their stroke, and their breathing patterns. Each element is not necessarily broken down into a sequence of actions, but instead is consciously reflected on at moments in practice.

58. Scholars have offered a variety of terms to clarify this distinction, including "proprioceptive awareness," "embodied knowledge," and "sensory awareness." Examples of these distinctions can be found in Janna Parivianan and Johanna Aromaa, "Bodily Knowledge Beyond Motor Skills and Physical Fitness: A Phenomenological Description of Knowledge Formation in Physical Training," *Sport, Education and Society* 22, no. 4 (2017): 477-–92; Wolf E. Mehling, Judith Wrubel, Jennifer J. Daubenmier, Cynthia J. Price, Catherine E. Kerr, Theresa Silow, Viranjini Gopisetty, and Anita L. Stewart, "Body Awareness: A Phenomenological Inquiry into the Common Ground of Mind-Body Therapies," *Philosophy, Ethics and Humanities in Medicine* 6, no. 6 (2011), http://www.peh-med.com/content/6/1/6; Barbara Montero, "Does Bodily Awareness Interfere with Highly Skilled Movement?" *Inquiry* 52, no. 2 (2010):105–22.

59. "How Upright Works," UPRIGHT GO, accessed May 2020, https://www.uprightpose.com/how-it-works/

60. Erin Manning, *Relationscapes: Movement, Art, Philosophy* (MIT Press, 2009), 44.

61. The Apple Watch run program does allow individuals to look at their heart rate during the run. However, this information requires lifting the wrist to activate the screen. Moreover, the size of the font on the screen, combined with a great deal of other statistical data, makes it incredibly hard to simply glance at the screen to get a heart rate reading. Apple Watch does provide pacing push notifications on completing a mile of a run.

62. Some examples of these programs can be found in the following apps: "Couch to 5K," Apple App Store, https://apps.apple.com/us/app/couch-to-5k-run-training/id448474423; "Nike Run Club," Apple App Store, accessed May 2020,

https://apps.apple.com/us/app/nike-run-club/id387771637; "Runkeeper," Apple App Store, accessed May 2020, https://apps.apple.com/us/app/runkeeper-gps-running-tracker/id300235330

63. Another way to understand the unconscious movements of runners is through the concept of "habitus." First introduced by Marcel Mauss, habitus refers to embodied pre-reflexive forms of knowledge. Nick Crossley builds on Mauss to note that habitus often involves "body techniques" that do not efface the body but are instead actions that often "work back upon the body so as to modify, maintain, or thematize it in some way." Crossley, *Reflexive Embodiment*, 104.

64. Hockey, "Sensing the Run," 188.

65. Hockey, "Sensing the Run," 189.

66. Moov, Inc., "Moov Coach and Guided Workouts," vers. 5.2.4809.52, accessed May 2020.

67. Moov, Inc., "Moov Coach and Guided Workouts."

68. Moov, Inc., "Moov Coach and Guided Workouts."

69. Sensoria, Inc., "Sensoria," vers. 2.3.0, accessed May 2020.

70. Sensoria, Inc., "Sensoria."

71. Leder uses the term "incorporation" to describe the way habits require careful attention to movement, sensation, and cognitive information. Leder, *The Absent Body*, 30.

72. Leder, *The Absent Body*, 32.

73. Hockey, "Sensing the Run," 189.

74. Hockey, "Sensing the Run," 189.

75. Allen-Collinson and Hockey, "Feeling the Way," 337.

76. Manning, *Relationscapes*, 54–55.

77. Manning, *Relationscapes*, 19.

78. Hockey draws on David Howes's concept of "emplacement" to describe how the body is understood not as a discrete entity but as one located within a sensuous environment. Hockey, "Sensing the Run," 187; David Howes, *Sensual Relations: Engaging the Senses in Culture and Social Theory* (University of Michigan Press, 2005), XVII.

79. Allen-Collinson, "Feeling the Way"; John Hockey and Jacquelyn Allen-Collinson, "Grasping the Phenomenology of Sporting Bodies," *International Review for the Sociology of Sport* 4, no. 2 (2007): 115–31.

80. Ninitha Maivorsdotter and Mikael Quennerstedt, "The Act of Running: A Practical Epistemology Analysis of Aesthetic Experience in Sport," *Qualitative Research in Sport, Exercise, and Health* 4, no. 3 (2012): 362–81.

81. Hockey and Allen-Collinson, "Feeling the Way," 337; Paul Rodaway, *Sensuous Geographies: Body, Sense and Place* (Routledge, 1994), 48.

82. "Moov Now," Moov, accessed May 2020, https://welcome.moov.cc/moovnow; "Homepage," Sensoria, Inc., accessed May 2020, https://www.sensoriafitness.com/

83. Svenaeus, *Hermeneutics of Medicine*, 92.

84. Svenaeus, *Hermeneutics of Medicine*, 95.

85. "The unhomelikeness of illness is consequently a certain form of senselessness, an attunement of, for instance, disorientedness, helplessness, resistance, and despair." Svenaeus, *Hermeneutics of Medicine*, 97, 115.

86. Svenaeus concedes that this "unhomelike" experience of being can be extended to non-illness-related conditions, such as imprisonment. However, he is less concerned about how the *physical* surroundings of an environment may appear unfamiliar to an individual and more concerned about how the embodied experience of those surroundings disrupts being-in-the-world itself. Svenaeus, *Hermeneutics of Medicine*, 117.

87. Svenaeus, *Hermeneutics of Medicine*, 118.

88. Svenaeus's definition also helps clarify that health can be discussed in relation not only to illness and disease but to conditions that alter one's homelike being-in-the-world. For example, he uses the diabetic, whose "healthy state" relies on daily fluctuations in blood sugar levels and disruptions through monitoring processes. For the diabetic, the homelike sense of being may shift along the spectrum of health and illness as the day goes on. Thus, to describe their experience as "healthy" or "ill" would be inadequate. Svenaeus, *Hermeneutics of Medicine*, 96–100.

89. This issue has also been discussed extensively in the edited collection *Against Health*, which argues that present definitions of health are based on difference: "The result explicitly justifies particular corporal types and practices, while implicitly suggesting that those who do not play along suffer from ill health." Jonathan M. Metzl and Anna Kirkland, *Against Health* (New York University Press, 2010), 3; Svenaeus, *Hermeneutics of Medicine*, 115.

90. Svenaeus, *Hermeneutics of Medicine*, 95.

91. "Homelikeness here refers to the patterns of meaning of the existential (attuned, bodily, and articulated understanding), which make coherent transcendence of a self (person) into the world possible." Svenaeus, *Hermeneutics of Medicine*, 94, 114.

92. This discussion of health is indebted to phenomenologies of illness that advocate for a more diverse and nuanced understanding of health and illness that acknowledges the capacity to live with pain. For an example of this discussion, see James Brennan, "Transitions in Health and Illness: Realist and Phenomenological Accounts of Adjustment to Cancer," *Health, Illness and Disease*, edited by Havi Carel and Rachel Cooper (Routledge, 2014), 129–42; Antonio Cassado de la Rocha and Arantza Etxebrria, "Towards Autonomy-within-Illness: Applying the Triadic Approach to the Principles of Bioethics"; *Health, Illness and Disease*, edited by Havi Carel and Rachel Cooper (Routledge, 2014), 57–76.

93. Svenaeus, *Hermeneutics of Medicine*, 112.

94. It should be noted that Sara Ahmed has described race using the concept "home-like-being-in-the-world." She argues that it is incredibly difficult for people of color to feel at home in a culture of whiteness. Instead, they continually feel a sense of discomfort as they fail to "fit in" to the social norms. In the context of running wearables, this likewise brings up the discomforts that may arise from running through certain social and physical environments. Kurt Streeter's 2020 editorial "Running While Black" sparked conversation around the feeling of running through white spaces. He describes how social and political conditions ultimately shaped his "comfort" or "discomfort" in navigating certain neighborhoods. In other words, his editorial describes how his blackness prevented a "homelike-being-in-the-world" that was once available to him (before the Black Lives Matter movement). Ahmed and Streeter's work illustrates how the feeling of "homelikeness" in

health is likewise shaped by identity and social and political conditions. Through a focus on the relationship between environment and body, Svenaeus's phenomenological definitions of health can help incorporate these factors, as subjective questions of "comfort" or "fitting" come to the fore. Sara Ahmed, "A Phenomenology of Whiteness," *Feminist Theory* 8, no. 2 (2007); Kurt Streeter, "On Running While Black, More Hope Than Before," *New York Times*, 22 November 2020.

95. Svenaeus, *Hermeneutics of Medicine*, 101.

96. While I distinguish between skill and my experience with these devices, it should be noted that scholars have discussed athletic skill and environmental awareness. For example, Ingold argues that "Skill at sports (or indeed more generally) is not merely 'an isolated ability in a person's body,' but is better understood as a meshing of a person's intentions, through their abilities with the environment (including other people), already interrogated by a skillful person for significant information." Tim Ingold, *The Perception of the Environment. Essays on Livelihood, Dwelling and Skill* (London: Routledge, 2000), 353.

97. Health and wellness, in particular, are often associated with a feeling of "happiness." Attunement, by contrast, does not have negative or positive connotations but rather describes the relationship between self and world. Sveneaus, *Hermeneutics of Medicine*, 94.

98. "Ability" and attunement are also not necessarily related to how "disability" is understood. As in his definition of health, Svenaeus is interested in how individuals experience attunement, not in defining universal or standardized thresholds for ability or health. In other words, the same sense of ability I describe could be experienced by those who are differently abled. What is important is the feeling of ability or capacity, not a specific physical skill such as running. However, it remains to be seen whether these devices can open up reflexive spaces for those with physical disabilities that prohibit certain forms of movement.

99. Allen-Collinson and Owton demonstrate the importance of sound for sporting bodies more generally. In their study of running and scuba diving, they argue, "sound is often integral to sporting experience; we listen in order to assemble important auditory information, including in relation to our respiratory patterns." Allen-Collinson and Owton, "Take a Deep Breath," 596.

100. Svenaeus, *Hermeneutics of Medicine*, 94.

101. Svenaeus, *Hermeneutics of Medicine*, 115.

Bibliography

Adams, Mary Louise. "Step-Counting in the 'Health-Society': Phenomenological Reflections on Walking in the Era of the Fitbit." *Social Theory & Health* 17 (2019): 109–24.

Adams-Hillard, Paula J., and Marija Valjic Wheeler. "Data from Menstrual Cycle Tracking App Informs Knowledge of Menstrual Cycle in Adolescents and Adults." *Journal of Pediatric and Adolescent Gynecology* 30 (April 2017): 268–74.

Ahmed, Sara. "A Phenomenology of Whiteness." In *F non, Phenomenology, and Psychology*, edited by Leswin Laubscher, Derek Hook, and Miraj U. Desai, 229–46. Routledge, 2021.

Aiello, Giorgia. "Theoretical Advances in Critical Visual Analysis: Perception, Ideology, Mythologies, and Social Semiotics." *Journal of Visual Literacy* 26, no. 2 (2006): 89–102.

Ajana, Btihaj. "Digital Health and the Biopolitics of the Quantified Self." *Digital Health* 3 (2017): 2055207616689509.

Allan, Patrick. "Five Ways to Cheat Your Way to 10,000 Fitbit Steps Every Day." Lifehacker, October 28, 2016. https://lifehacker.com/five-ways-to-cheat-your-way-to-10-000-fitbit-steps-ever-1788302045

Allen-Collinson, Jacquelyn, and John Hockey. "Feeling the Way: Notes toward a Haptic Phenomenology of Distance Running and Scuba Diving." *International Review for the Sociology of Sport* 46, no. 3 (2011): 330–45.

Allen-Collinson, Jacquelyn, and Helen Owton. "Take a Deep Breath: Asthma, Sporting Embodiment, the Senses and 'Auditory Work.'" *International Review for the Sociology of Sport* 49, no. 5 (2014): 592–608.

American Psychiatric Association. *Diagnostic and Statistical Manual of Mental Disorders*, 5th ed., 2013.

American Psychological Association. "Relax, Take a Deep Breath." 21 June 2017. https://www.psychiatry.org/news-room/apa-blogs/apa-blog/2017/06/relax-take-a-deep-breath

App Advice. "Breathesync." Accessed February 2018. https://appadvice.com/app/breathesync/722304193

Apple. "Apple Announces Three Groundbreaking Health Studies." 19 January 2023. https://www.apple.com/newsroom/2019/09/apple-announces-three-groundbreaking-health-studies/

Apple. "Close Your Rings," Accessed February 2023. https://www.apple.com/watch/close-your-rings/

Apple. "IOS—Research App." Accessed July 2022. https://www.apple.com/ios/research-app/

Apple. "Track Your Trends in the Activity App." 19 October 2019, accessed May 2020. https://support.apple.com/en-us/HT210343

Apple. "Your Heart Rate. What It Means, and Where on Apple Watch You'll Find It." 4 December 2017. https://support.apple.com/en-us/HT204666

Apple App Store. "Clue Period Tracker." Apple App Store. Accessed April 2019. https://itunes.apple.com/us/app/clue-period-tracker-ovulation/id657189652?mt=8

Apple App Store. "Couch to 5K." Accessed May 2020. https://apps.apple.com/us/app/couch-to-5k-run-training/id448474423

Apple App Store. "Flo Period and Ovulation Tracker." Accessed April 2019. https://itunes.apple.com/us/app/flo-period-ovulation-tracker/id1038369065?mt=8

Apple App Store. "Lioness: Sexual Health Tracker." Accessed May 2021. https://apps.apple.com/us/app/lioness-sexual-health-tracker/id1177248589

Apple App Store. "Nike Run Club." Accessed May 2020. https://apps.apple.com/us/app/nike-run-club/id387771637

Apple App Store. "Runkeeper." Accessed May 2020. https://apps.apple.com/us/app/runkeeper-gps-running-tracker/id300235330

Apple Watch. "Activity," vers. 14.6, 2021. Accessed June 2021.

Ardell, Donald B. *High-Level Wellness: An Alternative to Doctors, Drugs, and Disease*. Union Institute and University, 1977.

Ardell, Donald B. *The History and Future of Wellness*. Kendall/Hunt Publishing Co., 1985.

Armstrong, David, and Elizabeth Metzger Armstrong. *The Great American Medicine Show: An Illustrated History of Hucksters, Healers, Health Evangelists, and Heroes from Plymouth Rock to the Present*. Prentice Hall General, 1991.

Ayers, Toni, Maggi Rubenstein, and Carolyn Haynes Smith. *Masturbation Techniques for Women*. San Francisco: Multimedia Resource Center, 1972.

Baird, Karen L., Dana-Ain Davis, and Kimberly Christensen. *Beyond Reproduction: Women's Health, Activism, and Public Policy*. Fairleigh Dickinson University Press, 2009.

Banner, Olivia. *Communicative Biocapitalism: The Voice of the Patient in Digital Health and the Health Humanities*. University of Michigan Press, 2017.

Bardzell, Jeffrey, and Shaowen Bardzell. "Pleasure Is Your Birthright: Digitally Enabled Designer Sex Toys as a Case of Third-Wave HCI." In *Proceedings of the SIGCHI Conference on Human Factors in Computing Systems*, 257–66. 2011.

Barker, Leslie. "Do You 'Fit' the Heart Rate Equation?" Orangetheory Fitness, n.d. https://www.orangetheoryfitness.com/apps/blog/post/661

Barker, Leslie. "We Have a Heart: The 'Why' Behind Our Heart Rate Monitors." Orangetheory Fitness, n.d. https://www.orangetheory.com/en-au/articles/the-why-behind-our-heart-rate-monitors/

Barrica, Andrea. *Sextech Revolution: The Future of Sexual Wellness*. Lioncrest Publishing, 2019.

Bartram, Sean. *High Intensity Interval Training for Women*. DK, 2016.

Beilock, Sian. *Choke: What the Secrets of the Brain Reveal about Getting It Right When You Have To*. Simon and Schuster, 2010.

Beilock, Sian L., and Thomas H. Carr. "From Novice to Expert Performance: Memory, Attention and the Control of Complex Sensori-Motor Skills." In *Skill Acquisition in Sport*, 333–51. Routledge, 2004.

Bellour, Raymond. "The Unattainable Text." *Screen* 16, no. 3 (1975): 19–28.

Benner, Patricia. "The Phenomenon of Care." In *Handbook of Phenomenology and Medicine*, 351–69. Springer, Dordrecht, 2001.

Benson, Herbert, and Richard Friedman. "Harnessing the Power of the Placebo Effect and Renaming It Remembered Wellness." *Annual Review of Medicine—Selected Topics in the Clinical Sciences* 47 (1996): 193–200.

Benson, Herbert, and Miriam Z. Klipper. *The Relaxation Response*. Morrow, 1975.

Bhasin, Manoj K., Jeffery A. Dusek, Bei-Hung Chang, Marie G. Joseph, John W. Denninger, Gregory L. Fricchione, Herbert Benson, and Towia A. Libermann. "Relaxation Response Induces Temporal Transcriptome Changes in Energy Metabolism, Insulin Secretion and inflammatory Pathways." *PloS One* 8, no. 5 (2013): e62817.

BioWink. "Clue." vers. 5.13., 2019. Accessed November 2020.

BioWink, "Clue," vers. 103.0. Accessed February 2023.

Bobel, Chris. *New Blood: Third-Wave Feminism and the Politics of Menstruation*. Rutgers University Press, 2010.

"Bodysex | Betty Dodson & Carlin Ross." n.d. Accessed May 2021. https://dodsonandross.com/

Boston Women's Health Book Collective. *Our Bodies, Ourselves*. Atria Books, 2011 reprint.

Bowerman, William J., and W. E. Harris, *Jogging*. Charter Books, 1967.

boyd, danah, and Kate Crawford. "Critical Questions for Big Data: Provocations for a Cultural, Technological, and Scholarly Phenomenon." *Information, Communication & Society* 15, no. 5 (2012): 662–79.

Braun, Erik. "Mindful but Not Religious." In *Meditation, Buddhism, and Science*, edited by David L. McMahan and Erik Braun, 173–97. Oxford University Press, 2017.

Breathesync. "Homepage." Accessed February 2018. https://www.breathesync.com/

Brennan, James. "Transitions in Health and Illness: Realist and Phenomenological Accounts of Adjustment to Cancer." In *Health, Illness and Disease*, 141–54. Routledge, 2014.

Brody, Stuart. "The Relative Health Benefits of Different Sexual Activities." *Journal of Sexual Medicine* 7, no. 4, Part 1 (2010): 1336–61.

Brook, Robert D., Lawrence J. Appel, Melvyn Rubenfire, Gbenga Ogedegbe, John D. Bisognano, William J. Elliott, Flavio D. Fuchs, et al. "Beyond Medications and Diet: Alternative Approaches to Lowering Blood Pressure: A Scientific Statement from the American Heart Association." *Hypertension* 61, no. 6 (2013): 1360–83.

Brown, Dalvin. "Doctors Say Most Metrics Provided by Your Apple Watch, Fitbit Aren't Helpful to Them." *USA TODAY*, 14 August 2019. https://eu.usatoday.com/story/tech/2019/08/14/how-doctors-really-feel-data-your-apple-watch-fitbit/1900968001/

BWHI Staff. "I've Got What? Figuring Out Endometriosis." Black Women's Health Imperative, 25 July 2017. https://bwhi.org/2017/07/25/ive-got-figuring-endometriosis/

Cacchioni, Thea. "Heterosexuality and 'the Labour of Love': A Contribution to Recent Debates on Female Sexual Dysfunction. *Sexualities* 10, no. 3 (2007): 299–320.

Carel, Havi. *Phenomenology of Illness*. Oxford University Press, 2016.

Cawthon, Nick, and Andrew Vande Moere. "The Effect of Aesthetic on the Usability of Data Visualization." In *2007 11th International Conference Information Visualization (IV'07)*, 637–48. IEEE, 2007.

Cederström, Carl, and André Spicer. *The Wellness Syndrome*. John Wiley & Sons, 2015.

Centers for Disease Control. "Leading Causes of Death." Updated 17 March 2017. Accessed 16 July 2020. https://www.cdc.gov/nchs/fastats/leading-causes-of-death.htm

Centers for Disease Control. "Move More; Sit Less," June 2, 2022. https://www.cdc.gov/physicalactivity/basics/adults/index.htm

Centers for Disease Control. "Physical Activity: Why It Matters." Accessed 11 January 2022. https://www.cdc.gov/physicalactivity/about-physical-activity/why-it-matters.html

Centers for Disease Control. "The Surgeon General's Report on Smoking and Tobacco." Accessed July 2020. https://www.cdc.gov/tobacco/data_statistics/sgr/index.html

Chaari, Lotfi. *Digital Health Approach for Predictive, Preventive, Personalised and Participatory Medicine*. Vol. 10. Springer, 2019.

Chapman-Clarke, Margaret A. *Mindfulness in the Workplace: An Evidence-Based Approach to Improving Wellbeing and Maximizing Performance*. Kogan Page Publishers, 2016.

Charitsis, Vassilis. "Survival of the (Data) Fit: Self-Surveillance, Corporate Wellness, and the Platformization of Healthcare." *Surveillance & Society* 17, no. 1/2 (2019): 139–44.

Charnetski, Carl J., and Francis X. Brennan. *Feeling Good Is Good for You: How Pleasure Can Boost Your Immune System and Lengthen Your Life*. Rodale Books, 2001.

Chrisler, Joan C. "2007 Presidential Address: Fear of Losing Control: Power, Perfectionism, and the Psychology of Women." *Psychology of Women Quarterly* 32, no. 1 (2008): 1–12.

Chrisler, Joan C., and Paula Caplan. "The Strange Case of Dr. Jekyll and Ms. Hyde: How PMS Became a Cultural Phenomenon and a Psychiatric Disorder." *Annual Review of Sex Research* 13, no. 1 (2002): 274–306.

Chrisler, Joan C., and Jenifer A. Gorman. "The Menstrual Cycle: Attitudes and Behavioral Concomitants." In *Routledge International Handbook of Women's Sexual and Reproductive Health*, 55–69. Routledge, 2019.

Clarke, Adele E., Laura Mamo, Jennifer Ruth Fosket, Jennifer R. Fishman, and Janet K. Shim, eds. *Biomedicalization: Technoscience, Health, and Illness in the US*. Duke University Press, 2010.

Clarke, Tainya C., Patricia M. Barnes, Lindsey I. Black, Barbara J. Stussman, and Richard L. Nahin. *Use of Yoga, Meditation, and Chiropractors among US Adults Aged 18 and Over*. US Department of Health and Human Services, Centers for Disease Control and Prevention, National Center for Health Statistics, 2018.

Clue. "Do Menstrual Cycles Sync? Unlikely, Finds Clue Data." Updated 8 March 2017. Accessed November 2020. https://helloclue.com/articles/cycle-a-z/do-menstrual-cycles-sync-unlikely-finds-clue-data

Clue. "Homepage." Accessed November 2020. https://helloclue.com/period-tracker-app

Clue. "New in Clue: Our Sex Icons Got a Makeover." Updated 8 January 2018. Accessed November 2020. https://helloclue.com/articles/about-clue/new-in-clue-our-sex-tracking-icons-got-makeover

Clue. "What to Know about Clue's Cycle Analysis Feature." September 13, 2022. https://helloclue.com/articles/about-clue/introducing-enhanced-analysis-understand-what-your-period-is-telling-you

Colman, Felicity, Vera Bühlmann, Aislinn O'Donnell, and Iris van der Tuin. Ethics of Coding: A Report on the Algorithmic Condition [EoC]. H2020-EU.2.1.1.1—INDUSTRIAL LEADERSHIP—Leadership in Enabling and Industrial Technologies—Information and Communication Technologies. Brussels: European Commission. 0732407, https://cordis.europa.eu/project/rcn/207025_en.html. (2018): 1–54.

Comella, Lynn. *Vibrator Nation: How Feminist Sex-Toy Stores Changed the Business of Pleasure*. Duke University Press, 2017.

Cooper, Kenneth H. *Aerobics*. Bantam, 1968.

Cooper, Kenneth H. *The New Aerobics*. Bantam, 1970.

Cornfeld, Li. "Videotape and Vibrators: An Industry History of Techno-Sexuality." *Feminist Media Historie* 6, no. 4 (2020): 94–120.

Cranz, Alex. "Hands On with the Vibrator that Wants to Be the Smartest Sex Toy in the World." *Gizmodo*. 16 August 2017. https://gizmodo.com/hands-on-with-the-vibrator-that-wants-to-be-the-smartes-1797868452

Crawford, Kate, Jessa Lingel, and Tero Karppi. "Our Metrics, Ourselves: A Hundred Years of Self-Tracking from the Weight Scale to the Wrist Wearable Device." *European Journal of Cultural Studies* 18, no. 4–5 (2015): 479–96.

Crawford, Paul, Brian Brown, Charley Baker, Victoria Tischler, Brian Abrams. *Health Humanities*. Palgrave Macmillan UK, 2015.

Crawford, Robert. "Healthism and the Medicalization of Everyday Life." *International Journal of Health Services* 10, no. 3 (1980): 365–88.

Crossley, Nick. *Reflexive Embodiment in Contemporary Society*. Open University Press, 2006.

Crossley, Nick. "The Circuit Trainer's Habitus: Reflexive Body Techniques and the Sociality of the Workout." *Body & Society* 10, no. 1 (2004): 37–69.

Daily Telegraph. "Fitbit Devices Could Be Harmful to Heart Patients, Researchers Warn." *Daily Telegraph*, 17 August 2020.

Dame. "About Us." Accessed April 2021. https://www.dameproducts.com/pages/about-us

Dame. "What Is the Pleasure Gap?" 4 April 2019. https://swell.damewellness.co/what-is-the-pleasure-gap/

Dame. "Workshops." Accessed April 2021. https://damewellness.co/pages/workshops?utm_source=swell&utm_medium=blog&utm_campaign=nav

da Rocha, Antonio Casado, and Arantza Etxeberria. "Towards Autonomy-Within-Illness: Applying the Triadic Approach to the Principles of Bioethics." In *Health, Illness and Disease*, 69–88. Routledge, 2014.

Daston, Lorraine, and Peter Galison. *Objectivity*. Princeton University Press, 2007.

Dekkers, Wim. "Pain as a Subjective and Objective Phenomenon." In *Handbook of the Philosophy of Medicine*, 169–87. Springer, 2017.

Delaney, Janice, Mary Jane Lupton, and Emily Toth. *The Curse: A Cultural History of Menstruation*. University of Illinois Press, 1988.

Della Bianca, Laetitia. "The Cyclic Self: Menstrual Cycle Tracking as Body Politics." *Catalyst: Feminism, Theory, Technoscience* 7, no. 1 (2021).

Department of Health and Human Services. "History of Healthy People." Updated 2 December 2020. Accessed July 2021. https://health.gov/our-work/healthy-people/about-healthy-people/history-healthy-people

Department of Health and Human Services. *Physical Activity Guidelines for Americans*. 2nd ed. 2018. PDF.

Department of Health and Human Services. "Your Menstrual Cycle and Your Health." Office of Women's Health, Health and Human Services. 16 March 2018. https://www.womenshealth.gov/menstrual-cycle/your-menstrual-cycle-and-your-health

Dolezal, Luna, and Venla Oikkonen. "Introduction: Self-Tracking, Embodied Differences, and Intersectionality." *Catalyst: Feminism, Theory, Technoscience* 7, no. 1 (2021): 1–15.

Dominic, Anthony. "Orangetheory Fitness Exceeds 1 Billion in 2018 System-Wide Revenue." *Club Industry*, 4 February 2019. https://www.clubindustry.com/news/orangetheory-fitness-exceeds-1-billion-2018-system-wide-revenue

Dranove, David. *The Economic Evolution of American Health Care*. Princeton University Press, 2009.

Dudhwala, Farzana. "Redrawing Boundaries around the Self: The Case of Self-Quantifying Technologies." In *Quantified Lives and Vital Data*, 97–123. Palgrave Macmillan, 2018.

Elliott, Carl. *Better than Well: American Medicine Meets the American Dream*. W. W. Norton, 2004.

Elman, Julie Passanante. "'Find Your Fit': Wearable Technology and the Cultural Politics of Disability." *New Media & Society* 20, no. 10 (2018): 3760–77.

Epstein, Daniel A., Nicole B. Lee, Jennifer H. Kang, Elena Agapie, Jessica Schroeder, Laura R. Pina, James Fogarty, Julie A. Kientz, and Sean Munson. "Examining Menstrual Tracking to Inform the Design of Personal Informatics Tools." In *Proceedings of the 2017 CHI Conference on Human Factors in Computing Systems* (2017): 6876–88.

Epstein, Randi Hutter. "Can a Smartwatch Save Your Life?" *New York Times*, 26

July 2021. https://www.nytimes.com/2021/05/20/well/live/smartwatch-heart-rate-monitor.html

Esmonde, Katelyn, and Shannon Jette. "Assembling the 'Fitbit Subject': A Foucauldian-Sociomaterialist Examination of Social Class, Gender and Self-Surveillance on Fitbit Community Message Boards." *Health* 24, no. 3 (2020): 299–314.

Evans, Randolph W., and R. Couch. "Orgasm and Migraine." *Headache: The Journal of Head and Face Pain* 41, no. 5 (2001): 512–14.

Evenson, Kelly R., Michelle M. Goto, and Robert D. Furberg. "Systematic Review of the Validity and Reliability of Consumer-Wearable Activity Trackers." *International Journal of Behavioral Nutrition and Physical Activity* 12, no. 1 (2015): 1–22.

Fahs, Breanne, and Elena Frank. "Notes from the Back Room: Gender, Power, and (In)Visibility in Women's Experiences of Masturbation." *Journal of Sex Research* 51, no. 3 (2014): 241–52.

Fanon, Frantz. *Black Skin, White Masks*. London: Paladin, 1970.

Feehan, Lynne M., Jasmina Geldman, Eric C. Sayre, Chance Park, Allison M. Ezzat, Ju Young Yoo, Clayon B. Hamilton, and Linda C. Li. "Accuracy of Fitbit Devices: Systematic Review and Narrative Syntheses of Quantitative Data." *JMIR mHealth and uHealth* 6, no. 8 (2018): e10527.

Feldman, Henry A., Catherine B. Johannes, Andre B. Araujo, Beth A. Mohr, Christopher Longcope, and John B. McKinlay. "Low Dehydroepiandrosterone and Ischemic Heart Disease in Middle-Aged Men: Prospective Results from the Massachusetts Male Aging Study." *American Journal of Epidemiology* 153, no. 1 (2001): 79–89.

FIGO. "Period Syncing Myth Debunked." *FIGO: International Federation of Gynecology and Obstetrics*. 13 April 2017. https://www.figo.org/news/period-syncing-myth-debunked-0015541

Fisher, Linda. "The Illness Experience: A Feminist Phenomenological Perspective." *Feminist Phenomenology and Medicine* (2014): 27–46.

Fitbit. "About Us." Accessed 11 January 2022. https://www.fitbit.com/global/us/about-us

Fitbit, "Fitbit App," vers. 3.43.1. Accessed June 2021.

Fitbit "Fitbit Health Solutions." Accessed July 2021. https://healthsolutions.fitbit.com/researchers/

Fitbit. "What Should I Know about Fitbit's Relax Feature?" 18 November 2017, https://help.fitbit.com/articles/en_US/Help_article/2077

Fitbit. "Why Fitbit." Accessed May 2017. http://www.fitbit.com/whyfitbit

Fitbit Staff. "Here's Why You'll Love Relax, Fitbit's Guided Breathing Experience." Fitbit Blog, April 9, 2020. https://blog.fitbit.com/heres-why-youll-love-fitbits-new-+guided-breathing-experience/

Fit Tutor. "RPE Scale." Accessed May 2020. https://thefittutor.com/rpe-scale/

Flo. "Homepage." Accessed November 2020. https://flo.health/

Flo Health, Inc. "Flo," vers. 4.31. Accessed March 2019.

Flo Living. "MyFlo Period Tracker." 2023. Accessed February 2023. https://myflotracker.com/

Food and Drug Administration. "FDA Allows Marketing of First Direct-to-

Consumer App for Contraceptive Use to Prevent Pregnancy." FDA, 10 August 2018. https://wayback.archive-it.org/7993/20190207210732/https://www.fda.gov/NewsEvents/Newsroom/PressAnnouncements/ucm616511.html

Forberg, Sigrid. "Can a Fitness Tracker Save You Money on Your Health Insurance?" Yahoo Finance. 22 January 2021. https://finance.yahoo.com/news/heres-could-free-fitbit-insurance-151900485.html

Fors, Vaike. "Sensory Experiences of Digital Photo-Sharing—'Mundane Frictions' and Emerging Learning Strategies." *Journal of Aesthetics & Culture* 7, no. 1 (2015): 28237.

Fotopoulou, Aristea, and Kate O'Riordan. "Training to Self-Care: Fitness Tracking, Biopedagogy and the Healthy Consumer." *Health Sociology Review* 26, no. 1 (2017): 54–68.

Fox, Nick J. "Personal Health Technologies, Micropolitics and Resistance: A New Materialist Analysis." *Health* 21, no. 2 (2017): 136–53.

Fox, Sarah, and Daniel A. Epstein. "Monitoring Menses: Design-Based Investigations of Menstrual Tracking Applications." *Palgrave Handbook of Critical Menstruation Studies*, edited by Chris Bobel, Inga T. Winkler, Breanne Fahs, Katie Ann Hasson, Elizabeth Arveda Kissling, and Tomi-Ann Roberts, 733–50. Palgrave, 2020.

Fox, Sarah E., Amanda Menking, Jordan Eschler, and Uba Backonja. "Multiples over Models: Interrogating the Past and Collectively Reimagining the Future of Menstrual Sensemaking." *ACM Transactions on Computer-Human Interaction (TOCHI)* 27, no. 4 (2020): 1–24.

Fox, Susannah, and Maeve Duggan. "Tracking for Health." Washington, DC: Pew Research Center Internet & American Life Project, 2013. http://www.pewinternet.org/2013/01/28/main-report-8

Frank, Robert T. "The Hormonal Causes of Premenstrual Tension." *Archives of Neurology & Psychiatry* 26, no. 5 (1931): 1053–57.

Freidenfelds, Lara. *The Modern Period: Menstruation in Twentieth-Century America*. JHU Press, 2009.

Freud, Sigmund. *The Freud Reader*. New York: W. W. Norton, 1989.

Freud, Sigmund. *Jokes and Their Relation to the Unconscious*. Penguin Books, 1975.

Frith, Hannah. *Orgasmic Bodies: The Orgasm in Contemporary Western Culture*. Springer, 2015.

Gadamer, Hans Georg. *The Enigma of Health: The Art of Healing in a Scientific Age*. Stanford University Press, 1996.

Gallop, Cindy. "What Is Sextech and Why Is Everyone Ignoring It?" HotTopics.ht, March 30, 2020. https://hottopics.ht/14192/what-is-sextech-and-why-is-everyone-ignoring-it/

Gambier-Ross, Katie, David J. McLernon, and Heather M. Morgan. "A Mixed Methods Exploratory Study of Women's Relationships with and Uses of Fertility Tracking Apps." *Digital Health* 4 (2018): 2055207618785077.

Gelles, David. "How to Meditate." *New York Times*, n.d. https://www.nytimes.com/guides/well/how-to-meditate

Gerhard, Jane. "Revisiting 'The Myth of the Vaginal Orgasm': The Female Orgasm in American Sexual Thought and Second Wave Feminism." *Feminist Studies* 26, no. 2 (2000): 449–76.

Gill, Rosalind. "Mediated Intimacy and Postfeminism: A Discourse Analytic Examination of Sex and Relationships Advice in a Women's Magazine." *Discourse & Communication* 3, no. 4 (2009): 345–69.

Gilmore, James N. "Everywear: The Quantified Self and Wearable Fitness Technologies." *New Media & Society* 18, no. 11 (2016): 2524–39.

Gimlin, Debra. *Body Work: Beauty and Self-Image in American Culture*. University of California Press, 2002.

Gitelman, Lisa, ed. *Raw Data Is an Oxymoron*. MIT Press, 2013.

Gleason, Brett Kyle. *A Phenomenological Investigation of Wellness and Wellness Promotion in Counselor Education Programs*. Thesis. Old Dominion University, 2015.

Glow. "Eve." vers. 2.15.5. Accessed November 2019.

Goldstein, Michael S. *The Health Movement: Promoting Fitness in America*. Twayne Publishers, 1992.

Goleman, Daniel. *The Meditative Mind: The Varieties of Meditative Experience*. Tarcher/Putnam, 1996.

Gorzelitz, Jessica, Chloe Farber, Ronald Gangnon, and Lisa Cadmus-Bertram. "Accuracy of Wearable Trackers for Measuring Moderate- to Vigorous-Intensity Physical Activity: A Systematic Review and Meta-Analysis." *Journal for the Measurement of Physical Behaviour* 3, no. 4 (2020): 346–57.

Green, Harvey. *Fit for America: Health, Fitness, Sport, and American Society*. Pantheon, 1986.

Greene, Liz. "The Labour of Breath: Performing and Designing Breath in Cinema." *Music, Sound, and the Moving Image* 10, no. 2 (2017): 109–33.

Gupta, Kristina. "'Screw Health': Representations of Sex as a Health-Promoting Activity in Medical and Popular Literature." *Journal of Medical Humanities* 32 (2011): 127–40.

Gupta, Kristina, and Thea Cacchioni. "Sexual Improvement as If Your Health Depends on It: An Analysis of Contemporary Sex Manuals." *Feminism & Psychology* 23, no. 4 (2013): 442–58.

Gurevich, Maria. "Rethinking the Label: Who Benefits from the PMS Construct?" *Women & Health* 23, no. 2 (1995): 67–98.

Haile, Luke, M. Gallagher, and Robert J. Robertson. *Perceived Exertion Laboratory Manual*. Springer-Verlag, 2016.

Haley, Bruce. "The Healthy Body and Victorian Culture." In *The Healthy Body and Victorian Culture*. Harvard University Press, 1978.

Halpern, Orit. *Beautiful Data: A History of Vision and Reason since 1945*. Duke University Press, 2015.

Hanich, Julian, and Christian Ferencz-Flatz. "What Is Film Phenomenology?" *Studia Phaenomenologica* 16 (2016): 11–61.

Hardman, Adrianne E., and David J. Stensel. *Physical Activity and Health: The Evidence Explained*. Routledge, 2009.

Harvey-Jenner, Catriona. "The Orgasm Gap Is REAL—Women Are Losing Out." *Cosmopolitan*, 25 March 2015. https://www.cosmopolitan.com/uk/love-sex/sex/news/a34410/female-orgasm-survey/

Hasson, Katie Ann. "From Bodies to Lives, Complainers to Consumers: Measuring Menstrual Excess." *Social Science & Medicine* 75, no. 10 (2012): 1729–36.

Hasson, Katie Ann. "Not a 'Real' Period? Social and Material Constructions of Menstruation." *Gender & Society* 30, no. 6 (2016): 958–83.

Healy, Rachael Louise. "Zuckerberg, Get Out of My Uterus! An Examination of Fertility Apps, Data-Sharing and Remaking the Female Body as a Digitalized Reproductive Subject." *Journal of Gender Studies* 30, no. 4 (2021): 406–16.

Heyes, Cressida J. *Self-Transformations: Foucault, Ethics, and Normalized Bodies*. Oxford University Press, 2007.

Hill, Kashmir. "'Deleting Your Period Tracker Won't Protect You,.'" *New York Times*, 2 July 2022.

Hockey, John. "Sensing the Run: The Senses and Distance Running." *The Senses and Society* 1, no. 2 (2006): 183–201.

Hockey, John, and Jacquelyn Allen Collinson. "Grasping the Phenomenology of Sporting Bodies." *International Review for the Sociology of Sport* 42, no. 2 (2007): 115–31.

Hogarth, Harriet, and Roger Ingham. "Masturbation among Young Women and Associations with Sexual Health: An Exploratory Study." *Journal Of Sex Research* 46, no. 6 (2009): 558–67.

Holly, Karen. "Pelvic Rehab Health—My One-Year Lioness Vibrator Experiment—Why Vibrators Matter." Updated 2019. n.d. Accessed May 2021. https://www.karenkholly.com/blog/pelvic-rehab-health-my-one-year-lioness-vibrator-experiment-why-vibrators-matter

Houck, Judith. *Hot and Bothered: Women, Medicine and Menopause in America*. Harvard University Press, 2006.

Houghton, Lauren C., and Noémie Elhadad. "Practice Note: 'If Only All Women Menstruated Exactly Two Weeks Ago': Interdisciplinary Challenges and Experiences of Capturing Hormonal Variation Across the Menstrual Cycle." *The Palgrave Handbook of Critical Menstruation Studies*, edited by Chris Bobel, Inga T. Winkler, Breanne Fahs, Katie Ann Hasson, Elizabeth Arveda Kissling, and Tomi-Ann Roberts, 725–32. Palgrave, 2020.

Howell, Jeremy, and Alan Ingham. "From Social Problem to Personal Issue: The Language of Lifestyle." *Cultural Studies* 15, no. 2 (2001): 326–51.

Howes, David. *Sensual Relations: Engaging the Senses in Culture and Social Theory*. University of Michigan Press, 2005.

Hudson Jones, Anne. "Literature and Medicine: Traditions and Innovations." *The Body and the Text*, edited by Bruce Clarke and Wendell Aycock, 11–24. Texas Tech University Press, 1990.

Hyperice. "Core." Accessed February 2023, https://www.hellocore.com/

Illich, Ivan. *Limits to Medicine: Medical Nemesis*. Marion Boyars, 1976.

Illich, Ivan, Irving K. Zola, John McKnight, Jonathan Caplan, and Harley Shaiken. *Disabling Professions*. Marion Boyars, 1977.

Ingold, Tim. *The Perception of the Environment. Essays on Livelihood, Dwelling and Skill*. Routledge, 2000.

iroha. "Concept." Accessed April 2021. https://iroha-tenga.com/en/concept/

iroha. "iroha+." Accessed April 2021. https://iroha-tenga.com/en/plus/

iroha. "iroha stick." Accessed April 2021. https://iroha-tenga.com/en/stick/

Irvine, Janet. *Disorders of Desire*. Temple University Press, 1990.

Irvine, Janice M. "From Difference to Sameness: Gender Ideology in Sexual Science." *Journal of Sex Research* 7, no. 1 (1990): 7–24.

Jackson, Theresa E., and Rachel Joffe Falmagne. "Women Wearing White: Discourses of Menstruation and the Experience of Menarche." *Feminism & Psychology* 23, no. 3 (2013): 379–98.

Jethani, Suneel. "Mediating the Body: Technology, Politics and Epistemologies of Self." *Communication, Politics & Culture* 47, no. 3 (2015): 34–43.

Johnston-Robledo, Ingrid, Jessica Barnack, and Stephanie Wares. "'Kiss Your Period Good-Bye': Menstrual Suppression in the Popular Press." *Sex Roles* 54 (2006): 353–60.

Jones, Therese, Delese Wear, and Lester D. Friedman, eds. *Health Humanities Reader*. Rutgers University Press, 2014.

Jons, Ryan. "Orangetheory Fitness Costs and Orangetheory Membership Costs." *Gym Price List*, 2022. https://gympricelist.com/orangetheory-fitness-prices/

Kennedy, Eileen, and Pirkko Markula, eds. *Women and Exercise: The Body, Health and Consumerism*. Vol. 5. Routledge, 2011.

Kennedy, Helen, and Rosemary Lucy Hill. "The Feeling of Numbers: Emotions in Everyday Engagements with Data and Their Visualisation." *Sociology* 52, no. 4 (2018): 830–48.

Kennedy, Helen, Rosemary Lucy Hill, Giorgia Aiello, and William Allen. "The Work that Visualisation Conventions Do." *Information, Communication & Society* 19, no. 6 (2016): 715–35.

Khidekel, Marina. "The Race to Hack Your Period Is On." *ELLE*, November 29, 2021. https://www.elle.com/beauty/health-fitness/a21272099/clue-period-app/

Kinsey, Alfred C., Wardell B. Pomeroy, and Clyde E. Martin. *Sexual Behavior in the Human Male*. New York: Harper & Row, 1972.

Kinsey, Alfred C., Wardell B. Pomeroy, Clyde E. Martin, and Paul H. Gebhard. *Sexual Behavior in the Human Female*. Indiana University Press, 1953.

Kissling, Elizabeth Arveda. "Bleeding Out Loud: Communication about Menstruation." *Feminism & Psychology* 6, no. 4 (1996): 481–504.

Kissling, Elizabeth Arveda. *Capitalizing on the Curse*. Lynne Rienner Publishers, 2006.

Kitchin, Rob. "Big Data, New Epistemologies and Paradigm Shifts." *Big Data & Society* 1, no. 1 (2014): 2053951714528481.

Klein, Wendy. *Bodies of Knowledge: Sexuality, Reproduction, and Women's Health in the Second Wave*. University of Chicago Press, 2010.

Klinger, Liz. "How Does Lioness Help Me Have Better Sex/Orgasms?" Lioness. Accessed May 2021. https://help.lioness.io/en/articles/3873563-how-does-lioness-help-me-have-better-sex-orgasms

Klinger, Liz. "How People Have Explored with Lioness." Lioness. 10 March 2019. https://lioness.io/blogs/sex-guides/how-people-have-explored-with-lioness-smart-vibrator

Koedt, Anne. "Myth of the Vaginal Orgasm." *Notes from the First Year*. New York Radical Feminists, 1968.

Komisaruk, Barry R., Carlos Beyer-Flores, and Beverly Whipple. *The Science of Orgasm*. Johns Hopkins University Press, 2006.

Kraus, François. "The Practice of Masturbation for Women: The End of a Taboo?" *Sexologies* 26, no. 4 (2017): e35–41.

Kressbach, Mikki. "Breath Work: Mediating Health through Breathing Apps and Wearable Technologies," *New Review of Film and Television Studies* 16, no. 2 (2018): 184–206. https://doi.org.10.1080/17400309.2018.1444459

Kressbach, Mikki. "Period Hacks: Menstruating in the Big Data Paradigm." *Television & New Media* 22, no. 3 (2021): 241–61. https://doi.org/10.1177/15274764 19886389

Kressbach, Mikki Ivan Martinez-Medina, and Thomas Streed. "Strategies for Teaching Ephemeral Media: Phenomenological Description." *Journal of Interactive Technology and Pedagogy* (12 October 2022). https://jitp.commons.gc.cu ny.edu/strategies-for-analyzing-ephemeral-media-phenomenological-descript ion/

Kuuru, Tiina-Kaisa, and Elina Närvänen. "Embodied Interaction in Customer Experience: A Phenomenological Study of Group Fitness." *ournal of Marketing Management* 35, no. 13–14 (2019): 1241–66.

Laird, Amanda. *Heavy Flow: Breaking the Curse of Menstruation*. Dundurn, 2019.

Lander, Louise. *Images of Bleeding: Menstruation as Ideology*. Hart Graphics, 1988.

Laqueur, Thomas. *Making Sex: Body and Gender from the Greeks to Freud*. Harvard University Press, 1992.

Larsen, Paul, and Martin Bucheit. *Science and Application of High Intensity Interval Training: Solutions to the Programming Puzzle*. Human Kinetics, 2019.

Laws, Sophie. *Issues of Blood: The Politics of Menstruation*. Springer, 1991.

Lazar, Sara W., George Bush, Randy L. Gollub, Gregory L. Fricchione, Gurucharan Khalsa, and Herbert Benson. "Functional Brain Mapping of the Relaxation Response and Meditation." *Neuroreport* 11, no. 7 (2000): 1581–85.

Leder, Drew. *The Absent Body*. University of Chicago Press, 1990.

Lee, Hyunho, and Youngseok Lee. "A Look at Wearable Abandonment." In *2017 18th IEEE International Conference on Mobile Data Management (MDM)*, 392–93. IEEE, 2017.

Lee, Janet, and Jennifer Sasser-Coen. *Blood Stories: Menarche and the Politics of the Female Body in Contemporary US Society*. Routledge, 2015.

Lieberman, Hallie. *Buzz: The Stimulating History of the Sex Toy*. Simon and Schuster, 2017.

Lieberman, Hallie, and Eric Schatzberg. "A Failure of Academic Quality Control: The Technology of Orgasm." *Journal of Positive Sexuality* 4, no. 2 (2018): 24–47.

Lindsey, Elizabeth. "Health within Illness: Experiences of Chronically Ill/Disabled People." *Journal of Advanced Nursing* 24, no. 3 (1996): 465–72.

Lioness. "Guide to Good Vibes with Lioness." 28 July 2018. https://blog.lioness .io/guide-to-good-vibes-with-the-lioness-vibrator-8d73962829e9?gi=256c4d6 a4cf4.

Lioness. "Homepage." accessed April 2021, https://Lioness.io

Lioness. "How Does Our Technology Work?" Accessed April 2021. https://lioness .io/pages/how-it-works

Lioness. "Research." Accessed May 2021. https://lioness.io/pages/user-faq-lioness -research-platform

Lioness, "Lioness Health and Sex Tracker," vers. 2.0.07. Accessed June 2021.

Lomas, Natasha. "Natural Cycles App Told to Clarify Pregnancy Risk." *Tech Crunch*, 17 September 2018. https://techcrunch.com/2018/09/17/natural-cycles-contraception-app-told-to-clarify-pregnancy-risks/

Lora Di Carlo. "About Us." Accessed April 2021. https://www.loradicarlo.com/about-us

Lora Di Carlo. "Homepage." Accessed April 2021. https://www.loradicarlo.com/

Lousada, Mike, and Elena Angel. "Tantric Orgasm: Beyond Masters and Johnson." *Sexual and Relationship Therapy* 26, no. 4 (2011): 389–402.

Lunney, Abbey, Nicole R. Cunningham, and Matthew S. Eastin. "Wearable Fitness Technology: A Structural Investigation into Acceptance and Perceived Fitness Outcomes." *Computers in Human Behavior* 65 (2016): 114–20.

Lupton, Deborah. "Beyond Techno-Utopia: Critical Approaches to Digital Health Technologies." *Societies* 4, no. 4 (2014): 706–11.

Lupton, Deborah. *Digital Health: Critical and Cross-Disciplinary Perspectives*. Routledge, 2017.

Lupton, Deborah. "The Digitally Engaged Patient: Self-Monitoring and Self-Care in the Digital Health Era." *Social Theory & Health* 11, no. 3 (2013): 256–70.

Lupton, Deborah. "The Diverse Domains of Quantified Selves: Self-Tracking Modes and Dataveillance." *Economy and Society* 45, no. 1 (2016): 101–22.

Lupton, Deborah. "How Does Health Feel? Towards Research on the Affective Atmospheres of Digital Health." *Digital Health* 3 (2017): 2055207617701276.

Lupton, Deborah. *The Quantified Self*. John Wiley & Sons, 2016.

Lupton, Deborah. "Quantified Sex: A Critical Analysis of Sexual and Reproductive Self-Tracking Using Apps." *Culture, Health & Sexuality* 17, no. 4 (2015): 440–53.

MacPherson, Erin. "How Accurate Are Apple Watch Calories? How to Make them as Accurate as Possible." iPhone Life, 17 May 2021. https://www.iphonelife.com/content/how-accurate-are-apple-watch-calories-how-to-ensure-theyre-accurate

Maguire, Jennifer Smith. *Fit for Consumption: Sociology and the Business of Fitness*. Routledge, 2007.

Mahar, Elizabeth A., Laurie B. Mintz, and Brianna M. Akers. "Orgasm Equality: Scientific Findings and Societal Implications." *Current Sexual Health Reports* 12 (2020): 24–32.

Maines, Rachel P. *The Technology of Orgasm: "Hysteria," the Vibrator, and Women's Sexual Satisfaction*. JHU Press, 2001.

Maivorsdotter, Ninitha, and Mikael Quennerstedt. "The Act of Running: A Practical Epistemology Analysis of Aesthetic Experience in Sport." *Qualitative Research in Sport, Exercise and Health* 4, no. 3 (2012): 362–81.

Manning, Erin. *Relationscapes: Movement, Art, Philosophy*. MIT Press, 2009.

Marksberry, Kellie. "Take a Deep Breath." American Institute of Stress, 12 August 2012. https://www.stress.org/take-a-deep-breath

Martin, Emily. *The Woman in the Body: A Cultural Analysis of Reproduction*. Beacon Press, 2001.

Martschukat, Jürgen. "The Age of Fitness: The Power of Ability in Recent American History." *Rethinking History* 23, no. 2 (2019): 157–74.

Masters, William, and Virginia Johnson. *Heterosexuality*. Harper Collins, 1994.

Masters, William, and Virginia Johnson. *Human Sexual Response*. Little Brown, 1966.

Mattke, Soeren, Hangsheng Liu, John Caloyeras, Christina Y. Huang, Kristin R. Van Busum, Dmitry Khodyakov, and Victoria Shier. "Workplace Wellness Programs Study." *Rand Health Quarterly* 3, no. 2 (2013).

Maude. "FAQs: Do You Offer Discrete Shipping?" Accessed April 2021. https://getmaude.com/pages/faq#products

McKenzie, Shelly. *Getting Physical: The Rise of Fitness Culture in America*. University Press of Kansas, 2013.

McMahan, David L., and Erik Braun. "Introduction: From Colonialism to Brainscans: Modern Transformations of Buddhist Meditation." In *Meditation, Buddhism, and Science*, edited by David L McMahan and Erik Braun, 1–20. Oxford University Press, 2017.

McPhate, Mike. "Just How Accurate Are Fitbits? The Jury Is Out." *New York Times*, 25 May 2016. https://www.nytimes.com/2016/05/26/technology/personaltech/fitbit-accuracy.html

Mehling, Wolf E., Judith Wrubel, Jennifer J. Daubenmier, Cynthia J. Price, Catherine E. Kerr, Theresa Silow, Viranjini Gopisetty, and Anita L. Stewart. "Body Awareness: A Phenomenological Inquiry into the Common Ground of Mind-Body Therapies." *Philosophy, Ethics, and Humanities in Medicine* 6, no. 1 (2011): 1–12.

Merleau-Ponty, Maurice. *Phenomenology of Perception*. Routledge, 2013.

Metzl, Jonathan. "Introduction: Why 'Against Health'?" In *Against Health*, edited by Jonathan Metzl and Anna Kirkland, 1–12. New York University Press, 2010.

Metzl, Jonathan, and Anna Kirkland, eds. *Against Health: How Health Became the New Morality*. New York University Press, 2010.

Meyers, Jane E., and Thomas J. Sweeny. *Counseling for Wellness*. American Counseling Association, 2005.

Migella, Jessica. "7 HIIT Mistakes You're Probably Making." Daily Burn, 7 August 2017. https://dailyburn.com/life/fitness/hiit-workout-mistakes/

Miller, James William. "Wellness: The History and Development of a Concept." *Heft* (2005): 84–102.

Millington, Brad. "Fit for Prosumption: Interactivity and the Second Fitness Boom." *Media, Culture & Society* 38, no. 8 (2016): 1184–200.

Millington, Brad. "'Quantify the Invisible': Notes toward a Future of Posture." *Critical Public Health* 26, no. 4 (2016): 405–17.

Mintz, Laurie B. "The Orgasm Gap: Simple Truth and Sexual Solutions." *Psychology Today*, 4 October 2014.

Moere, Andrew Vande, and Helen Purchase. "On the Role of Design in Information Visualization." *Information Visualization* 10, no. 4 (2011): 356–71.

Mol, Annemarie. *The Body Multiple: Ontology in Medical Practice*. Duke University Press, 2002.

Montero, Barbara. "Does Bodily Awareness Interfere with Highly Skilled Movement?" *Inquiry* 53, no. 2 (2010): 105–22.

Moov. "Moov Now." Accessed May 2020. https://welcome.moov.cc/moovnow

Moov, Inc. "Moov Coach and Guided Workouts," vers. 5.2.4809.52. Accessed May 2020.

Morley, James. "Inspiration and Expiration: Yoga Practice through Merleau-Ponty's Phenomenology of the Body." *Philosophy East and West* (2001): 73–82.

Moukheiber, Zina. "I Asked 20,000 Doctors about Fitbit and Apple's HealthKit, and Here's the Answer." *Forbes*, 24 November 2014. https://www.forbes.com/sites/zinamoukheiber/2014/11/24/i-asked-20000-doctors-about-fitbit-and-apples-healthkit-and-heres-the-answer/?sh=4bd4501251a7

Mularoni, Alessandra. "Feminist Science Interventions in Self-Tracking Technology." *Catalyst: Feminism, Theory, Technoscience* 7, no. 1 (2021).

Muse. "How It Works." Accessed May 2020. https://choosemuse.com/how-it-works/

Muse. "Muse Research." Accessed February 2020. https://choosemuse.com/muse-research/

Muse. "What Is Neurofeedback and Biofeedback?" Accessed July 2020. https://choosemuse.com/blog/what-is-neurofeedback-and-biofeedback/?store_id=ca&utm_source=google&utm_medium=cpc&gclid=Cj0KCQiAnL7yBRD3ARIsAJp_oLaCO0TnOoO9BFkbQJemfEwBupmoytKD3H5UuM-folMGSoOBJ6U0iK0aAgGfEALw_wcB

Muse. "What It Measures." Accessed May 2020. https://choosemuse.com/what-it-measures/

Muse. "Why Muse?" Accessed February 2020. https://choosemuse.com/why-muse/

Nafus, Dawn, and Jamie Sherman. "Big Data, Big Questions| This One Does Not Go Up to 11: The Quantified Self Movement as an Alternative Big Data Practice." *International Journal of Communication* 8 (2014): 1784–94.

National Wellness Institute. "Six Dimensions of Wellness." Accessed July 2020. https://nationalwellness.org/resources/six-dimensions-of-wellness/

Natural Cycles. "About Natural Cycles." Accessed November 2020. https://www.naturalcycles.com/about/

Natural Cycles. "Homepage." Accessed July 2021. https://www.naturalcycles.com/

Neff, Gina, and Dawn Nafus. *Self-Tracking*. MIT Press, 2016.

Negra, Diane, and Yvonne Tasker. *Interrogating Postfeminism*. Duke University Press, 2007.

Nelson, Alondra. *Body and Soul: The Black Panther Party and the Fight Against Medical Discrimination*. University of Minnesota Press, 2011.

Neuhaus, Jessamyn. "The Importance of Being Orgasmic: Sexuality, Gender, and Marital Sex Manuals in the United States, 1920–1963." *Journal of the History of Sexuality* 9, no. 4 (2000): 447–73.

Newton, Victoria Louise. *Everyday Discourses of Menstruation*. Palgrave Macmillan, 2016.

Nicolò, Andrea, and Michele Girardi. "The Physiology of Interval Training: A New Target to HIIT." *Journal of Physiology* 594, no. 24 (2016): 7169.

Nike Inc. "Nike Run Club," vers. 6.8.0. https://apps.apple.com/us/app/nike-run-club/id387771637

Noble, Bill, David Clark, Marcia Meldrum, Henk Ten Have, Jane Seymour, Michelle Winslow, and Silvia Paz. "The Measurement of Pain, 1945–2000." *Journal of Pain and Symptom Management* 29, no. 1 (2005): 14–21.

Novotny, Maria, and Les Hutchinson. "Data Our Bodies Tell: Towards Critical Feminist Action in Fertility and Period Tracking Applications." *Technical Communication Quarterly* 28, no. 4 (2019): 332–60.

OED Online. "aesthetic, n. and adj." Accessed December 2021. https://www.oed.com/view/Entry/3237

OED Online. "mindfulness, n." Accessed June 2020. https://electra.lmu.edu:5402/view/Entry/118742?redirectedFrom=mindfulness

Orangetheory Fitness. "Homepage." Accessed April 2020. https://www.orangetheory.com/en-us/

Orangetheory Fitness. "What Makes Orangetheory Work: Technology." Online video clip. Uploaded to YouTube 18 October 2018. https://www.youtube.com/watch?v=4n6hZzsXXOs

Ostherr, Kirsten. "Digital Medical Humanities and Design Thinking." In *Teaching Health Humanities*, edited by Olivia Banner, Nathan Carlin, and Thomas R. Cole, 245–60. Oxford University Press, 2019.

Parviainen, Jaana, and Johanna Aromaa. "Bodily Knowledge beyond Motor Skills and Physical Fitness: A Phenomenological Description of Knowledge Formation in Physical Training." *Sport, Education and Society* 22, no. 4 (2017): 477–92.

Perry, Shannon. "The Lioness Vibrator: Learn to Love Your Body." Gennev. 25 March 2021, https://gennev.com/education/lioness-vibrator-sex-toy

Peterson, Jake. "How To: Cheat Your Apple Watch Rings." Gadget Hacks, December 26, 2018. https://ios.gadgethacks.com/how-to/cheat-your-apple-watch-rings-0191261/

Pink, Sarah, and Vaike Fors. "Being in a Mediated World: Self-Tracking and the Mind–Body–Environment." *Cultural Geographies* 24, no. 3 (2017): 375–88.

Planned Parenthood. "Spot On Period Tracker." Accessed February 2023. https://www.plannedparenthood.org/get-care/spot-on-period-tracker

Porter, Jon, and Nick Statt. "Google Completes Purchase of Fitbit." *The Verge*, 14 January 2021. https://www.theverge.com/2021/1/14/22188428/google-fitbit-acquisition-completed-approved

Pratap, Abhishek, Elias Chaibub Neto, Phil Snyder, Carl Stepnowsky, Noémie Elhadad, Daniel Grant, Matthew H. Mohebbi, et al. "Indicators of Retention in Remote Digital Health Studies: A Cross-Study Evaluation of 100,000 Participants." *NPJ Digital Medicine* 3, no. 1 (2020): 1–10.

Precedence Research. "Fertility Market Size to Hit Around US$47.9 Billion by 2030." GlobeNewswire News Room, 10 February 2021. https://www.globenewswire.com/news-release/2021/02/10/2173389/0/en/Fertility-Market-Size-to-Hit-Around-US-47-9-Billion-by-2030.html

Prior, Jerilynn C. "The Menstrual Cycle: Its Biology in the Context of Silent Ovulatory Disturbances." In *Routledge International Handbook of Women's Sexual and Reproductive Health*, 39–54. Routledge, 2019.

Przybylo, Ela, and Breanne Fahs. "Empowered Bleeders and Cranky Menstruators: Menstrual Positivity and the 'Liberated' Era of New Menstrual Product Advertisements." In *The Palgrave Handbook of Critical Menstruation Studies*, edited by

Chris Bobel, Inga T. Winkler, Breanne Fahs, Katie Ann Hasson, Elizabeth Arveda Kissling, and Tomi-Ann Roberts, 375–94. Palgrave, 2020.

Quantified Self. "Homepage." n.d. https://quantifiedself.com/

Quinlivan, Davina. *Place of Breath in Cinema*. Edinburgh University Press, 2012.

Ratcliff, Kathryn Strother. *Women and Health: Power, Technology, Inequality, and Conflict in a Gendered World*. Pearson, 2002.

Reich, Wilhelm. *The Function of the Orgasm*. Farrar, Straus and Giroux, 1973.

Reindell, Herbert, and Helmut Roskamm. *Ein Beitrag zu den physiologischen Grundlagen des Intervalltrainings unter besonderer Berücksichtigung des Kreislaufes*. Editions Médecine et Hygiène, 1959.

Riley, Sarah, Adrienne Evans, and Martine Robson. *Postfeminism and Health: Critical Psychology and Media Perspectives*. Routledge, 2018.

Roberts, Celia, and Catherine Waldby. "Incipient Infertility: Tracking Eggs and Ovulation Across the Life Course." *Catalyst: Feminism, Theory, Technoscience* 7, no. 1 (2021).

Rodaway, Paul. *Sensuous Geographies: Body, Sense and Place*. Routledge, 1994.

Røstvik, Camilla Mørk. "Crimson Waves: Narratives about Menstruation, Water, and Cleanliness." *Visual Culture & Gender* 13 (2018).

Røstvik, Camilla Mørk. "Mother Nature as Brand Strategy: Gender and Creativity in Tampax Advertising 2007–2009." *Enterprise & Society* 21, no. 2 (2020): 413–52.

Rowland, Katherine. *The Pleasure Gap: American Women and the Unfinished Sexual Revolution*. Hachette UK, 2020.

Ruckenstein, Minna. "Visualized and Interacted Life: Personal Analytics and Engagements with Data Doubles." *Societies* 4, no. 1 (2014): 68–84.

Ruckenstein, Minna, and Natasha Dow Schüll. "The Datafication of Health." *Annual Review of Anthropology* 46 (2017): 261–78.

Ruff, Tessa. "An App Is Not Birth Control: Natural Cycles' Approval Raises Serious Questions." *Women's Health Activist* 44, no. 1 (January-February 2019): 6.

Ruffino, Paolo. "Engagement and the Quantified Self: Uneventful Relationships with Ghostly Companions." In *Self-Tracking*, edited by B. Ajana, 11–25. Palgrave Macmillan, 2018.

Ryan, Samantha, Jane M. Ussher, and Janette Perz. "Women's Experiences of the Premenstrual Body: Negotiating Body Shame, Self-Objectification, and Menstrual Shame." *Women's Reproductive Health* 7, no. 2 (2020): 107–26.

Saks, Mike. "Medicine and the Counter Culture." In *Medicine in the Twentieth Century*, edited by J. V. Pickstone, 113–23. Taylor & Francis, 2020.

Sanders, Rachel. "Self-Tracking in the Digital Era: Biopower, Patriarchy, and the New Biometric Body Projects." *Body & Society* 23, no. 1 (2017): 36–63.

Sarbacker, Stuart Ray. *Tracing the Path of Yoga: The History and Philosophy of Indian Mind-Body Discipline*. State University of New York Press, 2021.

Sawh, Michael. "How to Calibrate Your Fitbit for Better Accuracy." Wareable, November 28, 2022. https://www.wareable.com/fitbit/how-to-calibrate-fitbit-3031

Scanlin, Amy. "Expanded Use of De Novo Pathway Offers Opportunity for Device Manufacturers." *MedTech Intelligence*, April 16, 2018. https://www.medtechintell

igence.com/feature_article/expanded-use-of-de-novo-pathway-offers-opportunity-for-device-manufacturers/

Scarry, Elaine. *The Body in Pain: The Making and Unmaking of the World.* Oxford University Press, 1987.

Schechner, Sam, and Mark Secada. "You Give Apps Sensitive Personal Information. Then They Tell Facebook." *Wall Street Journal*, 22 February 2019. https://www.wsj.com/articles/you-give-apps-sensitive-personal-information-then-they-tell-facebook-11550851636

Segerståhl, Katarina, and Harri Oinas-Kukkonen. "Designing Personal Exercise Monitoring Employing Multiple Modes of Delivery: Implications from a Qualitative Study on Heart Rate Monitoring." *International Journal of Medical Informatics* 80, no. 12 (2011): e203–13.

Sensoria, Inc. "Homepage." Accessed May 2020. https://www.sensoriafitness.com/

Sensoria, Inc. "Sensoria." vers. 2.3.0. Accessed May 2020.

Sharon, Tamar. "Healthy Citizenship beyond Autonomy and Discipline: Tactical Engagements with Genetic Testing." *Biosocieties* 10, no. 3 (2015): 295–316.

Sharon, Tamar, and Dorien Zandbergen. "From Data Fetishism to Quantifying Selves: Self-Tracking Practices and the Other Values of Data." *New Media & Society* 19, no. 11 (2017): 1695–709.

Shephard, Roy J. *A History of Health & Fitness: Implications for Policy Today*. Springer International Publishing, 2018.

Sherman, Jamie. "Data in the Age of Digital Reproduction: Reading the Quantified Self through Walter Benjamin." *Quantified: Biosensing Technologies in Everyday Life* (2016): 27–42.

Slingerland, Edward. *Trying Not to Try: The Art and Science of Spontaneity*. Crown Publishers, 2004.

Smith, Gavin J. D. "Surveillance, Data and Embodiment: On the Work of Being Watched." *Body & Society* 22, no. 2 (2016): 108–39.

Smith, Gavin J. D., and Ben Vonthethoff. "Health by Numbers? Exploring the Practice and Experience of Datafied Health." *Health Sociology Review* 26, no. 1 (2017): 6–21.

Smith, Stephanie. "5 Ways to Know You're Going Hard Enough with HIIT." Fitbit Blog, 7 December 2017. https://blog.fitbit.com/5-ways-know-youre-going-hard-enough-hiit/

Sommer, Barbara. "How Does Menstruation Affect Cognitive Competence and Psychophysiological Response?" In *Lifting the Curse of Menstruation*, edited by Sharon Golub, 53–90. Routledge, 2017.

Soto-Vásquez, Arthur D. "Moving with Fitbit: Body Narratives, Fit Subjectivities, and Racialized Discipline." *Communication Studies* 72, no. 6 (2021): 1112–28.

SpireHealth. "Homepage." Accessed July 2020. https://spirehealth.com/pages/stone

SpireHealth. "Science." Accessed February 2018. https://spirehealth.com/pages/science-behind-spire

Srinivasan, Ramesh. *Whose Global Village? Rethinking How Technology Shapes Our World*. New York University Press, 2018. Kindle ebook.

Starling, Mary Summer, Zosha Kandel, Liya Haile, and Rebecca G. Simmons.

"User Profile and Preferences in Fertility Apps for Preventing Pregnancy: An Exploratory Pilot Study." *Mhealth* 4 (2018).

Streeter, Kurt. "On Running While Black, More Hope Than Before." *New York Times*, 22 November 2020.

Sveen, Hanna. "Lava or Code Red: A Linguistic Study of Menstrual Expressions in English and Swedish." *Women's Reproductive Health* 3, no. 3 (2016): 145–59.

Svenaeus, Fredrik. *The Hermeneutics of Medicine and the Phenomenology of Health: Steps Towards a Philosophy of Medical Practice*. International Library of Bioethics. Springer, 2000.

Svenaeus, Fredrik. "The Phenomenology of Health and Illness." In *Handbook of Phenomenology and Medicine*, edited by S. Kay Toombs, 87–108. Kluwer Academic Publishers, 2001.

Sweeney, Thomas J., C. S. Gill, C. B. Minton, and J. Myers. "Five Factor Wellness Inventory." *Adultspan Journal* 14, no. 2 (2015): 66–76.

TEDx Talks. "Breathe to Heal: Max Strom." Uploaded to YouTube 7 December 2015. https://www.youtube. com/watch?v=4Lb5L-VEm34

TEDx Talks. "The Power of Breath: Christian De La Huerta." Uploaded to YouTube 23 April 2013. https:// www.youtube.com/watch?v=VLAziEkvUT8

TEDx Talks. "What Is Your Breath Telling You? Neema Moraveji." Uploaded to YouTube 22 December 2014. https://www.youtube.com/watch?v=tRAg7YfCpGc

This American Life. "Episode 681: Escape from the Lab Transcript." Accessed March 2021. https://www.thisamericanlife.org/681/transcript

Thomas, Gareth M., and Deborah Lupton. "Threats and Thrills: Pregnancy Apps, Risk and Consumption." *Health, Risk & Society* 17, no. 7–8 (2016): 495–509.

Thompson, Walter R. "Now Trending: Worldwide Survey of Fitness Trends for 2014." *ACSM's Health & Fitness Journal* 17, no. 6 (2013): 10–20.

Tiffany, Kaitlyn. "Period-Tracking Apps like Clue and Glow Are Not for Women." Vox, November 16, 2018. https://www.vox.com/the-goods/2018/11/13/18079458/menstrual-tracking-surveillance-glow-clue-apple-health

Till, Chris. "Commercialising Bodies: The New Corporate Health Ethic of Philanthrocapitalism." In *Quantified Lives and Vital Data*, edited by Rebecca Lynch and Conor Farrington, 229–49. Palgrave Macmillan UK, 2018.

Till, Chris. "Exercise as Labour: Quantified Self and the Transformation of Exercise into Labour." *Societies* 4, no. 3 (2014): 446–62.

Tin, Ida. "5 Unexpected Benefits of Period Tracking." Clue. 22 January 2019. https://helloclue.com/articles/cycle-a-z/5-reasons-you-should-pay-attention-to-your-period

Tomes, Nancy. *Remaking the American Patient: How Madison Avenue and Modern Medicine Turned Patients into Consumers*. UNC Press Books, 2016.

Toombs, S. Kay. *The Meaning of Illness: A Phenomenological Account of the Different Perspectives of Physician and Patient*. Vol. 42. Springer Science & Business Media, 2013.

Tremblay, Jean-Thomas. "Breath: Image and Sound, an Introduction." *New Review of Film and Television Studies* 16, no. 2 (2018): 93–97.

Tremblay, Jean-Thomas. *Breathing Aesthetics*. Duke University Press, 2022.

Tufte, Edward. *Visual Explanations: Images and Quantities, Evidence and Narrative*. Graphics Press, 1997.

Turrini, Mauro. "A Genealogy of 'Healthism.'" *eä Journal of Medical Humanities & Social Studies of Science and Technology* 7, no. 1 (2015): 11–27.

United States Office of the Assistant Secretary for Health. *Healthy People: The Surgeon General's Report on Health Promotion and Disease Prevention* 79, no. 55071. US Department of Health, Education, and Welfare, Public Health Service, Office of the Assistant Secretary for Health and Surgeon General; Washington, DC, 1979.

UPRIGHT GO. "How Upright Works." Accessed May 2020. https://www.uprightpose.com/how-it-works/

UPRIGHT GO. "The Benefits of Upright Posture." Accessed January 2023. https://www.uprightpose.com/en-nz/benefits/?afmc=1k

UPRIGHT GO. "Why Does Posture Matter?" Help Center. Accessed April 2020. https://help.uprightpose.com/en/articles/3346617-why-does-posture-matter

Upright Technologies. "UPRIGHT GO," vers. 1.8.0. Accessed April 2020.

Ussher, Jane M. *Managing the Monstrous Feminine: Regulating the Reproductive Body*. Routledge, 2006.

Ussher, Jane M., and Janette Perz. "PMS as a Process of Negotiation: Women's Experience and Management of Premenstrual Distress." *Psychology & Health* 28, no. 8 (2013): 909–27.

Ussher, Jane M., and Janette Perz. "Resisting the Mantle of the Monstrous Feminine: Women's Construction and Experience of Premenstrual Embodiment." In *The Palgrave Handbook of Critical Menstruation Studies*, edited by Chris Bobel, Inga T. Winkler, Breanne Fahs, Katie Ann Hasson, Elizabeth Arveda Kissling, and Tomi-Ann Roberts, 215–31. Palgrave, 2020.

Valencell. "National Wearables Survey Reveals Accelerating Convergence of Consumer Wearables and Personal Health & Medical Devices." 2018. https://valencell.com/news/national-wearables-survey-shows-convergence-of-wearables-and-health-devices/

Varvogli, Liza, and Christina Darviri. "Stress Management Techniques: Evidence-Based Procedures that Reduce Stress and Promote Health." *Health Science Journal* 5, no. 2 (2011): 74.

Vlajić Wheeler, Marija, Tabor Vedrana Högqvist, Kayleigh Teel, and Mike LaVigne. "The Science of Your Cycle: Evidence-Based App Design." Clue. 12 October 2015. https://helloclue.com/articles/about-clue/science-your-cycle-evidence-based-app-design

Vox Creative. "Women Are Having Fewer Orgasms. But Why?" Vox. 7 December 2020. https://www.vox.com/ad/21564023/women-pleasure-pornography-bellesa-streaming

Weeks, David J. "Sex for the Mature Adult: Health, Self-Esteem and Countering Ageist Stereotypes." *Sexual and Relationship Therapy* 17, no. 3 (2002): 231–40.

Weigel, Gabriella. "Coverage and Use of Fertility Services in US." *Women's Health Policy*. 15 September 2020. https://www.kff.org/womens-health-policy/issue-brief/coverage-and-use-of-fertility-services-in-the-u-s/#:~:text=Many%20fertility%20treatments%20are%20not,others%20(e.g.%2C%20IVF)

Wernimont, Jacqueline. *Numbered Lives: Life and Death in Quantum Media*. MIT Press, 2019.

Wheatley, John R., and David A. Puts. "Evolutionary Science of Female Orgasm." *The Evolution of Sexuality* (2015): 123–48.

Whipple, Beverly, and Barry R. Komisaruk. "Brain (PET) Responses to Vaginal-Cervical Self-Stimulation in Women with Complete Spinal Cord Injury: Preliminary Findings." *Journal of Sex &Marital Therapy* 28, no. 1 (2002): 79–86.

"White Paper on Connected Health: The Case for Medicine 2.0." Withings Health Institute, n.d.

White, Philip, Kevin Young, and James Gillett. "Bodywork as a Moral Imperative: Some Critical Notes on Health and Fitness." *Loisir et societe/Society and Leisure* 18, no. 1 (1995): 159–81

Whitson, Jennifer R. "Foucault's Fitbit: Governance and Gamification." *The Gameful World: Approaches, Issues, Applications*, edited by Steffen P. Walz and Sebastian Deterding, 339–58. MIT Press, 2014.

Whorton, James C. *Crusaders for Fitness: The History of American Health Reformers*. Princeton University Press, 1982.

Wolf, Christiane, and J. Greg Serpa. *A Clinician's Guide to Teaching Mindfulness: The Comprehensive Session-by-Session Program for Mental Health Professionals and Health Care Providers*. New Harbinger Publications, 2015.

World Health Organization. "Frequently Asked Questions." *World Health Organization*. Accessed July 16, 2020. https://www.who.int/about/who-we-are/frequently-asked-questions

World Health Organization. "Physical Activity." Accessed 11 January 2022. https://www.who.int/news-room/fact-sheets/detail/physical-activity

World Health Organization, "Seventy-First World Health Assembly WHA71.7 Agenda Item 12.4 26 Digital Health." 2018. https://apps.who.int/gb/ebwha/pdf_files/WHA71/A71_R7-en.pdf

Young, Iris Marion. *On Female Body Experience: "Throwing Like a Girl" and Other Essays*. Oxford University Press, 2005.

Index

Note: Page numbers in italics indicate figures.

Printed and bound by CPI Group (UK) Ltd, Croydon, CR0 4YY

09/06/2025

14686126-0001